T0135411

böhlau

ZÜRCHER BEITRÄGE
ZUR GESCHICHTSWISSENSCHAFT BAND 8

HERAUSGEGEBEN VOM
HISTORISCHEN SEMINAR DER UNIVERSITÄT ZÜRICH

THE HIDDEN PATIENTS

North African Women
in French Colonial Psychiatry

VON
NINA SALOUÂ STUDER

2016
BÖHLAU VERLAG KÖLN WEIMAR WIEN

Das E-Book wurde publiziert mit Unterstützung des Schweizerischen Nationalfonds zur Förderung der wissenschaftlichen Forschung.

Die vorliegende Arbeit wurde von der Philosophischen Fakultät der Universität Zürich im Herbstsemester 2012 auf Antrag von Prof. Dr. Gesine Krüger und Dr. habil. Jan-Georg Deutsch als Dissertation angenommen.

Bibliografische Information der Deutschen Nationalbibliothek:
Die Deutsche Nationalbibliothek verzeichnet diese Publikation in der Deutschen Nationalbibliografie; detaillierte bibliografische Daten sind im Internet über http://portal.dnb.de abrufbar.

Umschlagabbildung:
»Dortoir d'alitement du pavillon Sérieux de l'Hôpital pour maladies mentales de la Manouba.« Die Abbildung wurde entnommen: M. Raoul Vadon: L'Assistance Médicale des Psychopates en Tunisie. Med. thesis, University of Marseille 1935, zwischen S. 42 und 43.

Korrektorat: Rebecca Wache, Castrop-Rauxel
Gesamtherstellung: WBD Wissenschaftlicher Bücherdienst, Köln
Gedruckt auf chlor- und säurefreiem Papier
Printed in the EU

ISBN 978-3-412-50201-0

Table of Content

Acknowledgements

This book is based on my doctoral dissertation in history, which I was able to write at the Universities of Zürich and Oxford thanks to a scholarship from the Swiss National Science Foundation (SNF), who also generously supported the publication of this book. I would also like to thank my supervisors, Prof. Dr. Gesine Krüger, from the History Faculty of the University of Zürich, and Dr. habil. Jan-Georg Deutsch, from the History Faculty of the University of Oxford. Both have given me invaluable support during the process of researching and writing this book, and have helped me with their critical questions, their always helpful suggestions and their patience as I developed the tone, structure and framework. I wish to thank them both for having been great professional and personal mentors to me. Additionally, the seminars that both of them offered to doctoral students provided me with a vital opportunity to present and discuss preliminary findings to a group of peers. I would also like to express my sincere gratitude to all my friends and colleagues with whom I have discussed my project in Zürich, Oxford and at various conferences, and who have helped shape this book with their suggestions.

There have been so many esteemed researchers from such diverse fields as psychiatry, Islamic sciences, the history of medicine, colonial history and gender studies who patiently discussed my questions and findings with me, that it is impossible to name them all here, but I am most grateful to all of them for the precious assistance that they have given me. I would, however, like to personally thank the eminent Moroccan psychiatrists and psychoanalysts Rhita El-Khayat and Jalil Bennani for giving me the chance to discuss my project with them in summer 2011, and all the participants of my colloquium on colonial psychiatry in the Maghreb ("Madness in North Africa: Gender, Race and Religion in the Writings of French Colonial Psychiatry") at the Historical Institute of the University of Zürich in Spring 2013. The lively, intelligent and critical discussions in this colloquium helped me map out the difficult areas in this field and have demonstrated that there is a broader interest in this topic.

I am intensely grateful to the staff at those archives and libraries that I visited in Oxford, London, Paris, Rabat, Basel, Geneva and Zürich, for their assistance during my research. I must express my special gratitude to the ever-helpful staff at the Zentralbibliothek Zürich, who humoured even my strangest requests and who have been truly phenomenal in helping me find source material based on obscure references, and to the staff at the Bibliothèque Nationale du Royaume du Maroc in Rabat, who were unbelievably accommodating and cooperative.

Thanks are also due to Research Network Reconfigurations at the University of Marburg, and especially Dr. Achim Rhode, who kindly allowed me to work on the final draft of this book during my Visiting Research Fellowship there.

I would also like to thank all three of my parents, Christoph, Monique and Marc, for their endless loving support, without which this book would never have been possible. This work is inherently influenced by my mother who, as a descendant of French colonisers in Morocco and Algeria and as a midwife, fostered my interest both in the history of medicine and in the colonial Maghreb. I am aware how much I owe all three of them, both as an academic and as a person. I would also like to thank Darren's parents, Margaret and Alan, for their much appreciated support and belief in me, especially during the hardest times while writing this book. Finally, I would like to thank my partner Darren, for putting up with me at these most stressful moments of this project, for his unwavering, invaluable support, and, above all, for tirelessly proofreading the various drafts of this book and always providing insightful comments and highly appreciated suggestions.

Introduction

"I have found it more difficult to certify sanity than insanity."[1]

Thus wrote the British psychiatrist John Warnock in 1924, summarising a lifetime of professional experience with colonised patients. Although Warnock was writing about Egypt, where for twenty-eight years he was the main – and, for a long time, only – working psychiatrist, the quotation above also encapsulates the experiences of many French colonial psychiatrists working in the Maghreb and the difficulties they faced, or believed they faced, in their everyday professional lives. Warnock's quote hints at the significant complications presented by such factors as geography, culture, language and religion in the process of diagnosis; fears concerning an enormous number of "hidden", potentially dangerous insane that European methodologies were ill-equipped to identify; and, most pertinently for the subject of this book, the difficulties early colonial psychiatrists had in locating insanity within the local populace.

Warnock gave two very specific reasons for his statement. Firstly, he was referring to family members who wanted to be rid of a difficult, housebound patient and therefore alleged "all sorts of insane conduct on the part of the testator", which made it difficult to "separate the truth from the false". This situation seems to have seldom arisen in the colonial Maghreb, as was shown by concerns and theories about low Muslim patient numbers. His second reason, however, could be directly transposed into the discourse on North African "insanity", carefully built up by generations of French colonial psychiatrists. Warnock stated: "Often the patient is an old lady who understands very little about business, and of course, cannot read or write, and being in the Hareem knows scarcely anything of what goes on in the outside world, and one has to make the standard of intelligence low in these cases."[2] According to Warnock, this specific context of being confronted with an uneducated, segregated Muslim woman made the "diagnosis" of sanity extremely difficult. This professional unease when it came to assessing potential female Muslim patients can be found in many of the texts written by French colonial psychiatrists. The seemingly genuine confusion over what constituted "sanity" and "insanity" in Muslim North Africans in general, and the women in particular, and the question of whether Muslim women really were so uneducated as to make authoritative diagnosis almost impossible were two of the main preoccupations of French colonial psychiatry.

---

1 Warnock, Twenty-Eight Years, 586.
2 Ibid.

The Fascination with Insanity

French colonial psychiatrists were not the only ones fascinated with the question of North African forms of "insanity". Practically from the beginning of the French colonisation of the Maghreb,[3] many colonial authors showed an interest in issues which would be interpreted as psychiatric problems today. The scandalous particularities of cases of "insanity" and the possible dangers of "madmen" freely roaming the streets engendered concerns about – largely imaginary – social problems while providing a sensationalist appeal to European observers. As a result of this extensive public interest, "insanity" ended up being discussed in a wide range of French publications: from those with strictly legal or medical content to those which appealed to a broader audience, such as the colonial press, socio-anthropological publications and even literary texts.[4] The colonial psychiatrists writing on their Muslim patients were therefore only one strand in this discursive net on "insanity" among the colonised North Africans. Even though the French colonial psychiatrists often deplored this state of affairs and claimed that they were the only ones who could write authoritatively about the subtleties of the topic, they were influenced by the fears and wishes expressed in publications written outside their profession – especially when it came to the threats posed to settler societies by "madmen".

Both in the popular discourse and in the psychiatric texts, it was usually "madmen" and almost never "madwomen" who were seen as dangerous and problematic. In the psychiatric theories from the 19th and the early 20th centuries, it was believed that certain groups among the general population had a particular predisposition to madness. It was therefore one of psychiatry's main duties to define the morbid predispositions different groups of society embodied, in metropolitan as well as in colonial contexts.[5] During colonial psychiatry's initial contact with North Africans,

---

3   French control over the Maghreb started with the conquest of the Algerian coast in 1830. However, it took the French army until 1857, the year of the fall of Kabylia, to completely conquer Algeria. See for example: Lorcin, Rome and France, 299. On the conquest of Algeria, see also: Ageron, Histoire de l'Algérie contemporaine. Compared with Algeria, the colonisation of Tunisia and Morocco had been at once more informal – with both countries officially being "protectorates" and not conceived as part of *la Grande Nation* – and considerably shorter. Tunisia became a French "protectorate" in 1881 and Morocco in 1912, and both remained under French rule until their independence in 1956.

4   The literary fascination with insanity did not, of course, end with the independence of the Maghreb states. For a discussion on "female insanity" in postcolonial Algerian (and Lebanese) literature, see: Mallem, Folie féminine.

5   In the colonies, this morbid predisposition was believed to be influenced by diverse factors, such as the climate, lifestyles, professions, diets, the stages of evolution and the dangers of heredity. Most of these explanations for insanity will be discussed in the following chapters.

Muslims seemed to be less susceptible to mental problems and Muslim women even appeared to be almost excluded from these risk groups. This is shown by an early quote from the eminent French psychiatrist Louis Delasiauve, who wrote in 1865 that, in Algeria, "we notice that insanity prevails particularly among Europeans and men."[6] With Muslim women being neither predisposed to mental problems by gender[7] nor by "race",[8] many colonial psychiatrists accepted the presence of significantly fewer female Muslim patients in the colonial mental institutions as self-evident.

Other French colonial psychiatrists were convinced that insanity had to exist among Muslims in general and Muslim women in particular, but that it was somehow hidden from colonial perception, with the interned Muslim patients merely being the tip of the iceberg, while the vast bulk of "invisible patients", far exceeding those treated in the hospitals, lay hidden beneath the surface.[9] This led to the conclusion that a dauntingly large number of potential Muslim patients was, for some reason, evading the registration and care of colonial psychiatry. It was felt by many colonial psychiatrists that France, with its ideals of a *mission civilisatrice*,[10] had a moral duty to find, save, look after and – if possible – cure these neglected patients. In 1908 Louis

---

6   Delasiauve, Review of Collardot, 118. On the prevalence of male patients in the colonies, see also, for example: Jobert, Projet, 61; Reboul/Régis, Assistance, 199. The French sources have been translated into English, but both the intricacies of the original French, with single sentences being subdivided into complex, interlaced structures with clause after clause, and the complicated terminology of the psychiatric sources made it difficult to produce a translation that is accurate without being too literal, and which conveys the sense of the text without sacrificing too much of the idiom.

7   Not all French psychiatrists agreed with this statement. Many believed that, in the European context, women were more likely to become insane than men. The findings in Algeria therefore pointed to an apparent reversal of the European situation, which was also observed in other colonial contexts. Sally Swartz, for instance, wrote about the situation in the Cape colonies in 1999: "The fact that more men than women were incarcerated in Cape colonial asylums, a pattern which has been sustained throughout the 20th century, suggests that these asylums may have had a social function somewhat different from those in Europe and America, where more women than men were incarcerated. This is a topic that needs further research." Swartz, Lost Lives, 153.

8   The theory that less civilised "races" presented fewer cases of insanity, that insanity was, in fact, a "disease of civilisation", will be discussed in detail in Chapter 1.

9   On the popular analogy of the "iceberg" in the history of psychiatry, see for example: Porter, Wahnsinn, 117.

10 For a discussion of the concept of a *mission civilisatrice*, see for example: Conklin, Mission to Civilize, 1–9; Keller, Colonial Madness, 5 f. French colonial doctors and psychiatrists saw themselves and the benefits they brought to North Africa as both components and prototypes of this mission. See for instance: Bouquet, Médecine et colonisation, ii; Piessac, Devoir social, i; Aubin, Brèves réflexions, 8.

Margain, for instance, expressed his perceived humanitarian obligation as a French psychiatrist involved in colonisation projects as saving these "madmen", which were allegedly ignored by their own societies: "But I felt too heavily the importance of this question and the urgent interest that existed to create a movement of opinion in order to rescue from misery, from vagrancy, from death thousands of abandoned human beings, for me not to consent to courageously start to work."[11]

During this early colonial period, many French psychiatrists believed that the low numbers of Muslim patients could be partly explained through the lack of opportunity for appropriate care due to a lack of psychiatric institutions, which left them abandoned and at the mercy of – but not cured by – their traditional healing methods.[12] The most influential French colonial psychiatrist, Antoine Porot, for example, had no doubt in his first official report on North Africans in 1912 that Muslim patients would appear with the creation of French institutions.[13] And indeed, the numbers of both male and female Muslim patients rose after the construction of psychiatric institutions in the Maghreb in the 1930s. Yet despite rising numbers of female Muslim patients, Muslim "insanity" remained chiefly represented by men in the French perception. Photographic reproductions of the lived reality in these new model institutions, like the photograph used on the cover of this book,[14] for example, almost always depicted male and not female Muslim patients.

French colonial psychiatric interest in the Maghreb can be roughly divided into two periods, the dividing point between them being the building of psychiatric

---

11 Margain, Aliénation mentale, 87. This notion was part of the idea of a "moral conquest", in which France, the superior country militarily and morally, had an obligation to better the conditions in its colonies. Many doctors and psychiatrists felt that this improvement was best conducted through them. Victor Trenga, for example, wrote in 1913, after having attacked racism in Americans: "We, the French, are far from being of such an odious intransigency. If it pleased us no longer to be the educators of the world, the genius of our race would lose one of its purest characteristics. Our great originality is not to feel superior to other men; it is not wanting to keep our superiority to ourselves." Trenga, Âme arabo-berbère, 179.

12 In the French understanding of North Africa, the only possibilities open to people suffering from mental problems were the traditional Islamic asylums, so-called *māristāns*, which will be discussed in subsequent chapters. For historical analyses of the development of these *māristāns*, see: Issa Bey, Histoire; Bay, Islamische Krankenhäuser; Dols, Origins of the Islamic Hospital; Chakib et al., Maristane Sidi-Frej; Belkamel/Raouyane, Bimaristanes au Maroc; El Ayadi, Maristanes; Moussaoui/El Otmani, Introduction des hôpitaux. Arabic vocabulary that has not been adopted by European languages has been transcribed using the rules of the *Deutsche Morgenländische Gesellschaft*. See: Wagner, Regeln. The Arabic terms used in the sources have been compiled in a glossary. See p. 310.

13 Porot, Tunisie, 58.

14 The title page shows a ward for Muslim men at the Manouba Psychiatric Hospital in Tunisia, published by the psychiatrist Raoul Vadon in his 1935 dissertation.

institutions in the Maghreb in the 1930s. From 1845 to the 1930s psychiatric treatment of Muslim patients was mainly a metropolitan affair, with European and Algerian Muslim patients shipped to French asylums where metropolitan psychiatrists looked after these "colonial patients".[15] The first French medical experts on mental illness working on North African soil were mostly attached to hospitals as general doctors. Psychiatrists in the French asylums treating patients selected by these general doctors were dismissive of the latter's medical abilities, often remarking disparagingly upon their diagnoses.[16] The general doctors, by contrast, claimed that the psychiatrists in France could not possibly match their own understanding of the North African mentality.[17] These competing interpretations, this professional rivalry, were part of a broader struggle for authority over the field of mental illness, in which religious, legal and medical experts jostled.[18] The psychiatric profession was not consolidated until the end of the 19th century,[19] and in the context of North Africa, most general doctors included in their medical treatises paragraphs or even chapters on insanity among the colonised, even after this struggle had been decided in favour of the psychiatrists.

The Psychiatric Maghreb – a Unit of the Orientalist Imagination

The earliest French psychiatric investigation of an Arab Muslim population was written by Jacques-Joseph Moreau de Tours in 1843, who travelled, in his capacity as a personal psychiatrist, through the "Orient" with a private patient for a few years.[20] His psychiatric descriptions of the "Orient", published in France's foremost psychiatric

---

15 The term "colonial patients" is used to describe those who were not "metropolitan patients", i.e. Muslim, European and Jewish North Africans.

16 See, for example: Laurens, Contribution, 9; Peyre, Maladies mentales, 195.

17 Many psychiatrists also believed that a deeper understanding of Muslim "minds" or "mentality", indispensable for psychiatric practice, could only be gained by living in North Africa. The French psychiatrist Levet, for instance, wrote in 1909 that it was impossible to treat "Arab patients" without having experienced life in the Maghreb: "The insanity of Arabs presents special forms, which confuse the clinician; and I believe that to properly penetrate these patients, not only extensive experience of [treating] mad Arabs is needed, but also a perfect knowledge of the life, the normal native milieu, knowledge which doctors in the metropolitan asylums cannot have, who, for the most part, have only had the occasion to know Algeria through a quick pleasure trip." Levet, Assistance, 239.

18 For the concurrence between the medical and religious professions in the treatment of the insane in 19th century France, see: Dowbiggin, Inheriting Madness, 20 f., 38; Goldstein, Console and Classify, 197 f.

19 See, for example: Fernando, Mental Health, 57.

20 He travelled through Malta, Egypt, the Levant and Asia Minor. Moreau, Recherches, 104–15.

journal, the *Annales Médico-Psychologiques*, were taken up by many later psychiatrists who specialised in the Maghreb.[21] It was seen as a founding text of French colonial psychiatry on North Africa, despite the fact that it concerned neither French colonies nor North Africa. This extrapolation was possible because, despite its cultural diversity and regional differences, most colonial psychiatrists viewed the Arab-Muslim world as homogeneous enough to permit information on one region to be applied to any other. In North Africa, this meant that most differences – whether ethnic, linguistic or cultural – were eclipsed by the one binding character trait that "all" inhabitants shared: Islam, both in terms of a religion and, more broadly, a culture.[22] The geographic focus of this book on Algeria, Tunisia and Morocco is therefore based on the colonial source material itself, which is somewhat contradictory when it comes to the complexities of the relationships between North Africans. While many colonial authors were obsessed with differentiating Algerians from Tunisians and Moroccans (and vice versa), as well as Arabs from Berbers,[23] it was generally supposed that these differences were negligible in the light of the many similarities they displayed as "North Africans", "Arabs" or even "Muslims". A Berber might prove to be very different from an Arab in the professional experiences of the psychiatrists, but as "Muslims", they were still similar enough to be compared to any other Muslim in the world.[24] While certain distinctions remained present in the descriptions of Muslim men,[25] Muslim

---

21 The psychiatrist Jean-Michel Bégué described in 1996 how Moreau de Tours' findings were used by French psychiatrists as authoritative evidence over fifty years after the publication of his article. Bégué, French Psychiatry in Algeria, 537.

22 Apart from the Jewish populations in North Africa, which formed, in the minds of many colonial doctors and psychiatrists, an intermediate step between civilised European and primitive Muslim. Henry Bouquet, for example, described in 1909 how Tunisian Jews had a conception of insanity which was not based on the supernatural, and was, therefore, much closer to European theories. Bouquet, Aliénés en Tunisie, 27 f.

23 French colonial sources often drew contrasting pictures of the two "distinct races" of Arabs and Berbers, with Berbers being clearly preferable. The French ethnologist Aug. Dilhan, for example, envisaged the following recipe for a functioning Tunisian society in 1873: "Many Berbers, a certain amount of Moors, as few Arabs as possible, 10% Jews, 10% Europeans." Dilhan, Ethnographie, 212.

24 The French psychiatrist Victor Trenga, for instance, wrote in 1913: "At present, the five million Muslim natives inhabiting Algeria may be considered as forming a single society, a homogeneous whole, despite the diversity of origins and of language (nearly seven hundred thousand Kabyles speak a separate language, so different from Arabic)." Trenga, Âme arabo-berbère, 12.

25 See for instance the distinction of Arab and Berber men in medical and psychiatric colonial publications: Lafitte, Contribution, 23; Richardot, Pratiques médicales, 6 f.; Sicard, Étude, 65; Gervais, Contribution, 47; Arrii, Impulsivité criminelle, 30; Montaldo, Mortalité infantile, 83; Sutter, Épilepsie mentale, 72. This has been discussed by other historians: Keller, Colonial Madness, 12.

women in the psychiatric source material appeared to be comparable and equatable across all possible geographic and ethnic divides.

This typically Orientalist imagining of a nebulous unity, somehow ingrained in those who were not European, can be found in texts by both psychiatric experts and laymen interested in psychological problems across the whole time period analysed in this book. The French author Raymond Charles, for example, wrote in his 1958 book on the "Muslim Soul" that Islam "presents a psychological and social structure which establishes among its followers a remarkable kinship despite biological or geographical obstacles."[26] Charles explained these deep-rooted mental similarities between all Muslims by appropriating (and corrupting) the Islamic concept of *'umma*, the idea of a supranational religious unity of all Muslims: "Admittedly, the forms of existence of an Indonesian, a Black African and a North African coincide: but a certain mental uniformity results from their obedience to a rigorous dogmatic and ritual unity."[27] According to Charles, all of these different colonial subjects not only had similar forms of existence, but their mere adherence to the religion of Islam reinforced these similarities.

This psychiatric unity of the Maghreb was uncritically accepted by most colonial psychiatrists. Étienne-Paul Laurens, for example, offhandedly explained in an article written in 1919 that information collected by his colleague Auguste Marie on psychiatric patients in Cairo could be easily applied to Algeria: "Although these are not, strictly speaking, Arabs from Algeria, we thought it useful to cite this work, which relates to Arabs who, in short, are in all respects similar to our natives of Algeria."[28] If the perceived similarities between Egyptians and Algerians allowed for such statements in clinical matters, it is not surprising that some psychiatric experts had no problems in formulating generalisations on "this North African race",[29] "the North African pathology"[30] or "the Muslim North African mentality",[31] based on their professional experiences in one of the three colonies in the Maghreb.

While these generalisations conform to modern stereotypes about Muslims, this assumption of "sameness" was both deeply problematic and inherently racist, as it was based on the Orientalist paradox of even the most sophisticated differences among "Orientals" disappearing when directly comparing them to allegedly superior Europeans. Somewhat surprisingly, this imaginary, single unit of the Maghreb in psychiatric matters remained unchallenged by many postcolonial psychiatric authors, and

---

26   Charles, Âme musulmane, 8.
27   Ibid., 150.
28   Laurens, Contribution, 18.
29   Porot/Arrii, Impulsivité criminelle, 588.
30   Sutter, Épilepsie mentale, 71.
31   Brissot, Propos, 500.

assertions of the cultural sameness of the Maghreb can be found in a number of postcolonial psychiatric publications. The French psychiatrist J.-J. Maupomé, for example,
described in 1970 the "common denominator" between the different ethnicities in
postcolonial Morocco, "[which] unites Morocco: Islam; Islam with its rigours, its
ritual, its severity."[32] This same simplistic worldview was even advocated by certain
Arab postcolonial psychiatrists.[33]

It was the popularity of this idea of a deep-rooted Muslim sameness that allowed
Moreau de Tours' 1843 psychiatric article on the "Orient" to turn into one of the founding texts of French colonial psychiatry. Yet despite the importance of Moreau de Tours'
seminal publication, the years following his article only saw infrequent publications
touching on the subject of psychiatry in North Africa – which, at that time, meant
French Algeria. Only in the 1860s did psychiatry begin its preoccupation with the
Algerian insane, and the first – ultimately unsuccessful – plans for constructing an
asylum in Algeria were proposed.[34] The 1880s and 1890s saw the first publications
of travel accounts written by French psychiatrists who visited Algeria and the newly
"protected" Tunisia[35] and who described, in a quasi-ethnological way, what and whom
they encountered on their journeys. In their capacity as psychiatrists, they surveyed
existing Muslim asylums and general hospitals in the colonies and described the miserable conditions in both sets of institutions. While some of these psychiatrists were
truly shocked by the conditions the Muslim mad endured in the traditional Islamic
māristāns and deplored the inhumane treatments administered there, these reports
must be seen as quintessentially colonial testimonies used to justify the concept of
a "civilising colonialism".[36]

---

32 Maupomé, Quelques aspects, 34.
33 The Iraqi psychiatrist Ihsan al-Issa, for example, declared in a 1989 article that "since the
    Algerian sociocultural background is similar to that of Morocco and Tunisia, many of the
    psychiatric findings and information could be generally applied to these countries." Al-Issa,
    Psychiatry in Algeria, 240.
34 See: Delasiauve, Review of Collardot; Jobert, Projet. These early projects, rejected due to
    budgetary concerns, were discussed in depth in Sauzay's 1925 dissertation on the "Assistance
    of Sane and Insane Psychopaths in Algeria". See also: Porot, Allocution, 29 f.; ibid., Assistance
    psychiatrique, 86; Desruelles/Bersot, Note sur l'histoire, 311 ff. The titles of French sources have
    been translated into English in the text – the original French titles can be found in the biblio-
    graphy.
35 Variot, Visite; L'hôpital arabe de Tunis; Voisin, Souvenirs. The French psychiatric journal
    Annales Médico-Psychologiques also published a translated account of two visits by British
    psychiatrists to Egyptian asylums in that same period. Dumesnil/Pons, Deux visites.
36 These reports showed a combination of horror and pity, yet they were too similar in struc-
    ture, phraseology and details, following an unacknowledged blueprint, to be seen as individ-
    ual, humanitarian texts, and usually did not add to the already existing "knowledge" of the

Due to World War I and budgetary cuts, general doctors, travelling experts and metropolitan psychiatrists remained responsible for the assessment and treatment of North African mental patients until the 1920s. In 1925 Antoine Porot, founder of what became known as the psychiatric *École d'Alger*, became the first professor of General and Medical Pathology at the Medical Faculty of the University of Algiers.[37] This was to be the starting point of psychiatrists living, working and studying in North Africa. By the 1930s the first psychiatric hospitals for Muslim patients were finally built in the Maghreb, ending patient transfers to France.[38] This allowed colonial psychiatrists to become more vocal and authoritative, and by the 1940s and 1950s the *École d'Alger* even came to dominate the psychiatric mainstream discourse in France.[39]

Framing the Title – "The Hidden Patients"

The title "The Hidden Patients" was chosen for three reasons, the principal one being that female Muslim patients were somehow "hidden in plain sight" – present in the colonial institutions, but ignored in the written sources. Colonial psychiatry's strong focus on criminal insanity on the one hand and Muslim normality on the other distorted the portrayal of the clinical reality[40] and resulted in certain topics being neglected despite the breadth of publications. The physical absence of psychiatric texts concerned with female Muslim patients effectively hid them from the eyes of readers of the academic literature.[41]

A second reason for the title was the colonial obsession with explaining the low number of Muslim female patients by claiming that no respectable Muslim family would allow their women to be brought to a "mixed" hospital, where they would be literally unveiled, examined and treated by men. In the colonial imagination, Muslim families preferred to look after these patients at home, actively hiding "insane" Muslim women from the appropriate colonial psychiatric institutions. This "appropriation" of gender segregation – through a very literal interpretation of Muslim ideals – gave

---

colonised mad. Reports written by British psychiatrists about the *māristāns* in Cairo are equally analogous. See for example: Urquhart, Two Visits, 47; Tuke, Two Visits, 49. Chapters 3 and 4 present an analysis of these colonial reports on the conditions in these traditional North African asylums.

37 Keller, Colonial Madness, 137 f.

38 This will be discussed at length in Chapter 3.2.5 "Psychiatric Hospitals in North Africa".

39 On this development see: Keller, Colonial Madness, 6 f.; ibid., Taking Science, 18; 26.

40 See Chapter 1 and Chapter 2 for analyses of the focus on "normality" and "criminal insanity" respectively.

41 The readers of psychiatric publications were predominantly other psychiatrists who were, by this silence on certain topics, influenced in their own thematic approach.

French psychiatrists an explanation for the absence of Muslim women from their care, but also the possibility to imagine the existence of female "hidden patients", languishing without proper care in urban harems and rural dwellings.

The third reason for the title alludes to one of the main explanations for the low numbers of female Muslim patients in the later colonial period. French psychiatry proposed that primitive Muslim sanity was too similar to Muslim insanity for manifestations of the latter to be noticeable by French-trained psychiatrists.[42] This notion was influenced by theories about "primitive mentalities", proposed by the leading French ethnologist Lucien Lévy-Bruhl in 1922.[43] Lévy-Bruhl excluded North Africans from his description of a pre-logic, primitive mentality, and while colonial psychiatric writers acknowledged the differentiation between monotheistic Muslims – who had lived through a glorious past, but whose societies were now in decay – and Lévy-Bruhl's "real primitives", they insisted on describing a slightly different, but still irrational and primitive, *mentalité indigène* of the North African populations.[44] Through this theory, all North Africans could be envisaged as dangerously close to insanity, which implied, in the colonial imagination, masses of undiagnosed potential patients out there, unrecognisable to French-trained psychiatrists accustomed to strict distinctions between sanity and madness, and hidden from colonial care through the pathological characteristics and ways of life of the "race".

Selection of the Chronological Scope

The temporal frame of this analysis of female Muslim patients in French colonial psychiatric texts covers the years 1883 to 1962, as this was the period in which French colonial psychiatry in North Africa was at its most active. In 1883 the French psychiatrist and criminologist Adolphe Kocher wrote the first treatise dedicated exclusively to the examination of an aspect of North African psychopathology. His dissertation, "Criminality among Arabs", related his personal experiences at the Civil Hospital of Mustapha in Algiers, where mental patients were processed before being sent to

---

42 This normal "primitive mentality", shared by all Muslims, will be examined in Chapter 1.

43 Lévy-Bruhl, Mentalité primitive. On the influence of Lévy-Bruhl's theory on French colonial psychiatry see for example: Louçaief, Manifestations hystériques, 34; Ammar, Ethnopsychiatrie (1970), 300; Razanajao/Postel, Vie et l'œuvre psychiatrique, 158; Jacob, Psychiatrie française, 371; Berthelier, Homme maghrébin, 98; Bennani, Psychanalyse, 74 f.; 80 f.; Macey, Algerian with the Knife, 164; Keller, Taking Science, 25.

44 For example: Porot/Sutter, 'Primitivisme', 226; 234; Taïeb, Idées d'influence, 24; Courbon, Review of Porot/Sutter, 440; Sutter, Review of Taïeb, 55; Susini, Aspects cliniques, 91; P., Review of Aubin, 93; Sutter et al., Aspects algériens, 892.

France.[45] In 1891 Abel-Joseph Meilhon, who was to write one of the founding texts of French colonial psychiatry in 1896, authored the first account of Algerian patients in the asylum in Aix-en-Provence, where he worked. Any one of these dates could have been selected as a starting point for the time frame of this book, but 1883 was chosen because it was the publication date of the first dissertation that focused solely on an aspect of North African psychopathology. Earlier texts will be referred to, but due to their scarcity and brevity, the main focus of this historical analysis is on the period introduced by Kocher's treatise. 1962 was chosen as the end of the period covered because a number of important texts, still essentially colonial, were published in the final year of the brutal war in Algeria. These 79 years saw a plethora of administrational, legal and social changes, which in turn deeply influenced the perception and alignment of the colonial psychiatrists. The most important of these changes, in the context of this book, were the development of a French settler mentality in North Africa – which the psychiatrists working there were part of – and the gradual realisation that France could never civilise North Africans and that the status of Muslim women was intrinsically linked to the "assimilability" of North Africans.

In Algeria, this settler mentality was largely established by 1883, with France being able to look back on half a century of control. By contrast, Tunisia had only just been occupied and Morocco remained uncolonised for another 30 years. By the time of Kocher's publication, French Algeria had in fact been construed, both legally and within the French national discourse, as being a section of the motherland instead of a mere colony and had been officially divided into three French departments in 1848 – Oran, Constantine and Algiers.[46] It was, however, only in 1870, forty years after the French army had landed on the Algerian coast, that its administration changed from one dominated by military concerns and actors to a civic administration,[47] aiding Algeria's transformation into a settler colony[48] and thereby assisting the development of a settler mentality.

---

45 The focus of Kocher's dissertation on criminality can be explained by the fact that he was a student of the eminent French criminologist Alexandre Lacassagne. Kocher's dissertation was followed, in 1889, by a book from another student of Lacassagne's, Lucien Bertholon, entitled "Outline of Criminal Anthropology of Tunisian Muslims", based on his experiences as a doctor working in Tunisia. Bertholon, Esquisse, 389 f.

46 Lorcin, Rome and France, 302.

47 See, for example: Collot, Institutions de l'Algérie, 7 f.; Lorcin, Imperial Identities, 6; ibid., Imperialism, 655. No purely military administration was ever introduced to either Tunisia or Morocco.

48 The 1870s and 1880s showed a dramatic increase in the numbers of European settlers in Algeria. The European population of Algeria rose from 217,990 in 1866 to 412,435 in 1881 – an increase of almost 200,000 European settlers in only 15 years. Maison, Population, 1082. The historian David Prochaska wrote in his 1990 book, however, that the consolidation of a settler society

Algeria, and to a lesser degree Tunisia and Morocco, received rising numbers of mainly *petits blancs* or "poor white" immigrants[49] from France and other Mediterranean states during their colonisation. These *petits blancs* settled there voluntarily[50] – and, in the case of Italians, Spaniards, Maltese and others, became French in the process. These Mediterranean workers immigrated to North Africa in order to escape the economic hardships they endured in Europe.[51] By the end of the 19th century, this medley of European settlers had gradually turned into *Algériens*, a colonial term which encapsulated the new settler mentality and which was rarely used for the Muslim populations of North Africa, who were instead described as *musulmans* or *indigènes*.[52]

The 1870 change from military to civic administration in Algeria was influenced by developments in France itself. The defeat of France by Prussia, the end of the Second Empire and the Civil War of 1870/1871 drove France's Third Republic to change its overseas policies.[53] The historian Alice Conklin argued in her 1997 book "Mission to Civilize" that after these developments, which were deeply problematic for the French self-understanding of France as a superior nation, the Third Republic tried to regain a sense of importance through the solidification of its existing colonies and the expansion of its overseas settlements, which allowed "the Republic to engage in the politics of grandeur".[54] Similarly, the historian Robert Aldrich argued in a 2007 chapter on the French "Colonial Man" that after 1870 a perceived "deficit of

---

in Algeria started in 1890. Prochaska, Making Algeria French, 206. On the development of the proportions of the different groups in Algeria over the colonial period, see also: Kamel, Population et organisation.

49   Prochaska, Making Algeria French, 124; 172. On the question of poor white settlers in other colonial contexts, see, for example: Arnold, European Orphans and Vagrants, 104 f.; ibid., White Colonization, 139; Ernst, Idioms of Madness, 173.

50   Clancy-Smith, Islam, Gender, and Identities, 155. Prochaska defined these European *petits blancs* communities as "European colonies within the French colony" in his 1990 book on settler colonialism in the Algerian city of Bône. Prochaska, Making Algeria French, 154.

51   However, Algeria was also used to dispose of political "undesirables" throughout the 19th century. Lorcin, Imperial Identities, 9.

52   Clancy-Smith, Islam, Gender, and Identities, 155. The often problematic vocabulary in the sources was translated into English terminology. In the following chapters, some racist or otherwise questionable French terms, adopted because of their common usage, will be marked with quotation marks, even when they demonstrate a general attitude and are not specific quotes. The French term *indigène*, for example, will be rendered as "native" in the text; the French term *aliéné* – used throughout most of the colonial period – rendered as either "insane", "mad" or even sometimes "patient", depending on the specific context.

53   Patricia Lorcin, for example, explained this administrative transformation of the Algerian colony by the fact that the 1870 losses discredited the authority of the military in France. Lorcin, Imperial Identities, 7.

54   Conklin, Mission to Civilize, 11 f.

manliness" triggered an urge for compensation, which in turn formed a new "colonial masculinity and its actions – conquest, pacification, the building of new countries, settlement, promotion of traditional virtues".[55] The climate in Algeria at the time of Kocher's doctoral research and the publication of his results was correspondingly one dominated by nascent settler concerns and France's reassertion of its self-awareness as a civilised, politically and culturally important country.

The period analysed in this book also saw ideological shifts in explaining and justifying colonialism, such as the move from the alleged final goal of "assimilation" of the colonised populations to that of mere "association".[56] The ideology of "assimilation" became important in justifying the conquest and control over colonies in the 19th century and was already present in the early psychiatric discourse on the colonial Maghreb. The notion that colonised populations could be "assimilated" into the French nation was part of the French *mission civilisatrice*, which saw France as the bearer of civilisation par excellence. Seeing itself as a true paragon of civilisation, France imagined itself to be able to lift evolutionarily backward people up a step or two on the ladder of progress. The theory of assimilation claimed that colonised populations could, by being subjected to French law, through Western education and the broader everyday contact with French culture, be turned into veritable Frenchmen. This policy lost its stringency sometime between the turn of the century and the end of World War I and was finally dropped in favour of "association" – which had, however, also been around since the beginning of the new colonial expansion under the Third Republic.[57]

This abandonment of "assimilation" was usually justified, in the eyes of the colonial agents, by claiming that "association" was preferable as it showed more respect for local customs, religious traditions and the existing elites.[58] There was, however, also a more direct argument for "association", advocated by colonial psychiatrists from the 1920s onwards, which claimed that the colonised populations in general, and North Africans in particular, were, both culturally and genetically, not "assimilable". This discussion about the applicability of "assimilation" and "association" was also connected to questions about gender. The historian Julia Clancy-Smith, for example, explained in a 1996 article on North African women that gender had not initially been used by the French as an argument against the assimilability of North Africans. For her, the French colonial discourse in the 19th century had been formed by its opposition to a construction of "an active, masculine, seditious Islam seen as

---

55   Aldrich, Colonial Man, 125.
56   See also Raymond Betts 1961 book on this ideological shift: Betts, Assimilation and Association.
57   Conklin, Mission to Civilize, 187.
58   See for example: Pedersen, 'Special Customs', 52.

posing the most insuperable obstacles to France's civilizing mission".[59] According to
Clancy-Smith, it was only after the turn of the century that the treatment of Muslim
women by Muslim men became the main symbol for North African backwardness;
a "racial" character trait through which the French were able to explain the distinct
lack of civilisation in North Africans, after 70 years of Muslims being tempted by the
government to assimilate into Frenchmen.[60]

Source Material and Existing Literature

As mentioned above, many different forms of colonial publications focused on questions of "insanity" among North Africans. The primary source materials used in this
book, however, are the texts written by psychiatrists for a psychiatrically trained
audience, and those by colonial doctors, particularly during the early period when
psychiatry was not yet truly seen as a separate field of medicine. It should be further
noted that some of those authors classified as "psychiatric experts" in the context of
this book were, strictly speaking, not psychiatrists but neurologists. The publications of neurologists have been included in this study because they often focused
on questions very similar to those debated by psychiatrists. The distinction between
neurology and psychiatry existed in French psychiatry, but it seems to have been less
clear-cut than, for example, in the English-speaking world.[61] Many colonial psychiatrists wrote about "neurological" problems, for instance in publications on such topics as neurosyphilis,[62] and psychiatrists and neurologists worked closely together, as
shown by the fact that the largest annual expert conference in the field was for both
"alienists" and "neurologists".[63] The psychiatric institutions built in North Africa in
the 1930s were called "neuropsychiatric" hospitals;[64] Antoine Porot was the first in a

---

59 Clancy-Smith, Femme Arabe, 53.

60 Ibid., Islam, Gender, and Identities, 155.

61 Bynum discussed the widely varying correlation between neurology and psychiatry in different
    European contexts, focusing mainly on Germany. Bynum, Nervous Patient, 89 f.

62 Neurosyphilitic disorders will be examined in Chapter 5.3 on general paralysis.

63 At the Congrès des Médecins Aliénistes et Neurologistes de France et des Pays de Langue française,
    both "neurological" and "psychiatric" topics were discussed by a mix of neurologists and psy-
    chiatrists. These annual meetings will be called Congress in the upcoming chapters.

64 For example: Benkhelil, Contribution, 26; Charpentier, Comptes Rendus, 478; Discussion du
    rapport d'assistance psychiatrique, 185; Donnadieu, Alcoolisme mental, 163; Susini, Aspects
    cliniques, 17; Manceaux et al., États mélancoliques, 270; Benabud, Aspects psychopathologiques,
    2; Fanon, Hospitalisation de jour, 1118.

series of professors of neuropsychiatry in Algeria;[65] and many others described their activities as neuropsychiatric.[66]

Especially in the 1930s to 1950s, during the heyday of the *École d'Alger,* the rate of publications among this group of colonial psychiatric experts was remarkable. They wrote profusely on new treatments,[67] on specific disorders[68] and on aspects of the newly defined "primitive mentality" of North Africans.[69] These published texts form a narrative net of the knowledge available to an expert public at the time, through which influences, plagiarisms and arguments can be traced like a multidimensional family tree. These sources were examined for female Muslim voices, for both medical and Orientalist topoi in the treatment and the descriptions of female Muslim patients, for influences of broader political and scientific theories on these topoi, and for changes in both topoi and theories over the period observed.

Richard Keller described in his 2007 book "Colonial Madness" the various shifts in the French colonial psychiatric discourse on the Maghreb.[70] His book analysed in great detail the opinions of different groups of psychiatrists in their historical contexts, showing the developments of theories and discourse over the colonial period, but if we look at the descriptions and comments on Muslim women in the same source material, these important nuances that Keller elaborated on seem to disappear. While not wanting to artificially homogenise the discourse, it has to be admitted that the sameness of the descriptions of women in the source material makes French colonial psychiatry seem almost separate from its historical context – which is in clear contrast with Keller's findings. The vocabulary and the images used to characterise both normal and abnormal Muslim women often failed to correspond to the individual experiences of the authors and therefore, in many instances, bore very little relation to the historical contexts of texts and authors. Instead, the same phrases and the same imagery were used repeatedly, in texts spanning the period between the 1830s and the 1960s, and could be used to describe any of the three colonies. The repetition of these almost ahistorical tropes and of anecdotal knowledge about Muslim women shows the intense influences and affinities between the groups of authors more than it depicts historical reality. It shows the persistence of what was "known" about Muslim women, which did not change all that much across the whole period. In addition,

---

65 Sutter, Leçon inaugurale, 443.

66 Abbatucci, Assistance, 653. See also: McCulloch, Empire's New Clothes, 49.

67 For a discussion of the colonial literature on new treatments, see Chapter 4.

68 For example: Maréschal/Chaurand, Paralysie générale; Sutter, Épilepsie mentale; Porot, M. et al., Tuberculose des aliénés.

69 Porot/Sutter, 'Primitivisime'.

70 On Keller's view of the different periods of French colonial psychiatry, see, for example: Keller, Colonial Madness, 4.

many of the sources studied did not mention Muslim women at all. Some, despite being classics of colonial psychiatry, only fleetingly mentioned female Muslims,[71] while others nominally set out to treat the whole of Muslim society, yet presented a reality that was clearly exclusively male.[72]

Postcolonial theories have criticised these publications and the ideals disseminated by the *École d'Alger*, and the definition ex negativo of the male North African inherent in most of these texts. Most famous among these critics of French colonial psychiatry is Frantz Fanon, in his capacity as a trained psychiatrist rather than a political activist,[73] who argued that people suffering from psychiatric problems in a colonial context were driven into their psychoses, manias and compulsions by the colonial situation, which degraded and dehumanised them. For Fanon, psychiatric troubles were among the few possibilities open to North Africans to protest against colonisation.[74] He criticised colonial psychiatry's often systematic denigration of Muslim societies as backwards and primitive,[75] but also emphasised the impact of colonial psychiatry on the perception of individual Muslims, turning them into "born slackers, born

---

71   While the psychiatrist Jean Sutter included Muslim women in the case studies of his 1937 dissertation on "Mental Epilepsy in the North African Native", his theoretical conclusions were all about Muslim men. He discussed the dangers posed by violent and criminal Muslim "mental epileptics" at length and only stated in his conclusions that mental epilepsy also occurred in women, albeit in a different form: "In women, who are not exempt from it [mental epilepsy], one notices less dangerous or criminal reactions, but a disordered agitation, which sometimes leads to self-mutilation." The fact that Sutter explicitly differentiated women in this quotation demonstrates that all the general conclusions preceding it applied not to Muslims in general but to Muslim men. Sutter, Épilepsie mentale, 215.

72   The French psychiatrist C. A. Pierson, for instance, wrote in 1955 that he had carefully chosen twelve case studies from different social, economic and educational backgrounds to represent the "Psychopathology of Morbid Impulse in North Africans". However, this cultural diversity, as depicted by Pierson, was exclusively male, as he included no case studies on Muslim women. Pierson, Paléophrénie réactionnelle, 644.

73   Fanon should be seen both as a source – in his capacity as a French psychiatrist working in North African psychiatric institutions during the French colonisation of the Maghreb – and as a leading theorist. On this dilemma, see also: Berthelier, Homme maghrébin, 112 f. On contextualising Frantz Fanon as a clinical psychiatrist, see: Butts, Frantz Fanon's Contribution, 1015; Keller, Clinician and Revolutionary, 833; Terranti, Fanon vu de Blida, 89.

74   Fanon, Damnés, 284 f.

75   An extreme example of this can be found in Boigey's 1908 text: "Westerners have always evolved within the orbit of civilisation. [...] Other people, foremost among which are placed the Islamic populations, have, on the contrary, never produced any great work, built no capital city, constructed no fleet, never thoroughly studied any science, embellished in a durable manner no place in the world. While the social state of the West is the culmination of an immense work of philosophical ideas, Islam is the result of a set of instincts, arrested in their natural expansion by the work of a great imposter, which is Muhammad." Boigey, Étude psychologique, 5 f.

liars, born thieves, born criminals"[76] and forcing them into laziness, criminality and violence as a form of protest against the French colonisation.[77]

For Fanon, colonial psychiatry had a distinct goal that was part of the ideology of the colonisation of North Africa. This premise is still valid today. During the entire colonial period, French psychiatry played an important political role. That is not to say that psychiatrists were actively involved in the policy-making processes in the administrations of the three colonial Maghreb states, but rather that their writings and their daily practice fulfilled a political function or could be used by the administrations to further their own ends.[78] In a 1994 article, the historian Megan Vaughan described colonial medicine as a "soft" political force, and suggested that the colonial discourse within the medical sources should be seen as a tool to analyse "both the power and the limitations of colonialism".[79] This "soft", often rather subtle, impact of colonial psychiatry on the whole community as well as on French colonial politics must be understood when attempting to analyse the colonial psychiatric sources and their importance. These political aspects of French colonial psychiatry influenced the way the colonial psychiatrists viewed – or, in the thematic context of this book, failed to view – the colonised populations, narrowing their focus from the whole population to those areas that promised to be of most utility to the civilising mission, such as differences between the colonisers and the colonised, institutionalisation with regard to settler security, or determining the efficacy of treatments in order to limit the expenditure.

The absolute authority claimed by colonial psychiatrists concerning definitions of madness and normality has been challenged, and Orientalist stereotypes and clichés about the "colonised mad" have been uncovered by a variety of different authors. However, many of these "debunked" colonial stereotypes about Muslim North African men remain very much present in modern-day France, and colonial clichés, now concerning descendants of North African immigrants instead of the "natives", are "still at work [...] in our collective imagination", in the words of the psychiatrist Robert Berthelier in a recent article.[80] Modern stereotypes of North African Muslims often

---

76   Fanon, Damnés, 285.

77   Ibid., 83; 284.

78   Jock McCulloch suggested in 1993 that the writings of certain colonial psychiatrists, among his examples the founder of the *École d'Alger*, "suggest that psychiatric research in the colonial setting could be used to fashion usable political tools [...]." McCulloch, Empire's New Clothes, 47. Megan Vaughan also warned in 2007 that it was simplistic to regard colonial psychiatry purely as a "tool of racist oppression". Vaughan, Introduction, 9 f.

79   Ibid., Healing and Curing, 288 f.

80   Berthelier, Fanon, psychiatre encore et toujours, 77. See also: Boucebci, Aspects du développement psychologique, 163; Macey, Algerian with the Knife, 162.

reflect notions consolidated by colonial psychiatry.[81] The results achieved by postcolonial authors in bringing these persistent colonial stereotypes to light raised one of
the principal questions of this book – if colonial psychiatry was one of the sources for
stereotypes about Muslim men, which in many cases still influence modern conceptions of North African males, then what did colonial psychiatry say about Muslim
women? What were the female Muslim stereotypes reinforced by colonial psychiatry, and are present-day notions of Muslim femininity still partly based on these
colonial prejudices?

Both the choice of the topic and the handling of the related sources and topoi
were influenced by the recent wave of historical analyses of colonial psychiatry[82] and
the interrelations between psychiatry and "race".[83] The historian Megan Vaughan
ignited this interest in 1983 with an article dedicated to colonial psychiatry in modern day Malawi,[84] and she remains one of the most important proponents of this field
of study. In her influential 1991 book on colonial medicine, "Curing their Ills", she
dedicated a chapter to the problems of colonial psychiatry and set out many of the
premises which still dominate the current historical discourse on it, e. g. the focus on
the normality of the colonised,[85] the morbidity of the language employed in descriptions,[86] and the pathologisation of the whole colonised population.[87] In the different
chapters of this book, Vaughan's British-based premises are used to contextualise the
information available in the sources, adapted – where necessary – to the colonial
reality encountered in French North Africa.

---

81 Richard Keller, for instance, wrote in 2007 that modern French prejudices against North
     Africans "drew on a lexicon established and scientifically backed by the work of the Algiers
     School [...]." Keller, Colonial Madness, 208. See also: Boucebci, Aspects du développement
     psychologique, 163; Bennani, Psychanalyse, 91.

82 For example: McCulloch, Empire's New Clothes; ibid., Colonial Psychiatry; Sadowsky, Psy-
     chiatry and Colonial Ideology; ibid., Imperial Bedlam; Mahone, Psychiatry in the East African
     Colonies; ibid., Psychology of Rebellion; ibid., East African Psychiatry; Swartz, Black Insane
     in the Cape; ibid., Lost Lives. In the context of colonial psychiatry, most historical research has
     been conducted on African countries, but secondary literature on other geographical areas,
     such as India and Indonesia, was also used for comparisons, e. g. Mills, Re-forming the Indian;
     ibid., Mad and the Past; ibid., History; Ernst, European Madness; ibid., Idioms of Madness;
     Pols, Development; ibid., Nature of the Native Mind.

83 In the context of the interrelation between psychiatry and "race", Suman Fernando's 1991 book
     "Mental Health, Race and Culture" influenced this book's content considerably.

84 Vaughan, Idioms of Madness.

85 Ibid., Curing their Ills, 101.

86 Ibid., 107.

87 Ibid., 101. See also: Sadowsky, Psychiatry and Colonial Ideology, 108.

While studies on colonial psychiatry have flourished in recent years, relatively few historians have, until now, dedicated their analytical efforts to the French colonisation of North Africa. A number of French and North African psychiatrists and psychologists have worked on the history of psychiatry in North Africa, and their critical accounts have helped in interpreting clinical aspects, especially because many of them personally experienced its final days.[88] However, the most extensive critical analysis to date is Richard Keller's aforementioned fascinating book "Colonial Madness", which was published in 2007. In his interpretation of French colonial psychiatry, North Africa was framed by colonial psychiatrists as a "space of madness"[89] – but one lacking, for French observers, recognisable measures to cure patients.[90] Therefore, North Africa presented French colonial psychiatry with an opportunity to be innovative, modern and experimental both in theories and in the choices of treatments for the population.[91] Although Keller did not specifically address Muslim women, many of his findings have been used to formulate the hypotheses explored in this book.

Two articles on psychiatry and North African women have been vital in articulating problems specific to female Muslim psychiatric patients. One of these articles was written by the American historian Alice Bullard, entitled "The Truth in Madness", in which she focused on French colonial psychiatry in the Maghreb. The other, "Changing Attitudes towards Women's Madness in Nineteenth-Century Egypt", was authored by the Egyptian historian Hoda El-Saadi. Both analysed, among other things, female patient numbers,[92] male attitudes towards mental diseases in women,[93] and discrimination against female Muslim patients within both institutions and theories[94] – all major topics of the following chapters. Moreover, Bullard questioned the authority of the colonial psychiatric knowledge, based as it was on what she described as "paternal condescension allied to a racist condemnation of the entire civilization [...]."[95] She also proposed that Muslim women were "erased" by French colonial psychiatry and suggested that "only by tracing the boundaries of the French erasure of North African women can we begin to conceive what was erased; only by examining this male-centred theory of madness can we begin to ask questions about

---

88   For example: Ifrah, Maghreb déchiré; Aouattah, Ethnopsychiatrie maghrébine; Berthelier, Homme maghrébin; El-Khayat, Psychiatrie moderne; Jacob, Psychiatrie française; Bennani, Psychanalyse; Bégué, French Psychiatry in Algeria.
89   Keller, Colonial Madness, 3.
90   Ibid., 118.
91   Ibid., 84 f.
92   El-Saadi, Changing Attitudes, 301; Bullard, Truth in Madness, 121 f.
93   El-Saadi, Changing Attitudes, 298 f.; Bullard, Truth in Madness, 120.
94   El-Saadi, Changing Attitudes, 302; Bullard, Truth in Madness, 114; 127.
95   Bullard, Truth in Madness, 125 f. See also: McClintock, Imperial Leather, 43 f.

the female mad."[96] Both the questioning of colonial scientific "knowledge" and the notion of an almost intentional silence on the topic of female Muslim patients will be taken into account in the following chapters.

Finally, publications from the broader field of gender studies were consulted, analysing the situation of female psychiatric patients in Europe,[97] but also of women in Islamic and non-Islamic colonial societies. These gender-based historical analyses set important rules for the respectful handling of the delicate issues of colonised women. The "classics" of colonial gender studies were used in order to acquire a sensibility in understanding colonial hierarchies, descriptions of both colonised and colonising women, and the interrelations between different population groups. Ann Laura Stoler's writing, for instance, helped in contextualising the colonisers and the complex interrelationships within the heterogeneous hierarchy of settler societies,[98] which was relevant in order to better understand the position of the few female colonial psychiatrists working in North Africa. Stoler's descriptions of the fear of colonised men attacking white women[99] as a means of unifying settlers[100] and her emphasis on the colonial interest in the sexuality of the colonised[101] both proved useful. Similarly, Alice Conklin's criticism of the limitations of the French *mission civilisatrice* when it came to improving the status of colonised women[102] could also be applied to the study of the French colonial psychiatric discourse. The specific context of colonised women in colonial psychiatric sources adds new dimensions and nuances to these theories.

Chapter Outline

This book focuses on the various interests of French colonial psychiatry, including an examination of which Muslim women came within its scope and interest and finally made it into the published texts, and which remained concealed and hidden. The chapters of this book set out the different stages of psychiatric institutionalisation and follow the path of Muslim women through them. The chapters are therefore thematically organised, as opposed to chronologically or geographically. Additionally,

---

96 Bullard, Truth in Madness, 123.
97 E.g. Showalter, Female Malady; Busfield, Mental Illness; ibid.; Female Malady?; Prestwich, Family Strategies; ibid., Female Alcoholism; Ussher, Madness of Women.
98 Stoler, Rethinking Colonial Categories, 136; 150; ibid., Carnal Knowledge, 41. See also: McClintock, Imperial Leather, 15.
99 Stoler, Making Empire Respectable, 636; ibid., Carnal Knowledge, 24 f.; 59 f.
100 Ibid., Rethinking Colonial Categories, 138.
101 Ibid., Making Empire Respectable, 635; ibid., Carnal Knowledge, 43. See also: Clancy-Smith, Islam, Gender, and Identities, 162; Lorcin, Imperialism, 668 f.
102 Conklin, Mission to Civilize, 87 f.

each of these chapters is introduced by one of the more detailed colonial case studies on female Muslim patients found in the source material, in order to contrast the marked absence of Muslim women discussed in the chapters themselves with detailed evidence for their presence. While case studies of colonial patients are problematic in many respects – from practically nullifying the patients' personal experiences by using generalisations and anonymisation, to the direct or indirect disrespect towards them as both women and Muslims, to their cases being misused in order to prove an author's theories –, it is the only way of accessing, to however small a degree, the voices of the colonial patients themselves. In the context of the chapters, these case studies will serve either to illustrate a particular colonial trope or to highlight an exceptional situation, diagnosis or behaviour.

Chapter 1 concentrates on those Muslim women who were excluded from colonial psychiatric institutions and on French conceptions of female Muslim normality. It examines the notions colonial psychiatrists had of North African society in general and how these notions influenced both the actual treatment of female Muslim patients and also what was written about them. This chapter analyses what French colonial psychiatrists "knew" about female Muslim normality, and their interest in the masses of non-patients around them, in order to determine how conceptions of Muslim normality were used to explain the low numbers of female Muslim patients.

Chapter 2 considers the mechanisms through which Muslim women entered the institutions of colonial psychiatry.[103] It focuses on the selection of abnormal patients from among the masses of quasi-abnormal non-patients and on the effects these methods of selection had on the Muslim perception of French psychiatry. It concentrates on those women who appeared in the rather narrow field of vision of colonial psychiatry and who could, therefore, be treated as pathologically abnormal, and also on the group of experts responsible for the selection of the small number of female Muslim patients. The chapter questions whether the selection of patients was a purely medical affair or whether it was influenced by other motives.

Chapter 3 concerns those female Muslim patients admitted to French mental asylums and psychiatric hospitals. While female Muslim patients were neglected in both theories and case studies, they were present in some of the published statistics. Consequently, the presented statistics were analysed critically in order to find signs of the presence of female Muslim patients so often denied by the theories. It examines their numbers in these institutions and their ratios compared to other patient groups – mortality rates, percentage of patients released as cured, and the distribution of different psychiatric diagnoses among this patient group. It addresses the questions of the statistical evidence set forth by colonial psychiatrists for the absence of female

---

103 This was before notions of out-patient treatments took hold in psychiatry – throughout most of the period examined in this book, "treatment" meant automatic institutionalisation.

Muslim patients from colonial care, the classification of the symptoms colonial psychiatrists encountered in their female Muslim patients, and the psychiatric diagnoses they used to make sense of the symptoms they were confronted with.

Chapter 4 looks at what happened to Muslim women in these colonial institutions. It asks whether they received any medical treatment and, if so, what treatments were administered. The chronological order in which treatments were introduced is also examined. Most importantly, this chapter determines whether Muslim women were treated differently from the other patient groups.

Chapter 5 focuses on the question of why certain diseases, common in Europe, remained undiagnosed in Muslim women. This chapter, dealing with the absence of female Muslims in specific categories of diagnoses rather than with the broader context of colonial psychiatry itself, will take up many of colonial psychiatry's hypotheses, raised in earlier chapters, and analyse them in more depth.

As this book deals with a potentially confusing number of different colonial psychiatric authors, brief biographies of each of the important figures have been set out in Appendix A. Appendix B contains the statistics and graphs composed for a better understanding of the sources.

Chapter 1
Making Sense of Normality:
The Fascination with Non-Patients

1.1 Case Study on North African Superstitions and the Shift from "Abnormality" to "Normality"

In Suzanne Taïeb's dissertation on superstitions in psychiatric disorders in Algeria, published in 1939, she included a large number of reports on her female Muslim patients. Taïeb was an exception in this regard, as only a few French colonial psychiatrists published case studies on female Muslim patients, a methodological problem which will be discussed in detail in Chapter 3.[1]

One of her case studies concerned a 25-year-old Algerian woman who had been admitted to Blida Psychiatric Hospital on the 14th of March 1938, following a manic episode. Taïeb described her as "behaving like an agitated maniac at her admission, incoherent, hallucinating, she hears voices telling her lots of things that she cannot remember. This state lasted for about five months. In September, the patient gradually calmed down, became more lucid, [and] readily provided information about her background and illness. This [her illness] goes back to the eve of Ramadan of the previous year. [She] nursed her last born when she *saw a Jinn in human form coming towards her, who carried a wooden crate and threw it at her. She ducked, tried to escape, but felt paralysed.* Since that day, she did not feel any more like other human beings. She suffered fugues, she cried loudly, *fought against the Jinn who tormented her. In her dreams, the Jinn often appeared in the form of a skeleton; he did not speak, but he pursued her.* Her family consulted tolbas [plural of ṭālib, scholar; in this context: traditional Muslim doctors, specialising in "sorcery"[2]], but they were unable to exorcise him [the jinn], which is why she was hospitalised. A month ago the Jinn withdrew from her, she no longer sees him. 'He left me in peace', she said. She is, indeed, very calm, docile, handles the household, but she retains some convictions, because when she happens to suffer from a stomach ache, she declares that it is an Arab disease, about which the

---

1 Further, many case studies on female patients could not be used as source material because they were anonymised to the extent that the ethnicity of the individuals was not recognisable. More information on the figure of Suzanne Taïeb can be found in a 2012 biography, written by the anthropologist Laura Faranda: Faranda, Signora di Blida.

2 On the figure of the ṭālib, see also: Chapter 4.5 "Contextualising Progress", p. 174, FN 171.

doctor can do nothing. *'It is the Jinn in my stomach... Do not believe me crazy because of this.'* She refuses to be [further] examined."[3]

Suzanne Taïeb's case study is interesting for a number of reasons. First of all, it includes a brief allusion to the cured state of Muslim women, as the patient is depicted as "very calm", "docile" and "handling the household" once the jinn – or the manic episode, in Taïeb's interpretation of the situation – had disappeared. This account of an almost cured "normality" fits in with descriptions of female "normalities" found in the colonial psychiatric source material and analysed in this chapter. The context of the case study allows the reader to understand that it was the patient's illness which made her loud, agitated and difficult to handle. Additionally, descriptions of this shift from illness back to "normality" are rarely found in relation to female Muslim patients, based on the low success rates of French colonial psychiatry on the one hand and the scarcity of published case studies on the other. Secondly, Taïeb's case study gives an insight into both the Algerian interpretation of mental disorders – as the episode was produced by a querulous and deeply terrifying jinn, according to the patient herself – and North African healing methods, i.e. the attempted exorcism, both of which fell, in the colonial worldview, under the heading of "superstitions".[4] Finally, Taïeb's portrayal of her patient's expression of an "Arab disease" shows both the deep lack of mutual understanding and the difficulties in communication between colonial patients and psychiatrists, beyond the merely linguistic obstacles.[5]

This case study therefore introduces two premises, which will be taken up again in this chapter. The first premise is that the colonial sources described female North African "normality" as being symbolised by the absence of certain (aggressive) actions or dynamic character traits, thereby defining this "normality" by an allegedly innate passivity and meekness. This definition of female "normality" as lacking certain (either European or male) qualities will be examined below. The second premise is the colonial assumption that North African traditions directly translated as "superstitions", which in turn were taken to symbolise North African "normality". This equation between (a) Maghrebi culture, (b) a form of "abnormality" (as "superstitions" were perceived as both backwards and deeply unhealthy) and (c) North African "normality" will be analysed in this following chapter.

---

3 Taïeb, Idées d'influence, 87 f. Emphasis in the original.
4 This is also shown by the subtitle of Taïeb's dissertation – "On the Role of Superstitions". See also the subchapter on "Medieval Superstitions" for an analysis of the colonial handling of "superstitions" with regards to Muslim women.
5 The linguistic problems are discussed in Chapter 3.3.2, "North African Diagnoses", p. 135.

1.2 Female Muslim Normality in Psychiatric Theories

Colonial psychiatric definitions of North African normality must be taken into account when trying to contextualise what was written about abnormality, i. e. in this case about female Muslim patients. Psychiatric interest in the normality of the colonised was based on the assumption that "healthy" normality was essentially European.[6] The colonised normality might have little in common with this European normality, and required experts to describe and explain the way of life of a different ethnic, cultural, social, religious and (importantly for this work) gender group.

In the eyes of French colonial psychiatrists, differences between normality and abnormality in Muslims paled in comparison to differences to European normality.[7] In his 1883 dissertation on the "Criminality of Arabs", the psychiatrist Adolphe Kocher wrote: "Fatalistic, enemy of all progress, the indigenous Muslim is still what he was before 1830; faded by defeat, he lost his native pride, and, from our civilisation, he only took the vices. It seems that an insurmountable barrier stands between us and him. It [the barrier] exists indeed, unwavering: the Qur'an."[8] The psyche of Muslims, soaked in the Qur'an, was imagined to be fundamentally different from Europeans, unchanging and inadaptable to modernity. This self-evident primacy of European normality, and the subsequent labelling of everything differing from this normality as abnormal, is omnipresent in the sources. Another example can be found in the 1909 psychiatric dissertation on the "Alienated in Tunisia" by Henry Bouquet: "There would be material for a very interesting chapter of compared mental pathology in this country, where it is difficult to find a normal psychological standard."[9] By alluding to the abnormalities of non-patients, Bouquet suggested that among Tunisians, European-style "normality" was difficult to find: instead of normality, he found a form of pathology in the character traits and customs of normal Muslims.[10]

Though influenced by modern theories about academic and social "othering", and a post-Foucauldian awareness of the social exclusion of all "abnormality" in search of

---

6 The basis of any psychiatric definition of "normality" was the European male, invariably those living a "civilised", modern, urban life. See for example: Boucebci, Aspects de la psychiatrie, 175.

7 Megan Vaughan's insight that, in the colonial context, indigenous populations were already excluded as a whole, distinctive from the colonisers through their ethnicity and their social status, and that, therefore, no further "othering" of mental patients was required is important in this chapter. Vaughan, Curing Their Ills, 107.

8 Kocher, Criminalité, 1 f.

9 Bouquet, Aliénés en Tunisie, 17.

10 John Warnock's quote on the difficulty of "diagnosing sanity" in Egypt, discussed in the introduction, referred to the same problem. Warnock's statement that he found it "more difficult to diagnose sanity than insanity" must be seen in the context of colonial psychiatrists struggling to identify colonised "normalities". Warnock, Twenty-Eight Years, 586.

a definition of normality, this chapter is mainly based on the interest of the colonial psychiatrists in "abnormal normality" that one encounters repeatedly in the colonial sources. The question of whether "Muslim normality" deserves such a prominent place when one specifically analyses the "psychopathology", the mental "deviance", the "abnormality" of female Muslims in North Africa is answered by the context of the sources themselves – French colonial psychiatrists had a deep-seated interest in the pathological normality of the "natives", as the publications clearly show. They saw both the "normal" and the "pathological" psychology of the indigenous population as within their field of expertise, and typical publications included chapters or paragraphs on normal behaviour, lifestyle and traditions as much as on a specifically Muslim psychopathology or on diseases and symptoms they had in common with Europeans.[11] In their discussions on North African normality, general terms such as Muslim personality, Muslim customs and Muslim culture were used almost synonymously and interchangeably. In their narrow conceptualisation of the Maghreb, North African culture not only dictated the minutiae of normal Muslim life, but, as the French psychiatrist Robert Berthelier argued in 1994, it also regulated the forms and frequency of mental diseases.[12]

But how can it be explained that the French experts, whose authority was based on their knowledge of "abnormality", took such an interest in the everyday aspects of indigenous life? The British medical historian Megan Vaughan wrote extensively about this focus of colonial psychiatry, and in her opinion the descriptions, explanations, and interpretations of indigenous normality, expressed by colonial psychiatrists, were more influential than what they wrote about their insane patients.[13] In the introduction to the book "Psychiatry and Empire", which she published with Sloan Mahone in 2007, Vaughan (referring to Mahone's article on colonial psychiatrists in East Africa in this edited volume[14]) wrote: "As in so many other cases, this influence was felt through their speculations, not so much on the psychopathology of their patients as on their theories of the 'abnormal' state of the 'normal' natives' mind [...]."[15]

This colonial assumption of an "'abnormal' state of the 'normal' natives' mind" forms the basis of this chapter, which looks at the colonial psychiatric definitions of male and female indigenous normality and maps out the generalisations and contradictions of the source material. The Muslim femininity perceived as normal in the colonial

---

11 One example is the 1926 dissertation of Don Côme Arrii on the "Criminal Impulsivity of Indigenous Algerians". Arrii juxtaposed Muslim normality and abnormality in what he called a *"sketch of the normal and pathological psychology of the natives"*. Arrii, Impulsivité criminelle, 15. Emphasis in the original.

12 Berthelier, Homme maghrébin, 34.

13 Vaughan, Curing their Ills, 100 f.

14 Mahone, East African Psychiatry, 41–66.

15 Vaughan, Introduction, 8.

sources is in many ways one-dimensional and ahistorical, with French psychiatrists not differentiating between the individual Muslim women they wrote about and making no distinction between their patients and those of their predecessors. They did, however, notice two distinct social "classes" in the Muslim societies they encountered, changing over time under French influence, but the differences between these strata and the class development during colonialism seemed, as portrayed by the colonial authors, to have no influence on the psyche of Muslim women. *The* Muslim woman was essentially the same whether born into a family of nobles or beggars.[16]

Colonial psychiatrists confused and melded notions from all strata in their picture of normal Muslim femininity. Muslim women were caged and languid, as if stepping out of Orientalist paintings, like the wives, daughters and sisters from the upper classes, with no man outside the family ever setting eyes on them. Muslim women worked hard and aged fast, like the wives of Muslim peasants, who worked the fields alongside the animals of their shared master. Muslim women were deeply sexual and unsatisfiable in their lust, locked away in harems, constantly plotting and hiding their countless affairs from their murderously jealous husbands and male family members. Muslim women were married at a prenubile state, suffered marital abuse, and could not, legally or socially, defend themselves against the "legitimate" attacks of their husbands. These opposing narratives – composed of contrasting imagery from the harem and the "douar", the North African village[17] – co-existed in the colonial imagination, forming, regardless of their inherent contradictions, a single picture, detached from time and geography.[18]

Looking at the context of this fascination with North African normality, one comes across two sets of psychiatric theories, both connected to the important question of why there were fewer mental patients in North Africa than in France. The (chronologically) first theory – civilisation leads to madness – was used by early French psychiatrists, such as Abel-Joseph Meilhon in 1896, while the second – Muslim normality is quasi-pathological – became more popular after 1918 with the rise of the *École d'Alger*, although both theories co-existed.

---

16 The alienation between European observers and Muslim women was further aggravated by comparing poor Muslim women from the countryside unfavourably with the French urban middle classes, rather than French rural women. Lorcin, Imperial Identities, 66 f.

17 The word "douar" is now part of the French vocabulary and comes from the Arabic *dawwār*.

18 See also: Clancy-Smith, Islam, Gender, and Identities, 164. Orientalist harem fantasies influenced this imagined female Muslim normality. In 1922, for example, Renée Lacascade wrote in her medical dissertation "Childcare and Colonisation" that "Muslim women live enclosed in the harem at the disposal of their husband, lord and master, by turns indifferent, demanding, meddlesome, always despotic, only considering his personal pleasure when it comes to women [...]." Lacascade, Puériculture et colonisation, 13. For a discussion of the imagery of the harem, see for example: Marsot, Revolutionary Gentlewomen, 265; Ahmed, Western Ethnocentrism, 524 ff.; Massad, Desiring Arabs, 9; Amster, 'Harem Revealed', 299.

1.2.1   Civilisation Leads to Madness

This theory held that Muslims were too primitive to become insane because insanity was a burden of civilisation. In this explanation, the low-level civilisation, the "primitive normality", of all Muslims, but particularly the even less enlightened Muslim women, afforded an instinctive protection against mental diseases. In 1868, for example, the psychiatrist Jobert compared the numbers of Algerian and French patients and explained: "This difference is due to the climate and the way of life of the Arabs, which causes less disorder in brains un-tormented by thought."[19]

This concept had its origins in the French Revolution. As Richard Keller stated: "Following the Rousseauist notion that madness marched in step with modern progress – that departure from one's true place in nature meant alienation from one's mental nature as well – psychiatrists such as Pinel and Brierre de Boismont proposed that madness was the price Europeans paid for living in civilization; psychological well-being, by contrast, appeared to be the privilege of so-called primitive populations."[20] This correlation between the level of civilisation and the numbers of mental patients, with lesser civilisations suffering from fewer disorders, was obvious to many French psychiatrists in different colonial contexts.[21] One of them, Paul Borreil, who worked on Senegalese mental patients in French hospitals, wrote in his 1908 dissertation: "in general, we can say that the frequency of psychopaths in a country is proportional to the degree of advancement *in civilisation* [...]."[22] Through this theory, early French colonial psychiatrists could easily explain the low numbers of "indigenous" mental health patients encountered in North Africa.

However, this theory sat uncomfortably with some of the core ideals of French colonialism: if civilisation was the goal that justified the colonisation of the barbarian North African region, then the French *mission civilisatrice*, through its introduction of modernity and civilisation, was the factor causing more mental diseases in the colonised populations. The possibility of steadily rising numbers of patients, stemming from the infectiousness of civilisational insanity, was a problem for colonial psychiatry, and therefore both the "normal" indigenous primitivity and the consequences of civilisation had to be analysed. The question of whether the primitivity that originally protected North Africans from mental diseases could, under certain

---

19   Jobert, Projet, 13.
20   Keller, Taking Science, 23. Keller referred to Françoise Jacob's 1994 article, in which she proposed that before 1850, French psychiatrists firmly believed insanity to be a disorder of civilisation. Jacob, Psychiatrie française, 366.
21   See also: Moreau, Recherches, 124; La civilisation est-elle cause des maladies nerveuses, 505.
22   Borreil, Considérations, 10. Emphasis in the original.

circumstances, be a positive force that merited France's moral and financial support needed to be answered.

The overall numbers of North African patients in general, and Muslim women in particular, were significantly lower than those of French patients. It was argued that Muslim women had so little contact with colonial officialdom, being segregated and held in ignorance by oppressive fathers and husbands, that fewer suffered from this disease of civilisation. In 1939 the psychiatrists Desruelles and Bersot, for example, quoted a personal communication sent to them by the founder of the *École d'Alger*, Antoine Porot. In it, Porot had explained the low proportion of female Muslim patients: "By her passivity, by her humble domestic duties, I believe the Arab woman [to be] much less exposed to insanity than men; her reduced and modest life, without agitation and external conflict, has to make her less vulnerable and less exposed to the vicissitudes and the anxieties of life."[23] From Porot's point of view, Muslim women were forced to lead a brutally secluded life, which, however, offered them a special immunity. More contact with colonialism, through education or more rights, could potentially eradicate this seclusion-based immunity. This immunity fascinated many colonial psychiatrists, especially since "emancipated" French women were seen to be suffering in greater numbers than Frenchmen.[24]

The connection between civilisation and the gendered distribution of patients seemed self-evident to many colonial psychiatrists, including one of the few female psychiatrists working in colonial North Africa, the aforementioned Suzanne Taïeb, who expressly explained the Muslim gender proportions among the patient numbers in her 1939 dissertation as depending on the level of civilisation: "The difference between women and men is of the same nature as that between an evolved subject and one that is less so [...]."[25]

In order to understand the exact pathological impact of civilisation, French colonial psychiatrists therefore tried to define the facets of daily life that made Muslim women less evolved than Muslim men. The French doctor Witold Lemanski, one of the few psychiatric experts writing extensively on Muslim women,[26] attempted to explain the low incidence of insanity among Muslim women in 1913 through their characters and lifestyles: "We have to necessarily search for the causes in the way of life, habits of temperance, absence of heredity, religious customs, conception of fatalism, absence of any physical or moral overwork, ignorance of eccentricity, and neurasthenia."[27]

---

23 Desruelles/Bersot, Assistance aux aliénés en Algérie, 593, FN 1.
24 Compare to Chapter 3, p. 124.
25 Taïeb, Idées d'influence, 79.
26 With articles and chapters in his book dedicated to the psychology of Muslim women such as "On the Rarity of Madness in Arab Women" or "Psychology of the Arab Woman".
27 Lemanski, Mœurs arabes, 108.

Among those reasons, however, the main explanation for the immunity of Muslim women was sought in the segregated, calm life Muslim women were forced to lead, just as Antoine Porot had told Desruelles and Bersot in 1939.[28] Abel-Joseph Meilhon, for example, wrote in his 1896 article on "Mental Alienation in Arabs" that he objected to the idea that the immunity of Muslim women to mental illness was due to them being more easily controllable than Muslim men: "With reason, we prefer to assign it [the immunity of Muslim women] to the living conditions of the native woman, systematically removed from any company."[29]

The physical segregation from company, entertainment, distraction and stimulation was seen to play an important role in this protection mechanism, which was understood to be almost innate and not socially conditioned. Raymond-Joseph Matignon mentioned the total segregation of Muslim women in his explanation for their immunity in his 1901 medical dissertation on "Medical Art in Tunis", alongside many of the tropes of Muslim normality analysed below: "Neuroses seem infrequent in Tunisia, which should probably be attributed to the profound apathy of the Arab, a consequence of his doctrinal fatalism; to the absence of any intellectual or moral over-excitement, the cerebral functions being reduced to their minimum work for the benefit of the vegetative and sensual life; to the kind of solitary existence and degrading practices that are imposed on women. She lacks the most common opportunities for hysteria: the reading of novels with tragic situations and lascivious descriptions, mundane courtships, rivalries of ambitions, wounds of self-esteem, intellectual overwork, fatigues of the workshop, worries about the future and disappointments in love."[30]

The hard life normal Muslim women led in this novel-free, unromantic, emotionally sterile bubble, imposed by segregation, was healthy in its simplicity, stark primitivity and unsophistication, lacking the many dangers French women faced, who tried to find their place in a male world. These dangers of civilisation were, in Matignon's eyes, symbolised in French women's passion for fashionable novels, work and various mundanities.

The goal of France's *mission civilisatrice* in North Africa was evidently not this form of feminine, over-educated and unhealthy civilisation, but rather a romanticised

---

28 Desruelles/Bersot, Assistance aux aliénés en Algérie, 593, FN 1.

29 Meilhon, Aliénation mentale, part 1, 25.

30 Matignon, Art médical, 84. While patriarchy started to weaken in France, the psychiatrist Raoul Vadon wrote about the comparatively healthy patriarchal lifestyle in Tunisia to which he credited the low numbers of insane in the country in his dissertation "Medical Assistance of Psychopaths in Tunisia" as late as 1935: "This is especially true of Muslim women who still live in a state of semi-confinement and who are not easily exposed to emotional shocks, sudden changes of life and environment, which certainly favour cerebral derangements, mental troubles of constitutional defectives and psychasthenic states in the countries more advanced in civilisation." Vadon, Assistance, 43 f.

simple and wholesome lifestyle. The same idea was taken up by Witold Lemanski in 1913, who wrote in his book "Arab Morals": "As everyone knows, it is a very close relationship between insanity and way of life: the natural character of the Arab woman, through her placidity, her restraint, her calmness, her equanimity, does not predispose to the strenuous work of the brain. She does not care for business, or politics, or religious controversy; she is engaged in her daily work, summarily accepting her destiny. No disappointments, no vexations, no grief disturbs her usual calm: also, we would only with difficulty find the common aetiological causes of insanity there. Eccentricity, originality, lucid insanity, in a word, of those civilised to excess, are rare in the harem: on the contrary, there is a perfect adaptation of the individual to the milieu, without clashes or violent shocks."[31]

In this context, one should ask if the focus on the immunising effect of segregation, simplicity of life, and acceptance of patriarchy and given status was not a social comment on the liberating effects of the emancipatory struggle in Europe. Another quote by Lemanski focuses directly on the question of the psychiatrically harmful consequences of emancipation: "Emancipation does not exist in Arab women, it is easy to conceive. It seems that the unique role that she should play in life is that of wife and mother. There are, in female Arab society, none of these rebellious or independent [women] who seem to forget the weakness of their sex and enter violently into the struggle of existence."[32] The careful descriptions of the normal lives of Muslim women mirrored, from a psychiatric point of view, the problems newly faced by French women in Europe: Muslim women knew and accepted their role in society and therefore were safe, while in France this balance was unsettled, with some women being forced to work while others, "civilised to excess",[33] tried to obtain a social status which was inherently unhealthy for them.[34] It is clear that in these contexts the descriptions of Muslim female normality must be read as a form of criticism of French female normality. The descriptions therefore did not necessarily express a reality, but a state that was secretly seen to be more desirable than that in France. In this context, the descriptions of normal Muslim femininity, despite their harshness, must be seen as an idealised version of desirable global femininity.

---

31 Lemanski, Mœurs arabes, 108 f.

32 Ibid., 27.

33 Lemanski used this expression more than once to describe European women. For example: "She [the Muslim woman] is not like that [woman] civilised to excess [...]." Ibid., 104.

34 Witold Lemanski seemed to be obsessed with European women. In his 1913 book he praised Muslim women for not being either as exaggeratedly religious as Catholic women, whose religiosity he saw as another reason for the high frequency of insanity in Europe, or as shockingly unreligious as female atheists, which he deemed to be equally unhealthy. Ibid., 99; 114 f.; 116; 181 f.

It was, however, not only the spatial distance from "civilised life" and their primitive, healthy lifestyle that protected Muslim women from insanity. Even if Muslim women suffered from mental illnesses, their primitively low status in North African social hierarchies, as understood by the French, hindered their family members from voluntarily surrendering them to colonial care. The famous psychiatrist Alexandre Brierre de Boismont wrote in an 1866 article: "The limited social importance of women in the Orient also provides a rational explanation for the very restricted number of this sex in the numbers of mental alienation."[35] The reasoning behind this peculiar hypothesis seems to be, at least partly, that a Muslim man would never permit his wife to be looked after by a colonial psychiatrist, not because of the strict segregation of the sexes, but rather the little value, emotionally and economically, of Muslim women. With his wife in hospital, a Muslim man would, at one stroke, be deprived of a womb for future sons, a "beast of burden" and an "instrument of pleasure",[36] his wife being nothing more than a personification of these "objects" to him.

1.2.2   Normality is Quasi-Pathological

The second theory asserts that Muslim normality was already "almost pathological" and is a reaction to the civilisational theories described above. The idea of North Africans being infected by the *mission civilisatrice* was attacked, the concept of Muslim immunity refuted, and the theory of Muslim normality being a protection against insanity replaced by Muslim normality being quasi-morbid in itself. Following this explanation, it was difficult for early French colonial psychiatrists to find patients, especially females, amongst Muslim populations, because they could not identify the insane – Muslim normality was so close to European psychopathology as to be unrecognisable. Symptoms of insanity in Europeans were part of Muslim normality – a point of view stated by the psychiatrist Raoul Vadon, who described this professional difficulty in his 1935 dissertation: "On the other hand, the violence of language, the hyperactivity natural to Oriental races, make reactions, which would seem to border on manic agitation in a Frenchman or a European, go unnoticed in a Tunisian."[37]

Equipped with their knowledge of European psychiatry, suited to specifically European normalities and abnormalities, French psychiatrists initially failed in locating the Muslim insane, and even if they found them, the North African mentality was so exotic that translating Muslim symptoms into clear French diagnoses was daunting. The psychiatrist Michèle Chappert described both linguistic and cultural difficulties

---

35   Brierre de Boismont, Rapport, 75.
36   See p. 48 and p. 58.
37   Vadon, Assistance, 44.

as late as 1962 in her dissertation on puerperal psychoses: "To this purely linguistic difficulty is of course added all that differentiates the European from the North African Muslim on religious, social and cultural levels; the phenomena of inner life, the very processes of thought, the modes of reaction separate them; despite his efforts, the doctor is often baffled, while the patient is unable to effectively cooperate with him."[38]

This theory of a North African "primitive mentality", propagated by the École d'Alger, explained the failure to locate the indigenous insane by maintaining that Muslim normality was quasi-pathological, making it impossible to find anything comparable to European normality. French colonial psychiatrists, at least in the later years of the École d'Alger, with their "race-based" theories already somewhat discredited, insisted that Muslim normality was not defined by the morbidity of the "race", but purely by the "primitive mentality" of North African Muslims.[39] This division was artificial, with no bearing on the reality of their explanation – the "primitive normality" of North Africans was still defined by "race" and by adherence to Islam. Even if they claimed that the "normality" of Muslims was determined by their "primitive mentality", this still meant that "normality" was indirectly determined by "race". Jean Sutter, Yves Pélicier and Porot's son, Maurice Porot, carefully differentiating between North African primitivity and the "real" primitivity of other "races", wrote in 1959: "These are the common conditions which, although difficult to define, have a much greater influence than racial or climatic factors in giving the 'native mentality' a set of fairly constant features, which puts them [...] halfway between the mental structure of the 'civilised' European and the 'primitive mentality' studied by [Charles] Blondel and [Lucien] Lévy-Bruhl. From the latter, it [the mentality of North Africans] acquires its fatalism, its mystic, or more often magical, conception of causality, its very subjective notion of time (which makes the chronological classification of elements of a story so often impossible), its usual ineptitude at accuracy and abstraction, its knowledge remaining steeped in emotion, the assertive character of its beliefs, [and] the empiricism of its ethical notions."[40]

This inherent difference between these manifestations of a normal "primitive mentality" and the French textbook cases caused considerable problems for the French-trained psychiatrists who tried to work with North African patients. Antoine Porot himself mentioned this in an article on the "'Primitivism' of North African Natives", written together with one of his students, Jean Sutter, in 1939, clearly with some exasperation: "These facts also introduce major difficulties in analysing, in the native, the development of mental processes, the character of the association of

---

38 Chappert, Contribution, 18.
39 See for example: Frey, Évolution, 247.
40 Sutter et al., Aspects algériens, 892. For the lack of understanding of time, see also: Fribourg-Blanc, État mental, 138.

ideas; we must know that *the absence of what we are used to call logic* is not, at least in many cases, a morbid sign."[41] The psychiatrist Humann cited in an 1934 article on the "Mental Troubles of the Natives in the Algerian Sahara" a similar, somewhat more general warning to other psychiatrists, unused to North African normalities: "It is understandable that such conceptions [belief in jinn etc.], which obviously offend common sense and the judgement of the European observer, but which are supported in the indigenous milieu with equal faith and certainty by healthy as well as alienated men, somewhat confuse the psychiatrist, for whom it is often difficult to establish the boundary between normal and pathological, to isolate the delusion from what conforms to the normal understanding of the indigenous community."[42] The confusion of normality with abnormality was fatal in this context, because it was both expensive and bad for the prestige of colonial psychiatry, if normal Muslims were hospitalised. French colonial psychiatric literature was, in a way, a literature of warning. Established psychiatrists wanted to warn "new" psychiatrists about traps when interpreting the minds and comportment of North African Muslims, to point out potential problems in understanding them and to clear up professional uncertainties.

The theory that Muslim normality was so pathological as to be almost abnormal finds its most extreme incarnation in a 1908 article by the psychiatrist Maurice Boigey. He posited that a belief in the principles of Islam caused some form of insanity in all Muslims: "Its [Islam's] progress can be less explained through theology than through mental pathology. [...] This is somehow a true epidemic [of] madness, which the qur'anic hordes have spread, weapons in hand. The first disciples of the prophet were degenerates, and their doctrines, put into practice, have caused true mental lesions in those who followed them. In other words, Mahomet implanted in the brain of the Believers a true *neuropathic state*."[43] He went on to explain that there were six manifestations of Muslim insanity,[44] and that normal Muslims exhibited aspects of these different insanities, which made them abnormal (compared with European normality) without actually rendering them insane. "In short, the mental state of the majority of Believers is a mixture of insanities, to various degrees, of tangled delusions, hidden by an appearance of reason."[45] Unsurprisingly, the belief that Islam itself caused low-level

---

41 Porot/Sutter, 'Primitivisme', 230. Emphasis in the original. The same sentiment can be found in a second article by Porot, written with another of his students, Don Côme Arrii, in 1932. In it, they described the difficulty of measuring different stages of dementia in "subjects whose mental fund is already so low on the scale of debility!" Porot/Arrii, Impulsivité criminelle, 604.

42 Humann, Troubles mentaux, 1085.

43 Boigey, Étude psychologique, 7 f. Emphasis in the original.

44 Ibid., 8 f. Among these manifestations, Boigey listed the "folly of words", as allegedly shown in the repetitive nature of the Arabic language, and the "perversion of the sexual instinct [...]."

45 Ibid., 9. Capitalisation in the original.

insanity was contested, and there were a number of French psychiatrists who claimed that Islam had a beneficial influence on the development of mental disorders. Witold Lemanski was one of them, claiming in 1913, only four years after Boigey's article, that Islam "[...] is severe, but simple, calm, tranquil, without exaltation and mysticism. Never does it predispose to insanity."[46] However, Lemanski's praise of Islam must be seen in the context of his vehement anti-Catholicism.[47]

Whether their fascination with non-patients stemmed from the fear that their professional expertise would be challenged if they categorically misdiagnosed, or whether they supposed that some aspect of Muslim culture was pathogenic, it was nevertheless important to know more about Muslim normality. French colonial psychiatry needed to be able to identify "primitive mentality" in all its abnormal forms, to "measure" mental diseases and to clearly demarcate normal from pathological, not least to give itself the authority that came with establishing such definitions.

How was the low number of female Muslim patients explained in this theory? While insanity would eventually be recognised in most Muslim men, who were in daily contact with French settlers, Muslim women were usually hidden from French experts by the Islamic ideals of gender segregation. When these experts came into contact with normal Muslim women, they were so alien to them, so strange in behaviour, beliefs and customs, that insanity was not instantly recognisable. French psychiatrists learned to recognise the male Muslim madman by his aggressive behaviour and his alcohol and drug addictions. They needed equally unmistakable signals to help them separate the abnormalities of North African women from actual insanities.

1.3 Definitions of the Normality of Female Muslims

These two concepts – of civilisation causing madness and of a quasi-pathological normality – represented conflicting views, yet many colonial psychiatrists, seemingly unconscious of their inherent opposition, switched between them in their texts. There were, despite the obvious contradictions between those theories, also some profound similarities, based on underlying notions about Muslim normality, which allowed for interchange between both theories. Despite enormous differences in class, location, ethnicity and even historical period, the evaluation of Muslim femininity changed little – the Muslim women described in the psychiatric source material led a traditional, secluded, primitive life that somehow influenced their mental states. The development of the notion of "primitivity" being intrinsically linked with normal Muslim femininity is interesting in the context of both theories – the normal, deep-seated

---

46 Lemanski, Mœurs arabes, 115.
47 See for example: Ibid., 99 f.; 116.

primitiveness of female Muslims explained the absence of insanity in one case and showed its quasi-omnipresence in the other.

1.3.1   Shared Muslim Normality

Some of the character traits which, in the eyes of French colonial psychiatrists, defined the everyday life of female Muslims stemmed from a normality shared with Muslim men – both were, for example, repeatedly described as "childlike".[48] The basis of the psyche of all Muslims (normal/pathological, male/female, from all ethnic and "racial" backgrounds) was, for French colonial writers their adherence to Islam. Using Islam as an explanation for all findings in Muslim countries is what the Algerian sociologist Marnia Lazreg called the "religion paradigm", which, she claims, has trapped both colonial and modern feminist writers.[49] In the context of North African psychiatry, Megan Vaughan argues that Islam replaced the East African "tribe" as the mono-causal basis of all normality.[50] Therefore, it was assumed that Muslims had more in common with other Muslims, regardless of geography, than with the French living in the same country.[51]

The aspect of Islam wielding the biggest influence on the behaviour of patients and non-patients alike, in the eyes of French colonial officials, was "fatalism". In the colonial imagination it defined North Africans, so much so that the American historian Nancy Gallagher wrote: "By the beginning of the twentieth century two myths had become cornerstones of colonial history: the myth of Muslim fatalism and the myth of European medicine coming to the rescue."[52] From the very beginning, the experts on the Muslim psyche, colonial psychiatrists, discussed Muslim fatalism – i.e. fatalism as a psychiatric issue – at length. The "dogma of fatalism, this slavery, this submission to the absolute will of the One, that is to say, the abnegation of all moral dignity in matters of religion and politics (the great psychological fact of the Orient!)" had already been discussed in the first French psychiatric article on Muslims – "Research

---

48   See for example: Arène, Criminalité, 137; Lemanski, Mœurs arabes, 79; 166; Porot, Notes, 382 f.; Arrii, Impulsivité criminelle, 33; Fribourg-Blanc, État mental, 138; Porot/Sutter, 'Prim-itivisme', 229; Olry, Paralysie générale, 83; Alliez/Decombes, Réflexions, 154; Pierson, Paléo-phrénie réactionnelle, 646; Igert, Milieu culturel marocain, 651.

49   Lazreg, Feminism and Difference, 86; ibid., Eloquence of Silence, 13. See also: Tucker, Prob-lems, 326.

50   Vaughan, Introduction, 7.

51   In 1909, for example, the psychiatrist Henry Bouquet wrote in his dissertation that "Muslims are essentially religious: they are united, even more than by bonds of race or country, by reli-gious ties." Bouquet, Aliénés en Tunisie, 19.

52   Gallagher, Medicine and Power, 96.

on the Alienated in the Orient" by Jacques-Joseph Moreau de Tours, published in the *Annales Médico-Psychologiques* in 1843.[53]

French colonial experts suspected a direct connection between Muslim fatalism and the low numbers of indigenous mental patients in North Africa.[54] In this explanation, Muslims, believing that they had no real influence on their lives, as everything lay in the hands of God, neither suffered from feelings of guilt nor worried as much about the future as individualist Europeans. Étienne-Paul Laurens wrote in his 1919 dissertation on nervous syphilis in Algerian Muslims: "[...] we have to agree that the fatalism of the Natives often softens their worries as well as their sadness."[55] Fatalism gave North Africans a meaning in life, which hindered the development of mental diseases such as depression. Raoul Vadon wrote in his 1935 dissertation "Medical Assistance of Psychopaths in Tunisia": "How to explain the rarity of psychopathy [psychasthenia, neurasthenia, melancholia]. I asked myself; I believe that we should give this observation a cause, taken from the Mohammedan religion. There is, in all melancholics or psychasthenics, an exaggerated notion of nothingness, a particularly sharp sense of death. From birth, the Muslim despises death, this form of negation; and his philosophy of the future does not go beyond the 'mektoub' 'it was written.'"[56]

While fatalism had an influence on all North Africans, Witold Lemanski maintained in his 1913 book "Arab Morals" that Muslim women were even more fatalistic than Muslim men. "Precisely, the Arab woman knows how to live without desires and without complaints, surrounded by her husband and children. Her religious and disciplined spirit, respectful of traditions and customs, is perfectly adapted to the milieu. She reveres the word of God, revealed in the Qur'an; she does not rebel against misfortunes she cannot avoid; she submits herself. This does not go without some fatalism; but this confidence in the decrees of Providence constitutes a soothing doctrine for the mind. The *Mecktoub* (it is written), in its ineluctable brutality, destroys the will, but it also soothes the nervous system of those who cannot be resigned and who often fight in a sterile struggle."[57]

---

53 Moreau, Recherches, 121. Capitalisation in the original.

54 Abel-Joseph Meilhon wrote in his article "Mental Alienation in Arabs", published in 1896: "Thus, fanaticism, which destroys the sense of personality and makes a docile instrument of events out of man, adds to the absolute proscription of alcohol; what more effective barrier could be opposed to insanity?" Meilhon, Aliénation mentale, part 1, 26.

55 Laurens, Contribution, 45. Capitalisation in the original.

56 Vadon, Assistance, 45. Only a few doctors and psychiatrists disagreed with this conviction that Muslim life was dominated by fatalism. In 1907, for example, Abel Lévy-Bram wrote that, in his opinion, North Africans were not "hardened fatalists. The natives, mostly, are much more ignorant than fatalistic." Lévy-Bram, Assistance médicale, 22.

57 Lemanski, Mœurs arabes, 114. Emphasis in the original.

This fatalism caused passivity in both Muslim men and women, but from the perspective of the colonial psychiatrists, Muslim women were defined by it – they were brought to colonial care by others, hidden by their families, and mistreated by their husbands. These descriptions sprang from the conviction that Muslim women were always subjugated victims, never actively involved in their lives, whereas in reality, they performed many chores in the home and, especially among poorer classes, outside. In the context of questions of interest to colonial psychiatrists, "passive" Muslim women were the main carers for those sufferers of mental illness looked after at home.[58]

1.3.2   Characteristics of Muslim Women

While Islam and its concomitant fatalism were common to all Muslims in the colonial *weltanschauung*, some aspects of Muslim normality were stronger in, or exclusive to, Muslim women. Below, "clusters" in the definitions of female Muslim normality will be analysed, comprising groups of rather "outlandish", picturesque quotes. These widespread tropes, covering much of what was seen to be normal Muslim femininity, have been repeated throughout the period of French colonial psychiatry in the Maghreb, their authority stemming as much from their adaptability to different theoretical frameworks as from the referencing of past experts in both knowledge and idiom.

Muslim Women as Wombs

Comparable to the situation in Europe, Muslim women were depicted as biologically perfect mothers, who always desired further pregnancies.[59] This seemed obvious even to individuals who could under no circumstance be seen as experts on Muslim women. In 1875, Captain Charles Villot, working for the colonial administration in Algeria, wrote in his book "Morals, Customs and Institutions of the Natives in Algeria": "The woman, being destined to reproduce the human race, cannot escape her destiny. Islamic law does not admit monastic vows. The woman belongs to man and

---

58   Douki et al., Women's Mental Health, 187. As carers, it is probable that they determined when such domestic situations became untenable and the person had to be given over to colonial care. This agency of a group of women corresponds with Suad Joseph's definitions of patriarchy in the Arab world: Joseph defined patriarchy in 1996 as "prioritizing of the rights of males and elders (including elder women) and the justification of those rights within kinship values". Joseph, Patriarchy and Development, 14.

59   See for example: Lévy-Bram, Assistance médicale, 72 f.; Chappert, Contribution, 32; Mares/Barre, Quelques aspects, 48.

she cannot, under any pretext, abandon the role fixed on her in this world."[60] This quote makes it clear that the both biological and religious destiny of motherhood applied to French women too, while the only possible exception in Europe, i. e. religious celibacy, was not permissible in Islam. In Muslim societies, it was expected that all women should fulfil their biological potential.[61]

Witold Lemanski wrote profusely on Muslim women's genetic and social propensity to childbirth and childcare. He explained in 1913 that the simple and natural upbringing that Muslim women enjoyed "without aspirations towards a vague and romantic ideal" prepared them ideally for lives as wives and mothers,[62] ensuring they were not plagued by the mental disorders often associated with European motherhood: "Also puerperal insanity is very rare. Women have such a high conception of motherhood that their spirit becomes, if possible, even more phlegmatic and calm: their uncomplicated ideas do not get confused in the mazes of delusion."[63] In the colonial imagination, North African Muslim women were ideal for gestation (strong bodied, simple minded) and gained status through giving birth. In 1910 an expert in Muslim law, Louis Milliot, claimed that marrying a Muslim woman was motivated by two wishes: having "a servant and offspring".[64] He maintained that the second wish created the only emotional bond existing between husband and wife in Muslim countries.[65] This sentiment of worth through birth was echoed in 1959 in a late colonial article by Jean Sutter, together with Susini, Pélicier and Pacalis entitled "Some Observations on Nuptial Psychoses in Algerian Muslims". In it, they maintained that becoming a mother was the only possibility for a Muslim woman to overcome the abject status in which she was kept by her family and husband. "[...] Muslim women often acquire in practice a similar position to that of Western women, especially when she has become a mother, and it is not unusual to see her acquire, within the family, a major influence."[66]

---

60 Villot, Mœurs, 80.
61 Abel Lévy-Bram, for example, stated in 1907 that, "as in all societies [which have] retained a character of ancientness", Muslim society considered celibacy "as something bad, like a veritable crime." Lévy-Bram, Assistance médicale, 77.
62 Lemanski, Mœurs arabes, 89.
63 Ibid., 120. On this topic, see also Chapter 5.4 on "Puerperal Insanity: The Perfect Mothers".
64 Milliot, Étude, 245.
65 Milliot suggested that "pregnancy is a happy period for women. The Arab has an innate love of children, and, as crude and hard as he is, he has some consideration for his wife, through fear for the child, and gratitude to the mother." Ibid., 240.
66 Sutter et al., Quelques observations, 908.

Beasts of Burden

The French were convinced that normal Muslim femininity was largely defined by women being treated by their husbands as animals, "beasts of burden",[67] who worked in the house and in the fields like "slaves".[68] In the Orientalist imagination, the Muslim man had "complete domination" over the Muslim woman.[69] French colonial psychiatrists opposed and complained about this perceived abject status of women in Muslim societies and repeated these tropes of the subjugated "beast of burden" in their publications, always using the same formulaic phrases.[70]

French colonial psychiatrists saw the origin of this "natural" female servitude in Muslim lifestyles and therefore in normal Muslim femininity. In 1883, the psychiatrist Adolphe Kocher wrote in his dissertation on "Criminality in Arabs": "The father of the family is a despot, the woman is only a humble servant, sometimes queen one day, slave the next. This servitude of women is an atavistic fact, recalling their nomadic life of the past."[71] In the colonial imagination, the harsh nomadic life, with its almost biblical patriarchs, turned Muslim women into hardworking servants, their position in the family barely above that of an animal. Joseph-Marie-Fernand Lafitte described in his 1892 dissertation "Contribution to the Medical Study of Tunisia" the social status of Muslim women, and their thoroughly animal nature, by outlining the tragic biography of a "normal Muslim woman". He stated: "Received at birth into the family as an impediment – almost as a disgrace – she is brought up in the domestic hierarchy, in a rank below that of a foal or a heifer, vegetating, if she is robust, at the discretion of

---

67 This strange designation, "bête de somme", can be found in a plethora of psychiatric and medical texts and even in travel literature. For example: D'Arlach, Le Maroc, 48; Bertholon, Esquisse, 404; Lafitte, Contribution, 86; 118; Meilhon, Aliénation mentale, part 1, 24; 25; Abadie-Feyguine, Assistance médicale, 18; 67; Lemanski, Mœurs arabes, 218; Arène, Criminalité, 27; Lataillade, Coutumes, picture between pages 160 and 161.

68 The idea that Muslim women were treated as "esclaves" can be found in many of the sources. Bertherand, Médecine et hygiène, 198; Lafitte, Contribution, 23; Gomma, Assistance médicale, 111.

69 Sivan, Colonialism and Popular Culture, 35.

70 Describing Muslims in particular or the colonised in general as animals was part of the broader Orientalist discourse, as criticised by Fanon in the "Wretched of the Earth". Fanon, Damnés, 45. See also: Kabbani, Imperial Fictions, 27. In this context, it should be noted that French farmers and other workers in the countryside were also often described as living barely better than the animals they worked with in the 19th century. See for example: Taithe, Neighborhood Boys and Men, 70.

71 Kocher, Criminalité, 8. Don Côme Arrii repeats Kocher's phrasing in his 1926 dissertation, word by word, without acknowledging it. Arrii, Impulsivité criminelle, 31.

chance like a small animal, and abandoned only to the forces and instincts of nature."[72] Rejected and neglected, Tunisian women found socially accepted identities only as mothers, unable to step above their social status as a servant. Because menopause arrived early in Tunisian women, as many colonial authors claimed, even this period of fulfilling her destiny as a procreator was short. The Muslim woman returned to being only an animal. "She therefore does not serve anymore apart from turning the wheel, going about all the work in the house, doing all the chores outside, and even, if necessary, take place – as a beast of reinforcement – next to the donkey pulling the plough."[73] By ending on the picture of a post-menopausal woman pulling the plough alongside a donkey, which must have been recognisable to settlers and travellers to poor areas of the Maghreb, Lafitte explicitly likened Tunisian women to animals, while criticising Muslim men for doing the same thing.

This loss of humanity among females was echoed by Witold Lemanski in 1913, who saw Muslim women of nomadic tribes as "scarcely human", because of their treatment as "beasts of burden".[74] This blatant disregard for the Muslim woman, this disrespect for her rights, was even, in the eyes of the psychiatrist Don Côme Arrii, the cause for the high numbers of wife murders among Algerians. He wrote in his 1926 dissertation "Criminal Impulsivity in the Indigenous Algerian": "His [the Algerian man's] pride, the exclusive domain of men, reinforced by those conceptions specific to the Muslim world, which relegate women to the role of beast of burden, explains [...] a very special criminality in these primitive peoples. We want to speak about the cases, all too frequent, of the murder of the wife, of which we report four instances."[75] Discarding an old wife like an old animal seemed, in Arrii's argumentation, a logical conclusion to primitive Algerian men, after a lifetime of treating them as such.

For colonial psychiatric authors, it was clear that treating women as "animals" must have had some influence on these women's mental states, but the expected outcome – higher numbers of mental disorders – did not occur. Jean Sutter, for example, regretted in 1949 that Muslim women were treated as servants by all men in their lives, by their fathers as well as their husbands, but, paradoxically, went on to say: "The rigidity of such an organisation removes, one imagines, many psychological problems."[76] It was

---

72   Lafitte, Contribution, 115.
73   Ibid. As late as 1949, this notion of Muslim women as mere servants can be found in psychiatric texts: Jean Sutter wrote an article entitled "Some Aspects of Psychogenesis in the Indigenous North African Milieu". In it, he claimed that "[...] the woman's role is little better than that of a domestic and her attitude towards the men of the family reflects at all occasions the inferior character of her condition." Sutter, Quelques aspects, 215.
74   Lemanski, Mœurs arabes, 218.
75   Arrii, Impulsivité criminelle, 40.
76   Sutter, Quelques aspects, 215. See also: Brierre de Boismont, Rapport, 75.

suggested that being continually kept in a state of exhausted subservience affected Muslim women's psyches positively, as it made them not more fragile, psychiatrically speaking, but instead hindered the development of mental disorders by numbing their intellect. Lafitte speculated in 1892: "The precarious condition of the woman, her role as a slave, as a beast of burden, as a thing, to which she is condemned, are opposed to the development of mental faculties. There is a somewhat arrested development, an intellectual and moral atrophy."[77] Colonial psychiatrists suspected that the immunity of Muslim women's brains to mental problems stemmed, at least partly, from the lower status of Muslim women in traditional North African societies; their acceptance of their animal status anaesthetised their intellects and psyches, turned them into commodities, slaves, animals, incapable of developing mental health problems.[78]

Lack of Intellectual Overwork

Another aspect of female Muslim normality, the "lack of intellectual overwork",[79] was closely connected to the trope of Muslim women as animals, though it also applied to Muslim men. The main difference between these tropes was that this description of Muslim normality was not one observed and criticised in Muslim men, but, instead, one used by colonial psychiatrists to explain their findings. It was part of the theory, discussed above, that insanity was a disease of civilisation; life in Europe, with its constant "intellectual overwork" and mental overstimulation, was dangerous, from a psychiatric point of view. Too much thinking could make anyone go mad, for it changed the structure of the brain, making it more susceptible to mental disorders.[80]

Primitive peoples, with their primitively structured brains, were safe from such dangers, but had none of the benefits of civilisation. This theory can be found, for example, in Joseph-Marie-Fernand Lafitte's 1892 dissertation: "Diseases of the nervous system

---

77   Lafitte, Contribution, 86. Raymond-Joseph Matignon repeated Lafitte's phrase in 1901. Matignon, Art médical, 84. See also: Clancy-Smith, Islam, Gender, and Identities, 164.

78   Some later psychiatrists claimed that the picture of the North African women as "beasts of burden" was a misinterpretation of the colonial situation, for instance the psychiatrist Maurice Igert, who, in 1955, wrote an article on the "Moroccan Cultural Milieu and Neuroses": "Thus physically a slave, the woman is morally freer [than a Muslim man]." Igert, Milieu culturel marocain, 652.

79   The idea of a lack of "surmenage intellectuel" protecting North Africans is found in a wide variety of psychiatric sources. For example: Sicard, Étude, 86; Aboab, Contribution, 17; Benkhelil, Contribution, 59; Olry, Paralysie générale, 33.

80   Witold Lemanski, for example, explained in 1913 that "cerebral complications strike those whose organ is overworked in modern, excessively heated life; people whose civilisation is still simple have visceral accidents without tendency to a generalisation of the higher nervous centres." Lemanski, Mœurs arabes, 109.

are rare in Tunisia. We must, in my opinion, attribute this to the lower encephalic sensitivity in the Arab; to the absence of all intellectual or moral overwork or fatigue in him; to the generally peaceful individual existence and the natural indolence of the native; and finally to the doctrinal fatalism of his religion and the resignation which is the consequence of this."[81] The fertile combination of fatalism and a brain activity lower than that of Europeans effectively protected Muslims from nervous disorders.[82]

Some psychiatrists working on North Africa repeated, in this context, a sentence from an unspecified article by the French psychiatrist Gillot, who wrote, probably in 1902: "With regard to the nervous system of the Arabs, it has been seen to behave very differently to ours, from the pathological point of view. It is always in [a state of] moral rest. The Mohammedan does not have our cares, our sorrows, our intellectual overwork especially: if he does not know the exquisiteness of our mental joys, he on the other hand ignores our neurasthenic depressions."[83] Like Lafitte in 1892, Gillot explained the low numbers of nervous disorders through the essential differences between North Africans and Europeans; primitive, unthinking, uncaring Muslims could not possibly be expected to develop the same diseases of civilisation[84] as Europeans.

But the critique of Muslim intellects went further than just postulating that North Africans did not use theirs enough. Don Côme Arrii wrote in his 1926 dissertation on the "Criminal Impulsivity of Indigenous Algerians": "And when you consider the close relationship which unites our faculty to judge and our faculty to act, we understand that, in the native, the actions are conditioned, more frequently, by his habits of movement than by reflections and reasoning."[85] Following this hypothesis, it is clear that North Africans could never suffer from intellectual overwork, because they did, in Don Côme Arrii's worldview, not need to use their brains in their daily lives. In North African normality, only the "faculty to act" was vital – European "reflection and reasoning" were not needed.

---

81 Lafitte, Contribution, 85.

82 Even psychiatrists who did not believe in a Muslim immunity to mental illnesses usually agreed that North Africans never suffered from intellectual overwork. In 1907, for example, Georges Sicard wrote in his dissertation "Study on the Frequency of Nervous Diseases in Indigenous Muslims of Algeria": "The native does not offer a particularly resistant territory to nervous diseases. If he is less often touched, which is not proven, it is [due to] their lack of predisposing causes, alcoholism and intellectual overwork mainly." Sicard, Étude, 85 f.

83 Étienne-Paul Laurens implied in 1919 that this quote came from Gillot's 1902 article. Gillot, Quelques considérations. As quoted in: Laurens, Contribution, 16. This same sentence of Gillot's was also repeated by Goëau-Brissonnière and Benkhelil. Goëau-Brissonnière, Syphilis nerveuse, 31; Benkhelil, Contribution, 17.

84 In Europe, the disorder of neurasthenia was thought to be caused by the fatigues of civilisation. Stoler, Making Empire Respectable, 646.

85 Arrii, Impulsivité criminelle, 34.

Muslim women, who did not even have the dubious benefits of traditional Islamic schooling or everyday work experiences, were seen as even more primitive. It was believed that normal Muslim women's brains were reduced to almost complete torpor through the hardships of their unschooled and depersonalised lives. Adolphe Kocher claimed in 1883 that while Muslim men benefited from a certain immunity to mental illness due to their absence of thought, Muslim women, being at a lower level of evolution, were even better protected. Kocher argued, rather generally, that this protection stemmed from their segregated life, which could not stimulate their intelligence, so their brains atrophied: "The Qur'an came and regularised, it is true, the rights of women, but also condemned them to live confined in a harem and thus excluded them forever from the sanctuary of intelligence."[86]

Kocher claimed therefore that the peaceful, uneventful, secluded life of Muslim women in harems limited and simplified their brains to the point where mental illness became impossible – in the same way the hard treatment at the hands of their husbands did. These two Orientalist tropes, employed by French colonial psychiatrists to describe the normality of Muslim women, both contrasted with and, paradoxically, mirrored one another – the golden cage of the harem and the iron cage of the "beast of burden". Both extremes, however, had the same result on Muslim women in the colonial imagination.

Most colonial psychiatrists restricted their verdicts on the female Muslim intellect to conjuring up these images of caged femininity – only Witold Lemanski gave a deeper insight into the everyday life of Muslim women, trying to find the precise reason why their brains were less likely to develop insanities than Muslim men's, producing in the process an imaginative range of bizarre metaphors. In a 1900 article on the "Psychology of the Arab Woman", he likened the intelligence of North African women to a house, applying, as it were, the segregation in which a Muslim woman lived to the structure of her brain. "The intelligence of the Arab woman does not exceed the horizon of her house, forever closed in on her psychic development; she finds herself immured in a voluntary prison to which the acquisitions of her brain must be singularly restricted."[87] While gender segregation was usually understood to be imposed upon helpless Muslim women, Lemanski seemed to construe the restrictions of the house simultaneously as a choice – purely by coincidence one taken by all Muslim women – and as a form of confinement, thereby immediately denying the voluntariness of the choice. He also asserted that the enclosed and isolated houses of their brains were empty – no entertainment was available to divert

---

86 Kocher, Criminalité, 41.
87 Lemanski, Psychologie, 87. He repeated this sentence in his 1913 book. Ibid., Mœurs arabes, 62.

them; and this understimulation had "repercussions" on the "full development of their mental faculties".[88]

Apart from these architectural metaphors, Lemanski also employed a biological vocabulary, describing Muslim women as organisms, somehow detached from and almost working against the brain. In 1900 he described Muslim women as "deprived of all intellectual food", "vegetating rather than living",[89] and in 1913 he likened the way of life of Muslim women to a normality without brain activities.[90] Lemanski also used this quasi-biological vocabulary to criticise civilised French women: "Her [the Tunisian woman's] way of life, heredity, religion, morality do not create in her a fertile ground for psychoses: the particular instrument, which is this simple brain, proves to be less fragile than that of those [women] civilised to excess. At the very base of the character of Arab women, there are no latent germs of madness: this morbid culmination of moral disturbances is rare in beings whose tranquil life isn't a preparation for mental alienation."[91] In Lemanski's view, normal Muslim femininity was free of any "germ" that could potentially cause insanity. The houses of Muslim women's brains were so empty and clinically sterile as to destroy any pathological causes of insanity.

In the context of "lack of intellectual overwork" and its consequences for the brain, the following colonial contradiction, pointed out by the American historian Alice Bullard in 2001, is interesting. In 1896 Abel-Joseph Meilhon wrote that "the intellectual stagnation which results from this reclusive life obviously protects [Kabyle] women against moral deviations; among our 10 alienated women there is not one Kabyle, and we have seen that the fate of the Kabyle woman in the family places her well above the conditions of the Arab who is often only a beast of burden or an instrument of carnal pleasures."[92] In Meilhon's worldview, Kabyle women belonged to a more civilised society than Arab women.[93] This superior Kabyle civilisation did not express itself through female character traits, as Kabyle women were "intellectually stagnating", but through the intelligence of their husbands, who treated them better. Bullard argues that following the theory of civilisation causing mental turmoil, favoured by Meilhon, Kabyle women should have had more cases of mental diseases than their Arab contemporaries, while, in fact, there were no Kabyle women among Meilhon's

---

88   Ibid., Psychologie, 93.

89   Ibid., 93 f.

90   He claimed: "The organism evolves normally, without the brain, with its predominance of nervous work, hindering the general development." Ibid., Mœurs arabes, 98.

91   Ibid., 124.

92   Meilhon, Aliénation mentale, part 1, 25.

93   Meilhon repeatedly claimed that Kabyles and other Berbers were more civilised than Arabs, and that this had measurable psychiatric consequences. See for example: Ibid., part 1, 23 f.; part 3, 369.

patients.[94] In her argument, Bullard overlooks the complexities of the different, co-existing indicators of North African primitivity: both the "intellectual stagnation" of Kabyle women and the treatment of Arab women as "beasts of burden" were clear markers of the primitivity of North Africans for French contemporary readers, and while Kabyle men were, in Meilhon's eyes, more civilised than Arabs, the same cannot be assumed about Kabyle women. Analysing the tropes of "lack of intellectual overwork" and "beast of burden" reveals the real contradiction in Meilhon's theory – both the "intellectual stagnation" of Kabyle women and the "beast of burden" status of Arab women acted as a protection mechanism from insanity. Meilhon simply put the protection mechanism of "intellectual stagnation" of Kabyle women above the other by explaining their lower levels of insanity through it, and therefore classified "intellectual stagnation" as being more "primitive" than being treated as an animal.

Medieval Superstitions

In the French worldview, Muslim customs and superstitions dominated North African women's daily lives, a world commonly depicted as one of jinn, charms and magic.[95] Muslim customs and traditions were usually subsumed under the heading of "superstitions", whose persistence went against the enlightened ideals of the French *mission civilisatrice*.[96] In the context of colonial psychiatry, Muslim customs were described with a vocabulary of backwardness, stagnation and medievalism, and compared to French traditions of bygone times.[97] This feeling that the Muslim present could best be compared to the French past reflected a common Orientalist trope: Muslim societies were seen as stagnating, and the alleged medievalism of Muslim customs coloured the view French colonial psychiatrists had of the people conserving them. The differentiation between the French and the North Africans was partly based on this perceived lack of contemporaneousness. Muslims were denied the status of coevals because their lives seemed to be stuck in the exotic and unfamiliar

---

94 Bullard, Truth in Madness, 126.
95 Suzanne Taïeb described the world of North Africans in 1939 as follows: "We have seen the considerable role played by Jinn, Angels, Marabouts and Tolba [traditional Muslim doctors], Witches, the evil eye and other superstitions in the normal life of the native North African." Taïeb, Idées d'influence, 71. Capitalisation in the original.
96 L. Wolters, for example, wrote in his 1902 medical dissertation that "Arab medicine is today reduced to a few practices of gross superstition, a few remedies which would make the most backward women from our countryside laugh." Wolters, Rôle de l'instituteur, 44.
97 For example, in the text of the French psychiatrist Jean de Labretoigne du Mazel, where he described a traditional Moroccan asylum in 1922: "Moroccan society is at a stage of evolution which is close to our Middle Ages. There is certainly no need to go back to our Middle Ages to find the mad subjected to the rules of the cage and chains in France." Mazel, Visite, 15.

Muslim Middle Ages and thereby categorically deprived of the virtues of dynamism and development. In addition, many psychiatrists believed that North Africans had been essentially unchanged since the time of Muhammad and, as such, opposed progress.[98] Even those who avoided the comparison with either the European or Muslim Middle Ages usually acknowledged that, while Muslims had once had a golden past, their present state was one of degeneration and decay.[99] The sense of alienation felt by French observers when contrasting North Africans – medieval, backward, degenerate – with the French was complete.

The advances in sciences and art from this Muslims golden age had disappeared from common memory, and all that was left were traditions and superstitions. Observing and understanding these superstitions was therefore the psychiatric shortcut into the medieval psyche of Muslim culture. Suzanne Taïeb wrote in 1939: "Rational and scientific explanations do not exist for them; there are only emotional values, supernatural and mystic actions, which are not discussed or controlled, to which one is submitted and against which one has to find means of protection, when they are evil. If we add to this the passivity, the fatalism, the belief in predestination, which are other parts of their character, then we understand the important role of these influences in their mental life, normal and pathological."[100] Superstitions were the basis of the "primitive normality" of normal and abnormal North Africans and needed to be understood in order to avoid misdiagnoses, but they also were a major part of the character of the masses. In trying to define Muslim normality, French psychiatrists found that they had to recognise and categorise North African superstitions. Don Côme Arrii wrote in his 1926 dissertation: "The native lives in the past, a past filled with legends and tales of a childish fantasy. These stories are the basis, if not the totality, of his intellectual background."[101] A profession used to manias, psychoses and neuroses had to be aware that some "legends and tales of a childish fantasy" were part of the superstitious North African normality – and not a symptom of a disease –, and

---

98 Maurice Boigey, for example, wrote, in 1908, a definition of what it meant to be a Muslim: "He [the Muslim] is a man who has remained as he was at the beginning. He has the same passions, the same mannerisms, the same vices, the same extravagances, the same ardours, the same impulsions, the same intellectual horizon as those of his co-religionists who were contemporaries of Muhammad." Boigey, Étude psychologique, 6 f.

99 French psychiatrists agreed that the present state of degeneration influenced the psyches of North Africans. Victor Trenga, for example, wrote in 1913: "One imagines, when one is aware of the slow, but inevitable, ruin of all the abandoned splendours of North African Islam, a people of the living dead, destined to never escape their torpor." Trenga, Âme arabo-berbère, 44. See also: Lwoff/Sérieux, Aliénés au Maroc, 471.

100 Taïeb, Idées d'influence, 147.

101 Arrii, Impulsivité criminelle, 33.

this awareness could only be achieved by a deeper, more intimate knowledge of the superstitions present in the normal population.

The following article from 1911 on "Medicine in Morocco" seems to propose that some forms of mental disorder were not uncommon in North Africans precisely because of the superstitious preconditioning they all shared: "Hysterical manifestations are quite common among Muslims, but even more so among the Jews. They are also encouraged by the belief in the marvellous and the supernatural, by exaggerated religious practices, dear to different Moroccan groups [...]."[102] These "hysterical manifestations" were not symptoms of a serious mental disease in just a few North Africans, as they would be in rational, civilised Europe in 1911 – they were part of the normality of the masses, however abnormal they might have seemed to European observers at first sight.[103] In 1926, Don Côme Arrii also warned about confusing normal consequences of a superstitious upbringing with mental diseases: "The study of this native psychology, of this character with such curious pathological reactions, is explicable, partly, through the fact of this special imprint, marked on passive spirits, of very particular customs, morals, religion and superstitions."[104] This notion illustrated the professional fear of accidentally confusing a belief in "normal" superstitions with actual insanity. In the eyes of Don Côme Arrii, the dissemination of these superstitions was part of what made the distinction between normality and abnormality so difficult.

The idea of Muslim superstitions blurring the border between normality and abnormality for French psychiatrists armed with European symptoms and diagnoses was taken up by Antoine Porot and Jean Sutter. They maintained in 1939 that Muslims were so steeped in superstition that this effectively hid abnormalities from the European observers: "In the area of *perceptions*, for example, they are, even in the normal state, laden with a heavy emotional and mystical burden: also the natives do not react as we do to hallucinatory phenomena: they include them voluntarily in their usual life: hearing voices, seeing visions, there is nothing to shock directly the pre-logical conception they have of themselves and the outside world."[105] The professional warning to other psychiatrists in this passage was clear – even clearly pathological symptoms such as hallucinations were part of the primitive, pre-logical normality in the Maghreb and could therefore not be taken as signs of mental disorder.[106]

---

102 B., Médecine au Maroc, 382.
103 See also Chapter 5.5 "Hysteria: Disease of the 'Race'".
104 Arrii, Impulsivité criminelle, 38.
105 Porot/Sutter, 'Primitivisme', 229. Emphasis in the original.
106 A strikingly similar description of Arab Muslims, in this case Iraqi Muslims, can be found in a psychiatric text, written by an Iraqi psychiatrist and his Finnish wife in 1970: "A commonly held superstitious belief in magical powers, in the evil eye, in the Jinnee and many other para-religious ideas pose a problem when trying to determine normality without thorough knowledge

In the eyes of French colonial psychiatrists, no part of Muslim society showed the proverbial irrationality and obstinate rootedness in the past better than the traditions and superstitions preserved by Muslim women.[107] François Gomma wrote in his 1904 dissertation "Medical Assistance in Tunisia": "The condition of the Arab woman is known to everybody, and the sad existence to which she is reduced in the cities, behind the thick walls of the mysteriously impenetrable houses, the hard labour to which man submits her in the countryside, has been discussed everywhere. Still, those familiar with the Arabs are unanimous in proclaiming the influence of women in terms of the conservation of traditions and consequently of the indigenous mentality."[108] Being reduced to passivity by Muslim men and by their own lack of intellectual capacities, Muslim women found power in the world of traditions, a power that remained untouched by French influence, lying, as it did, beyond the colonial reach in those "mysteriously impenetrable houses" or the barbarous countryside.[109]

Muslim women were not only guardians of what French psychiatrists saw as traditions and superstitions – it was their own lives that were most deeply influenced by them. Suzanne Taïeb, writing in in 1939, linked superstitions to the segregated way of life Muslim women led in the colonial imagination: "Although the basis of superstitions is common to both native men and women, the latter, living isolated in harems, suffer more from it."[110]

---

of the cultural background. Behaviour which might elsewhere suggest psychotic mannerisms or preoccupation with hallucinations, and statements which sound delusional may well be in keeping with a particular local practice (religious or otherwise) or a mystic belief. It is sometimes noted in Iraq that auditory or visual hallucinations are not regarded as abnormal by the patient or his family." Al-Issa/Al-Issa, Psychiatric Problems, 18.

107 This trope can be found in texts from all genres. In this, Muslim normality conformed to European normalities – women were perceived to be superstitious and irrational in all societies. The psychiatrist Maurice Igert remarked in 1955, when writing about Moroccan women being the guardians of magic: "Isn't the woman everywhere the natural custodian of the rights of sentiments and the irrational?" Igert, Milieu culturel marocain, 651. See also: Thierry, Œuvre, 51.

108 Gomma, Assistance médicale, 105.

109 It was widely discussed whether North Africans would eventually be able to get rid of their backward "superstitions" through contact with France, pitching traditions against biomedicine in a bluntly colonial manner. Victor Trenga wrote in 1913: "The little people of Islam, on the contrary, though fanatical, although [they] found a significant dose of happiness and, above all, a reason for life in the ancestral beliefs and traditions, were quick to develop an interest in growing closer to us, finding very often, through our contact, moral and material well-being." Trenga, Âme arabo-berbère, 186 f. Later texts showed that modernisation did not cause these "superstitions" to disappear. Maurice Igert wrote in 1955: "However, these practices and beliefs [medical and magical] are unanimous among Moroccans, even developed [ones], even uprooted [ones]." Igert, Milieu culturel marocain, 650.

110 Taïeb, Idées d'influence, 78.

Genital Field

Another trope that French colonial psychiatrists repeated in their text is the idea that Muslim marriage was not a sacrament, as in Christianity, but a "contract",[111] through which a man bought access to a "champ génital", a "genital field". This is closely connected to the idea of Muslim women being nothing but an "instrument of pleasure" to their husbands.[112] In both images, North African women were passive, at the mercy of the strong sexuality of their husbands. Though there was never an allusion to the Qur'an in these quotes concerning "genital fields" acquired through marriage, the picture was probably the result of a literal interpretation of 2:223: "Your wives are a tilth for you, so go to your tilth."[113] Only Jean Coudray quoted (without naming) this sura in his 1914 dissertation. He did so without explicitly mentioning the "genital field" that women represented for their husbands or its sexual connotation, instead framing it as a general quote about the marital authority of the husbands over their wives.[114] This bizarre notion of the "genital field", detached from this qur'anic quote, can be found in many psychiatric texts.[115] As a phrase used to describe a "transaction" – Muslim women's "genital fields" were sold by their families in exchange for a dowry –, it remained strangely static over time and across literary genres.[116]

---

111 Don Côme Arrii wrote, for example, in 1926: "The husband buys his wife, who becomes his property." Arrii, Impulsivité criminelle, 41.

112 See, for example: Lévy-Bram, Assistance médicale, 76.

113 This sura was quoted in Raymond Charles's 1958 book "The Muslim Soul", even though he gave it an incorrect number. "Professor Schacht is not really sure about the reproductive significance of the symbol: 'Your women are your fields, go to your fields as you want' (IV, 231)." Charles, Âme musulmane, 236.

114 "[...] for our part, we do not often see young and pretty women in the [medical] consultation, because they are jealously guarded by their lords and masters, who have absolute authority over them: 'Your wives are your fields, you can go to your field as you like.'" Coudray, Considérations, 52.

115 The psychiatrist Sextius Arène, for example, wrote in 1913, quoting the French translation of Sidi Khélil by Seignette as the source of the sentiment: "By marrying, the woman sells a part of her person; in a market, one buys a commodity, in a marriage, one buys a 'genital field.'" Seignette, Code musulman, Vol. 2, 427. In: Arène, Criminalité, 77. For Sidi Khélil, see also p. 60, FN 121. Arène subsequently repeated the same sentiment but attributed it to Adolphe Kocher: "It can be said that the power of the husband is absolute, he does not get married, he buys a woman who becomes his property, his 'genital field', and he is the absolute master of it." Ibid., 81.

116 In 1875, Captain Charles Villot, working for the French administration in Algeria, wrote: "In a market, one buys a commodity; in a marriage, one buys the genital field of a woman." Villot, Mœurs, 70. The same sentence can be found in an 1889 article by the military doctor Lucien Bertholon: "The Muslim doesn't marry, he *buys* a woman. She becomes his property from this

Many French colonial psychiatrists deplored the fact that this "marriage contract" gave no rights to Muslim women on the one hand, while, on the other, women were not safe from the "contract" being terminated through repudiation and divorce or degraded by polygamy. Nevertheless, while condemning the degradation of femininity by reducing marriage to a base fulfilment of male lust, they still preferred the status of a married woman to that of a divorced or repudiated one.

The underlying notions of the aggressive sexuality of Muslim men can be found in countless other contexts.[117] It was generally agreed that male North African sexuality was omnipresent and guided their behaviour in many situations. Further, forms of "deviant" sexuality seemed to be part of North African normality.[118] This strong male sexuality had, in the colonial *weltanschauung*, serious consequences for the mental states of North Africans, insanity being one of them. But how could French colonial psychiatrists explain that Muslims, subjected to the unhealthy sexuality of their "race", produced fewer patients than the moderate French? Georges Lacapère explained this paradox in an article on the psychiatric consequences of syphilis,[119] published in 1918: "First comes *the absence of cerebral overwork*. This is obviously the great cause of the rarity of general paralysis which, in our country, affects almost exclusively individuals whose intellectual activity is considerable. If it is true that tabes [tabes dorsalis] is mainly due to genital overwork, one cannot invoke a similar reason to explain the rarity of this condition [i.e. general paralysis], because the Arab is perhaps more overworked than the European on this particular point. He escapes, however, the double intellectual and genital overwork, to which [Alfred] Fournier attached so much importance as an etiological factor of nervous syphilis."[120] While the overall "lack of intellectual overwork" was generally used to explain the absence of psychiatric disorders in North Africans, as discussed above, Lacapère further argued that there

---

moment, 'his genital field'. He is the absolute master of it." Bertholon, Esquisse, 432. Emphasis in the original. The jurist Louis Milliot wrote in 1910: "Marriage is a contract. It is a contract through which a woman, in exchange for a price which is the dowry, puts her 'genital field' to the disposition of a man." Milliot, Étude, 100. See also: Lévy-Bram, Assistance médicale, 77 f.

117 Antoine Porot and Don Côme Arrii wrote in their 1932 article: "The sexual instinct is so powerful in the male native, the woman an object of desire so jealously guarded, that the marauding of love sometimes takes a character of extraordinary boldness." Porot/Arrii, Impulsivité criminelle, 598.

118 In 1919, Étienne-Paul Laurens wrote about the "physical overwork" of male Algerians, by which he meant "sexual overwork": "[...] this overwork is certainly more intense among the natives than with us; we will not dwell on the practice of the coitus, of masturbation, in this population particularly inclined to it." Laurens, Contribution, 45.

119 The colonial psychiatric discussion on syphilis will be analysed in detail in Chapter 5.3 on "General Paralysis: Alcohol, Syphilis and Civilisation.

120 Lacapère, Vue d'ensemble, 147. Emphasis in the original.

were other psychiatric problems, in this case general paralysis, which could only be created by a combination of "intellectual and genital overwork". Through this construct, Lacapère was able to explain why their excessive sexuality alone did not lead to higher rates of insanity in North Africans.

Interestingly in this context of sexuality, French colonial psychiatrists believed that even insane Muslim women were married off – showing that the notion of "Muslim women as wombs" dominated all aspects of the North African societies. Adolphe Kocher quoted the 14th century Islamic scholar Khalil b. Ishaq, known in the Maghreb under the name of Sidi Khélil, in 1883: "The father has the right to impose marriage on his *insane* daughter, when the girl is an adult, pubescent, even if she has already been married and a mother; only if the madness has lucid intervals will a return to reason be awaited."[121] These marriages were horrific and deeply deplorable to most colonial psychiatrists, obsessed with Lamarckian theories of heredity and degeneration.[122] The traditional North African conceptualisation of mental illness, however, was not based on genetic or organic interpretations; therefore, the idea that insanity could be inherited was largely unknown. "Mentally unstable" women married and started new lives with their husbands and in-laws, everybody trusting that "demonic possessions" would disappear in time. In the colonial imagination, however, these marriages encouraged mentally "damaged" women to pass on their insanities to further generations.

Though the vocabulary concerning the "genital field" seemed to imply that North African women suffered greatly at the hands of their husbands, both in the marital bed and through the facility used to ban them from it, and even though allusions to this brutal aspect of female Muslim normality can be found in numerous psychiatric texts, it was never explained why this did not lead to higher rates of mental problems in Muslim women. Used to illustrate the backwardness of Muslim societies, the trope of the "genital field" with its implications about the status of Muslim women never prompted real psychiatric analysis. It is as if "knowledge" about Muslims – in

---

121 Kocher did not specify which translation of Sidi Khélil's text he was referring to. It could have been either Pierron's or Seignette's translation. Sidi Khélil, Vol. 2, 317. In: Kocher, Criminalité, 43. Emphasis in the original. Discussions of these marriages between the sane and the mad can be found in many colonial texts as especially the division of "nights" in polygamous families with an insane spouse preoccupied the colonial imagination. Bertherand, Médecine et hygiène, 95; Meilhon, Aliénation mentale, part 1, 21; Bouquet, Aliénés en Tunisie, 77; Milliot, Étude, 80; Livet, Aliénés algériens, 66; Porot, Tunisie, 59 f.; Arène, Criminalité, 79; Goëau-Brissonnière, Syphilis nerveuse, 72 f. See also: Arabi, Regimentation of the Subject, 278; Chaleby, Forensic Psychiatry, 42.

122 Dowbiggin, Degeneration, 188. These theories will be discussed in Chapter 4.3 "Morals and Degeneration".

this case their aforementioned immutability, stuck in a static, quasi-medieval state – effectively made further research unnecessary.

Sexualité Précoce[123]

The final trope analysed in this chapter concerns another aspect of indigenous sexuality that obsessed the French: the early and profound sexualisation of Muslim women. Whereas the trope of the "genital field" depicted Muslim women as completely passive, mere fields or instruments, suffering sexual assaults by their husbands, the trope of "precocious sexuality" turned female sexuality into an active, slightly dangerous and highly reprehensible character trait of normal Muslim women.[124] This duality of passive and active sexuality made it possible for the French observers to perceive Muslim women not only as eternal victims but also as only having themselves to blame for their hard fate.

The marriage of underage girls was seen as typical of Muslim societies and was heavily criticised by French colonial psychiatrists. In 1926 Don Côme Arrii blamed Muhammad himself for the continuation of this barbarous custom: "The law encourages him [the Muslim man] moreover to marry a virgin; and the native sees, in this prescription, an invitation to take all young girls. Muhammad himself, did he not lead the example by taking Aïcha as a fiancée, when she was six and by consummating the marriage with her as soon as she reached her ninth year? Driven by his ardent temperament, authorised by his beliefs and customs, the native commits thus, in the most legal fashion in the world, rape in marriage."[125] In the colonial interpretation, Muslims were legally allowed to marry prepubescent girls, following Muhammad's example, which showed the deeply primitive barbarity of their societies. This aspect of male sexuality was not seen as abnormal or as proof of a mental disorder but as a characteristic of normal male behaviour in the Maghreb. Maurice Boigey even claimed in a 1907 article that Muslim girls were married off before they were nubile

---

123 As in "dementia praecox", the early name for schizophrenia. By artificially pathologising this trope, I attempt to create a distance between this colonial construct and actual female sexuality.

124 The differentiation between active and passive sexuality serves to explain the different colonial tropes about female sexuality in North African countries. See also: Armand, Algérie médicale, 446; Amat, M'zab, 281; Brault, Pathologie et hygiène, 181; Boigey, Mariage, 1185; Sutter/Pélicier, Crise pubertaire, 516 f.

125 Arrii, Impulsivité criminelle, 41. The accusation that Islam condoned all forms of debauched sexuality, and by extension underage marriages, had been a cornerstone of Orientalist theories for centuries. Arrii relied on this tradition, without explicitly having to mention it. See, for example: Kabbani, Imperial Fictions, 36 f.

and voluntarily exposed to male sexuality, because they could not yet become pregnant and lose their beauty through pregnancies.[126]

This forced sexualisation of children was, understandably, deplored by French colonial writers, even though some French women implied that only women would truly be against marrying children off to middle-aged men.[127] French psychiatrists condemned the sexualisation of children as immoral and bad for the development of Muslim girls, and Muslim men indulging in such marriages were judged severely (socially, not legally).

Somewhat disturbingly, French colonial psychiatrists were simultaneously convinced that – due to climate, a special "racial" development and their "primitive mentality" – Muslim girls knew about, wanted and were physically ready for sexual intercourse at a time when French girls were still innocent children. Many medical experts claimed the early nubility of Muslim girls was the reason for their accelerated development and fast decay.[128] Discussions of this subject can be found, for example, in Kocher's 1883 dissertation: "The cause [for the early aging of Muslim women] does not escape us: married at the age of ten to twelve years, they undergo both the fatigues of marital approaches and those of childbirth early. But concerning Arab women, an important question remains to be solved: *at what age is she nubile?* Our personal observations, taken at the clinic in Algiers, the conversations that we have had on this subject, with old Algerian practitioners [i. e. with French doctors who had spent a long time in Algeria], without allowing us to give an absolute rule, has led us to the following results. The nubility of the indigenous woman is precocious. The first menstruation appears almost always between the extremes of ten and thirteen and a half years – very rarely is an Arab woman not menstruating at fourteen."[129]

It was not only that their young bodies were ready for childbirth – with early nubility came early lust. Kocher insisted that "young Arab girls, indeed, when the first signs of nubility appear in them, experience desires that they wish quite easily to

---

126 "In the Sahara, as almost everywhere in Africa, young girls are delivered to their husband before becoming nubile. As a result they are often exclusively mistresses and beasts of pleasure for three, four or five years, and it is only after this period that they become mothers." Boigey, Comment accouchent les Sahariennes, 377.

127 One such example can be found in the 1900 book "Arab Women in Algeria" by the French feminist Hubertine Auclert. In her book, she dedicated a whole chapter to this question, provocatively called: "The Arab Marriage is a Rape of Children". See: Auclert, Femmes arabes, 42. In this chapter, she wrote: "If women had their share of power in France, they would not allow to persist, on French ground, a law admitting the rape of children. Man tolerates this crime because he is solidary with those who profit from it." Auclert, Femmes arabes, 49. See also: Clancy-Smith, Femme Arabe, 60.

128 For example: Lafitte, Contribution, 115; Chellier, Voyage, 29.

129 Kocher, Criminalité, 37.

have appeased."[130] The notion of early sexualisation was connected with the conviction of Muslim women generally having loose morals. Active female sexuality was defined as a pathological condition of the entire female Muslim population, and the observation of a strong sexual impulse in women could therefore not be taken as a sign of abnormality. Not only did Muslim women become nubile earlier than European women, their sexuality was much stronger, showing little of the sexual restraint admired as a sign of true femininity.[131]

This early and, compared to French women, unnatural sexualisation of Muslim girls was seen as one of the defining aspects of North African societies, and the mental consequences of this "practice" on normal Muslim women were of interest to colonial writers. A phrase that colonial writers used in this context was that "Muslim girls became nubile before their sense of reason was developed".[132] While not mentioned in psychiatric writings, this explicit combination of early sexualisation and lack of reason in the texts of non-experts shows that a propensity for mental disorders was at least suspected in girls of that age and position.[133] Therefore, while deplorable, this early sexualisation and marrying of underage girls at least had the positive effect of protecting girls – apparently at a difficult, reasonless age – from mental diseases caused by sexual frustration and unfulfilled lust. It was claimed that a further positive effect of this early and deep sexualisation lay in the elimination of spinsterhood, which, in the logic of contemporary theories, created so much insanity in French women because they were denied their biological fulfilment, but did not exist in the Maghreb.[134]

---

130 Ibid., 185.

131 Charles, Âme musulmane, 229. The Orientalist notion of Muslim women being deeply sexual stands in marked contrast to modern psychiatric (and non-psychiatric) attitudes. In an article published in 2000, the psychiatrist Fakhr El-Islam wrote about "Mental Illness in Kuwait and Qatar" that Arab women "are expected not to show any interest in sex". El-Islam, Mental Illness, 123. See also: Al-Sawaf/Al-Issa, Sex and Sexual Dysfunction, 299.

132 Villot, Mœurs, 69; Milliot, Étude, 83.

133 Witold Lemanski, however, saw essential differences in the minds of North African women and French women. While French women at the point of nubility often experienced mental problems, Muslim women were safe: "[...] but never in the young Arab girl does one determine serious troubles of intelligence as in the European [girls]. Sexuality, vague at this time, does not appear under the forms of an ardent and passionate mysticism!" Lemanski, Mœurs arabes, 98 f.

134 See, for example: ibid., 183.

1.4　Gendered Processes of Pathologisation

All of these tropes expressed a French horror at the subjugation of the Muslim women they encountered in their North African colonies.[135] The focus on these specific tropes can be partly explained through the common notion that Middle Eastern and North African women endured a poor quality of life prior to Western influence,[136] which was used by colonial writers to criticise the backward Muslim societies these women lived in[137] and to justify the French colonisation of the Maghreb by focusing on the outrageously primitive and barbarous.[138] Nevertheless, while criticising the poor quality of Muslim women's lives, the French did not seek to actively change this situation. The focus of colonial psychiatry on the abject status of normal Muslim women in North Africa – in their descriptions of normal Muslim femininity – cannot be explained through a humanitarian interest to help them; their humanitarian effort, which undeniably existed, was focused on the treatment of abnormality.

French colonial psychiatrists wrote abundantly about normal Muslim women, but an analysis of their notions of normal Muslim femininity shows that all the topics they covered had been widely discussed by other colonial writers, and were, consequently, not in the least surprising to the contemporary public. Essentially, their findings did not extend beyond a repetition of Orientalist tropes and settler stereotypes. This uncertainty about the actual lives of Muslim women was connected with the difficulty of contacting Muslim women – both patients and non-patients. In an interview conducted in 2011, the Moroccan psychiatrist Jalil Bennani split the functions of colonial psychiatry along gender lines, dividing not only their methods but also the goal of their research into their treatment of Muslim men and Muslim women. In his eyes, French colonial psychiatrists were only "practitioners" when it came to Muslim men and "sociologists" when it came to Muslim women.[139] Definitions of the normality of male North Africans were often based on practical experiences with patients, and the normality of all North Africans was questioned by describing it with a vocabulary based on this everyday contact with patients. When experiences with male patients could be so easily adapted to define normality, one should ask whether, in the case of

---

135　While not specifically talking about psychiatrists, the historian Jeanne Bowlan pointed out how hypocritical the shock of French men at the situation of Muslim women in Algeria was, considering French women only gained the right to vote in 1944, whereas other Western European countries had introduced it after the First World War. Bowlan, Civilizing Gender Relations, 184.

136　Keddie, Problems, 226.

137　Mohsen-Finan, Condition des femmes au Maghreb, 81.

138　Adamson, Approaches, 23.

139　Interview with Jalil Bennani, Rabat, 20.07.2011.

Muslim women, psychiatrists hoped to draw conclusions about Muslim abnormality from their "sociological" descriptions of normality. Pathologising the whole population in one way or another (by applying experiences from their psychiatric practice to "normal men", and by using a pathologised vocabulary in their description of female normality) seemed a natural extension of their authority on psychopathology.

Megan Vaughan stated in 1991 that all colonial psychiatric theories "work backwards from psychopathology to 'normal psychology'",[140] and in the aforementioned introduction of "Empire and Psychiatry", while describing an article by the American historian Richard Keller, she stated that the "extensive contact with North African patients provided" the colonial psychiatrists with an "evidential basis on which to confirm some common-sense settler suspicions not only on the nature of 'Muslim madness', but also, more invidiously, on the pathological nature of the 'normal' North African mind."[141] Vaughan wrote about a normality described "backwards" from knowledge already formed on psychopathology – according to her and Keller, it was the "evidential basis" of the contact with Muslim patients which motivated the interest in abnormality and justified the focus on it. In the North African context, this was only the case when these French psychiatrists wrote about Muslim men, and this process seems to have been reversed when it came to Muslim women. In their case, the descriptions of normality had nothing to do with colonial psychiatrists' experiences with patients – the fascination with the exotic female "non-patient" eclipsed experiences of patients, resulting in a glaring gap between theories of North African women and actual practice in the asylums and hospitals.

The fact that so many colonial psychiatrists used the same formulations, detached from their historical and geographic context, and picturesque tropes without ever acknowledging each other points to the existence of these tropes in a pre-psychiatric definition of normal Muslim femininity. Colonial psychiatry did not "invent" the characteristics and the terminology of female Muslim normality – these were part of a canon of existing colonial prejudices –, but the authority of science conferred a validity which allowed these normative ideas to be adopted by a broader public. Colonial psychiatrists resorted to these settler tropes without questioning them or subjecting them to scientific scepticism – the mere fact that their psychiatric predecessors had already used them both verified the tropes and justified their continued usage. While French settlers had always suspected that Muslim women were incapable of causal thinking, psychiatry proved it by linking "intellectual overwork" to brain structures in a pseudo-scientific manner, raising it from an observed truth to an academic theory. The picturesque expression "beast of burden" needed no further explanation in a colonial context: French settlers in North Africa all "knew" what it meant and could confirm

---

140 Vaughan, Curing their Ills, 118.
141 Ibid., Introduction, 10.

it from personal experience. It had the advantage of instant recognition and acceptance in the settler community – for them, it was a rather banal truism. However, only psychiatrists, "experts of the human mind", were able to "explain" what being treated as an animal meant for Muslim women, and therefore justified – by the fact of their interest in it as much as by their theories – the usage of the term in a scientific context. The difference between these existing Orientalist tropes and the more "academic" psychiatric, if equally superficial, findings is a certain morbidity of language, which was in turn taken up – consciously or subconsciously – by other writers.[142]

The idea of Muslim women as perfect wombs was the basis of most of the other tropes analysed above – it was the underlying biological "truth" about both European and Muslim female normality, the lowest common denominator of all colonial psychiatric descriptions of Muslim women. The tropes of "lack of intellectual overwork" and "medieval superstitions" also applied to the normality of Muslim men but to a much lesser degree; whereas most men had no choice but to have some contact with the French, women were left in their natural, non-developed, and therefore superstitious and unreasonable, state of mind, which protected them so strongly from insanity.

The tropes of "beast of burden" and "genital field" concerned the suppression of Muslim women by Muslim men and conceptualised their status in North African societies as "things". Both of these aspects of the colonial imagery were contrasted with notions of idealised French femininity, which was conceived as genteel and moderate. The trope of "beast of burden" victimised Muslim women concerning their daily work, which was, in the eyes of the colonial observers, unnaturally hard,[143] and employed a vocabulary of "animals", "slaves", and "yokes". The trope of Muslim women as a "genital field" victimised Muslim women regarding male sexuality, employing a vocabulary of "instruments", "fields" and "watering". In the minds of the colonial psychiatrists, these two tropes were connected, and their combination encapsulated the suspicions of French psychiatrists that Muslim women were only used, by male Muslims, for hard work and sexual intercourse,[144] which had a direct effect on their

---

142 This adoption of a clearly pathological language in describing Muslim female normality makes for uncomfortable reading, for example, when one encounters phrases in feminist French writing clearly influenced by psychiatry. One can find the following statement in the 1931 book "Our Muslim Sisters", written by Marie Bugéja: "But what crazy ideas do not grow in the brains of Muslim women? The consequences [of this] are sometimes tragic." Bugéja, Sœurs musulmanes, 144.

143 This hard work had a negative influence on the biological goal of womanhood. Lafitte, for example, wrote in 1892: "It is easy to note that the Arab population in Tunisia decreases each year in considerable and really alarming proportions. Could it be otherwise in the deplorable conditions in which the woman is placed?" Lafitte, Contribution, 117.

144 One example of this combination can be found in the 1855 book by the French doctor Émile-Louis Bertherand, where he wrote that from an early age, Muslim women were used to being

intelligence. This reduction of Muslim women to a dumb "beast of pleasure or beast of burden" was heavily criticised by Marie Bugéja in 1931. In her eyes, this unfair and untrue reduction was due to Muslim women being described by French men, who had no access to Muslim women and who relied on unsafe information.[145]

This complete refutation of the authority of all male observers by Bugéja did not mean that some of the problems these colonial psychiatrists described – if not the conclusions they deduced from them – were not essentially true. The colonial tropes, chosen here to demonstrate a psychiatric interpretation of female Muslim normality, were based on actual social and legal – if somewhat misinterpreted – problems and on real human suffering. These observers being at a distance from the Muslim women they described, both ideologically and physically, did not automatically mean that the information they possessed was inherently wrong. The information was distorted, used to further political ends and dependent on "local informers", but it cannot be denied that there was some truth in both the misery described and the relative absence of female Muslim patients from colonial psychiatric care. This grain of truth in the colonial psychiatric interpretation of female Muslim normality is also shown through the fact that modern psychiatric descriptions of North Africa have returned to rely on in-depth knowledge about normality in order to understand both the development and particularities of mental problems from different cultural backgrounds. However, today female Muslim normality is used to explain the perceived high risk of Muslim women of developing psychiatric disorders.

For example, the distinguished Moroccan psychiatrist and feminist Rita El-Khayat wrote in 2005 that, today, Arab countries are defined by "three deficits", which cause mental problems in their populations: 1) "total ignorance"; 2) "the worst condition of women on the planet"; and 3) "the absence of human rights".[146] In this interpretation, Muslim women are, psychiatrically speaking, what they were during colonial times – potential victims. Yet, El-Khayat's vantage point, as a North African woman, is diametrically opposed to that of the colonial psychiatrists, and her criticism of these serious social problems cannot possibly be reduced to the colonial tropes discussed above. Nonetheless, these uneasy correlations between colonial and modern psychiatry must be critically scrutinised and addressed.

"abased to the role of slave and mere instrument of pleasure [...]." Bertherand, Médecine et hygiène, 198. See also: Meilhon, Aliénation mentale, part 1, 25; Collomb/Robert, Thème, 533 f. An analysis of the depiction of Algerian women as animals, work animals and sexual animals, can be found in: Gordon, Women of Algeria, 13 f.

145 Bugéja, Sœurs musulmanes, 81. Bugéja's defence of Muslim women was discussed by Marnia Lazreg in 1994. Lazreg, Eloquence of Silence, 95.

146 El-Khayat, Observations, 17. She also spells her name as Ghita El-Khayat.

Chapter 2
Discovering Deviance: The Criminalisation of Patients

2.1 Case Study on Alternative Modes of Admission

In an article published in 1896, the French psychiatrist Abel-Joseph Meilhon presented a collection of case studies on the 83 Muslim patients treated in the asylum in Aix-en-Provence during the year 1880. Among these patients were ten women, and Meilhon specified their disorders, descriptions of their behaviour and also the manner of their admission into psychiatric care. The admission of these female Muslim patients mostly followed the voluntary, administrative and judicial routes detailed in the chapter below. However, one of Meilhon's female Muslim patients was admitted in an uncommon way. The patient, a 40-year-old, single Arab woman, was admitted in November 1874, and Meilhon noted that "charged with arson, she comes from prison, where she was violent towards her fellow inmates; she knows the charge against her; but she denies it and assigns it to a cigarette, discarded by [some] Spaniards".[1]

Before being transferred to the mental asylum of Montperrin in Aix-en-Provence, this particular patient was admitted to another form of colonial "care" – the prison. This shows that her responsibility for the crime she had committed had not been questioned either by the police or in court. She had not been examined by a psychiatrist before being sent to prison. Instead, it was the physical threat she posed to her fellow inmates which made her psychiatric problems apparent to the French observers and which prompted her admission to psychiatric care. In Aix-en-Provence, however, the patient showed signs of confusion, agitation and megalomania, on which Meilhon specifically focused in his description. He described that she "takes the nurses for the sons of God, says that her daughter has had children, but that she herself has never had any. During her long stay in the asylum, we find reports of an intense, almost continuous, manic agitation, with incoherence, aggressive tendencies and hallucinations of sight and hearing. When we observed her [in 1880], we found her in a state of senile dementia; she rips [things] and becomes nasty at times; she answers us that she is 80 years old, [that she has] 80 children, that she has been designated by the Arabs to light fires; she says she is the daughter of God, but only on paper; she is very rich; at night, when she sleeps with closed eyes, eight women come to open them and to prevent her from sleeping."[2]

---

1 Meilhon, Aliénation mentale, part 2, 203.
2 Ibid., part 2, 203 f.

The confusion and distress of the patient is palpable in Meilhon's study. The initial reason for her arrest – the act of arson (which was not further elaborated on) that she claimed had been committed by some "Spaniards" – was of only secondary importance when Meilhon observed her after she had already been in Aix-en-Provence for six years. In 1880, at the age of only 46, she allegedly suffered from an aggressive form of senile dementia, which explained and justified her placement in colonial care. It is uncertain whether she suffered from this disorder when she was transferred to Aix-en-Provence from prison in 1874, or whether it developed during her stay in psychiatric care. It is also unclear whether her aggressive behaviour towards her fellow inmates, or, indeed, the crime itself, had been caused by an early onset of dementia or some other disorder, or whether this had instead been a display of protest, disobedience or fear.

This case study, detailing an exceptional mode of admission into colonial psychiatric care, was chosen as an introduction to this chapter because it illustrates a diversity in patient experiences that could easily, but should not, be neglected in an overview comprising almost 80 years of institutionalisation of North African women. Not all patients followed the same route through the colonial institutions, as shown in Chapter 2.6.4. Additionally, this case study allows for an initial critical look at the diagnosing process, which will be taken up again in Chapters 3 and 5.

2.2 Fascination with Criminality

French colonial psychiatrists, especially those belonging to the *École d'Alger*, frequently described male North Africans, including patients, as either dangerous or outright criminals in both their theories and their case studies,[3] but insisted the same could not be said for Muslim women because of the supposedly innate opposition of everything feminine to crime and brutality. Women, even if mad, were seen as docile and gentle, their behaviour perceived as having more in common with the idealised female normality discussed in Chapter 1 than with the actions of male Muslim patients. The argument that only the most dangerous insane were admitted into mental asylums, and that this basic criterion of admission – which, psychiatrists pointed out, did not come from them but from the "unreasonable traditions" of the local populations[4] – excluded women, was one of the explanations used by French psychiatrists for the low numbers of female patients in the psychiatric hospitals. One of the first psychiatrists focusing on North African patients at a time when they were still treated in France,

---

3 Keller, Colonial Madness, 208.

4 Even though it was entirely comparable to the situation in France, where the same focus on the danger posed by the patients dominated the processes of institutionalisation. See, for example: Guignard, Prémices de dangerosité, 35.

the aforementioned Abel-Joseph Meilhon, wrote on the low number of female Muslim patients in Aix-en-Provence in 1896: "One could perhaps say with some reason that the indigenous mostly sequestrate the dangerous insane, and that these rigorous measures become much rarer with regard to women, who, through their temperament, are less given to violence, and who can also be more easily mastered [...]."[5] Even though, on a theoretical level, colonial psychiatrists propagated the dogma of the violent male and the gentle female, there was, in reality, a strong criminalisation of female Muslim patients, the evidence for which can be found in the descriptions of the actions and the behaviour of these women in the case studies, as well as in the ways in which they were admitted to colonial psychiatric care.

Three "premises" will be analysed in order to introduce the main arguments of this chapter: a) definitions of criminality in a colonial context; b) French laws concerning asylums and the manners of internment these laws favoured; and c) the picture of the "violent Muslim man" and the "passive Muslim woman" in French colonial sources. In a second section, the three possible manners of internment in the colonial Maghreb – "voluntary placement", "administrative placement" and "judicial placement"[6] – will be examined. Descriptions of female patients – especially those defined as "prostitutes", "addicts" and "vagrants" – in published case studies will also be analysed in order to gain an insight into admission processes through the social classification of patients. It is important to note that most case studies did not feature extensive descriptions of the pre-institutional life of the patients, either because of the significant problems of communication between psychiatrist and patient[7] or because of a mutual absence of interest. Very often one can only find the most basic patient descriptions: name, often shortened in order to grant anonymity in publications, age, profession and ethnic group. These descriptions follow a strict format, specified according to what was deemed important by the hospital administration, in which the manner of admission was either so obvious that it need not be stated or so unimportant that it need not be recorded.

---

5 Meilhon, Aliénation mentale, part 1, 25. This was repeated, word for word, but without acknowledgment to Meilhon, in a 1908 dissertation on Senegalese patients shipped to France. Borreil, Considérations, 13.

6 While "placement volontaire" and "placement administrative" are colonial terms, the term "judicial placement" was chosen as an extension of the colonial vocabulary. It should be pointed out that traditional Islamic law was in fact very tolerant towards the insane and did not hold them responsible for their acts – judicial internment was therefore extraneous to Islamic law. See for example: Khiat, Essai, 128; Luccioni, Habous ou wakf, 48 f.; Chaleby, Forensic Psychiatry, 19; Pridmore/Pasha, Psychiatry and Islam, 383; Arabi, Regimentation of the Subject, 264; Dols, Insanity in Islamic Law, 81. Similarly, the popular interpretation of insanity as demonic possession meant that the insane were not believed to be answerable for their behaviour. See: Fanon/Sanchez, Attitude, 25.

7 The problems of communication will be looked at in Chapter 4 on the treatment of Muslim female patients. See p. 170.

The descriptions of female patients in the case studies were not static throughout the colonial period: psychiatrists more strongly "condemned" aggressive or immoral behaviour in their female patients in the early case studies, for example Meilhon in 1896, but much less so later on. During the period of these early publications, Muslim patients were still shipped to France from Algeria,[8] and the only contact with "Islam" these psychiatrists had was with the Muslim insane.[9] The high costs of transport and treatment in France meant that only the worst cases of mental problems were ever brought to the attention of French psychiatrists before the establishment of asylums on North African soil.

Changes in broader psychiatric theories (for example, the rise and fall of degeneracy), which one can find mirrored in the diagnoses and treatments administered to North African women, seem not to have been influential when it came to the admission processes of female patients. The manner of admission into psychiatric care – that is, the selection of patients through admission processes – did not evolve significantly in North Africa during colonial times.[10] The only notable change was the instalment of a "two line" psychiatric service under the *École d'Alger* in Algeria and, to a lesser degree, in Tunisia[11] and Morocco[12]. A "first line" of small psychiatric wards in the departmental hospitals (*première ligne*) looked after everyday cases, "curing" as many of them as possible[13] and only sending severe cases on to the "second line" hospitals (*deuxième ligne*).[14] It was hoped that the installation of a "two line" system would allow for more "voluntary placements" by having the "first line" look after less severe cases, thus attenuating the association with the unpleasant aspects of chronic insanity.[15] Despite the high hopes invested in the instalment of this system, no change was made to the admission processes themselves.

---

8 See Chapter 3.2.1 "Transported to France" for an in-depth analysis of these transfers.

9 The costs of the whole process – shipping the patients to France, their upkeep, and, in successful cases, their return journey to North Africa – was heavily criticised in colonial times. For example, by Meilhon in 1896: Meilhon, Aliénation mentale, part 6, 357.

10 Even though there was no major change in the types of admission during colonial times, many psychiatrists variously claimed that a change from "administrative" and "judicial placements" to "voluntary placements" had either already happened, like Gervais in 1907, or was surely about to happen, as asserted by Porot in 1943. Gervais, Contribution, 70; Porot, Œuvre psychiatrique, 362.

11 Ibid., Services hospitaliers, 794 f.

12 Ibid., Œuvre psychiatrique, 366 f.

13 Ibid., Services hospitaliers, 793.

14 Ibid., 794. See also: Rappel historique de l'assistance psychiatrique en Algérie, 815. Schwarz mentioned in his 1976 article that a third line for chronically ill and incurable patients was initially planned. Schwarz, Psychiatrie in Algerien, 88.

15 Desruelles/Bersot, Assistance aux aliénés en Algérie, 589.

2.3 Definitions of Criminality in a Colonial Context

Before looking at the administrative modes of admission into colonial psychiatric care, one must examine the colonial definition of indigenous criminality. Many French psychiatrists working on North Africa focused on the effects of criminality and criminal insanity on the general population. The first important work on Muslim criminality and its relation to insanity is the 1883 dissertation by the French psychiatrist Adolphe Kocher, "Criminality in Arabs from the Point of View of the Medico-Legal Practice in Algeria", which forms the starting point for this historical analysis of colonial psychiatry in the Maghreb. Even though Kocher had already researched "Arab criminality", the psychiatric obsession with North African criminality started under the influence of the *École d'Alger*. One of the first dissertations of the *École d'Alger*, dealing with the "Criminal Impulsivity in the Indigenous Algerian", was written in 1926 by Don Côme Arrii, who also published, together with his teacher Antoine Porot, an article under the same name in the *Annales Médico-Psychologiques* in 1932. Another of Porot's students, Charles Bardenat, wrote an important article about "Criminality and Delinquency in the Mental Alienation of Indigenous Algerians" in 1948, also published in the *Annales Médico-Psychologiques*.

Parallel to metropolitan interest in crimes committed by the "raving mad", as documented by countless sensationalist columns under the heading of "Aliénés en liberté" in the *Annales Médico-Psychologiques*, one can find reports about crimes committed by North Africans, both in North Africa and as immigrants in France.[16] Many colonial psychiatrists regretted that, mainly due to budgetary reasons, the systems of admission into colonial care were incomplete and allowed for potentially dangerous Muslim madmen to slip through the net.[17] Charles Bardenat, for example, exclaimed in 1948: "And how many psychopaths or abnormal natives still escape the control of the doctor!"[18]

Solomon Lwoff and Paul Sérieux encapsulated the colonial fear of the "unrecognised" indigenous mad in 1913 by stating that "thousands of unrecognised insane, these half-madmen, these degenerates of all sorts, [...] live in freedom, committing offences,

---

16 See, for example: Les aliénés en liberté, 173 f. On the crimes committed by uninstitutionalised "madmen", see also: Livet, Aliénés algériens, 43; Maréschal, Réflexions, 70. Don Côme Arrii summarised these fears in his 1926 dissertation on "Criminal Impulsivity in the Indigenous Algerian": "Too many madmen still roam free in the 'bled' [the countryside, from the Arabic word *balad*, which means country], free to indulge in all the deadly consequences of their impulsivity. In the absence of other means of assistance, families still sometimes impede them by chains on their feet, which are not always enough, however, to avert the danger of murder." Arrii, Impulsivité criminelle, 51.

17 See, for example: Susini, Quelques considérations, 27 f.

18 Bardenat, Criminalité, 318.

crimes, attacks of all sorts, participating in riots or even causing them, and from among whom many of the alleged fanatics, mystics and xenophobes are recruited."[19] French psychiatrists wanted to place the Muslim insane in asylums precisely because they feared that they all posed a hidden danger, and it greatly upset them to think that this total control was not possible.[20] It was this fear of the half-mad, of the hidden, of the seemingly normal which dominated the colonial treatment of the North African insane, and the idea that such crimes could also happen in France only made it all the more tangible. Porot and Arrii stated in their 1932 article on "Criminal Impulsivity" that one could find reports in France "every day" about the "crimes of these 'sidis' [here a derogatory designation for North African men, it is usually a respectful form of addressing someone; from Arabic *sayyid*, which means lord], newcomers in French criminality, who have rapidly found themselves playing a major role".[21]

The duty of psychiatrists therefore lay not only in recognising and diagnosing "danger" in the indigenous population, they also had to be able to contain it. This aspect of their duties gave considerable responsibility to colonial psychiatrists as, effectively, they had to protect the population.[22] In 1936, Porot quoted instructions from the then Governor-General of Algeria, Jules Gaston Henri Carde, about asylum regulations: a psychiatrist had the right to prohibit the release of any patient that he deemed dangerous – those who could "compromise the public order or the security of people" – even if the patient and his/her family demanded it.[23]

In 1883 Kocher studied the different medico-legal categories of indigenous criminality based on his experience of working at the Civil Hospital of Mustapha in Algiers.

---

19 Lwoff/Sérieux, Note, 695. Henry Reboul and Emmanuel Régis even claimed in their 1912 Congress report that "one could not exaggerate the role of the insane, in Muslim lands, as disruptors of the public order." Reboul/Régis, Assistance, 78.

20 Bardenat, Criminalité, 318.

21 Porot/Arrii, Impulsivité criminelle, 588. The same phrase can be found in Arrii's 1926 dissertation. Arrii, Impulsivité criminelle, 13. One of these authors, Antoine Porot, had written in 1912 that criminal acts committed by North African lunatics were "rare enough", basing this statement on "testimonials by the police [...]." This startling change in his opinion mirrors his deeper involvement in Algeria, slowly adapting to the mentality of French settlers, which is also shown in the scientific and biological racism of the *École d'Alger*. Porot, Tunisie, 71.

22 In 1911, for example, the psychiatrist Livet described the responsibility of psychiatrists in estimating the potential threats of patients. He recounted how a Muslim patient, released too early, had murdered a doctor in Algiers: "The assassin had stayed in Aix, had left unhealed, still deluded and hallucinating. On his return to Algiers, being denied entrance to the hospital, he waited, armed with an axe, at its door, for Dr Moutet and split his skull. It is obvious that this individual should not have left the asylum in Aix as early, or at least [that he should] have been carefully monitored after his release." Livet, Aliénés algériens, 43.

23 Carde, Jules Gaston Henri, Instruction, article 12. As quoted in: Porot, Services hospitaliers, 799.

His definition of criminality included offences that we would no longer classify as criminal, such as addictions[24] and various forms of sexuality, such as prostitution or homosexuality.[25] Through this broad definition of criminality, Kocher showed that he was part of the very popular movement of degeneration theorists, who saw, in the words of the historian Daniel Pick, "crime, suicide, alcoholism and prostitution" to be part of "social pathologies" that "endangered the European races".[26] In Kocher's categories, the "criminal" could be either sane or mad, and it was extremely difficult to authoritatively and scientifically differentiate between pure criminality and actual insanity. The distinction between criminality and criminal insanity was most often defined by the extreme violence of the act or by the breaking of unbreakable social norms. Kocher's dissertation portrayed the general fear of an intricate hidden relationship between criminality and insanity, which was also shown through one of the main duties of psychiatry being the identification of the "dangerous insane" before they had actually committed a crime – intercepting insanity to prevent it from evolving into criminality.[27]

2.4 French Laws on Placements in Asylums

A French law created on the 30th of June 1838 made it clear that the insane could only be kept in psychiatric asylums,[28] gradually eliminating all other forms of care that existed before and in parallel.[29] All mentally ill people, and also all those who disturbed the public order, could, under this law, be legally interned. The reason for this decision was not so much a genuine desire for better treatment of the insane than a deep-felt wish to protect the population from the perceived threat that the insane posed.[30] Soon after the passing of this law – that is, from the 1840s onwards –

---

24 Addictions were suspected to lead to violent forms of insanity in indigenous populations. Kocher, Criminalité, 135.

25 For example: Ibid., 161.

26 Pick, Faces of Degeneration, 21.

27 As late as 1961, L. Couderc explained that "the most distressing consequence of this state of affairs is the near impossibility, in most cases, of hospitalising and treating a mentally ill person before his condition has worsened to the point of making him dangerous, before he has come to the serious anti-social act, duly and officially recorded." Couderc, Conséquences, 253.

28 Keller, Colonial Madness, 25.

29 The French historian Hervé Guillemain wrote that prior to 1838, the three places where the "insane" were institutionalised in France were hospices, prisons and prison infirmaries. Guillemain, Malheur, 25.

30 Keller, Colonial Madness, 52 f.

only dangerous patients were admitted into psychiatric care in France due to serious overcrowding in existing asylums.[31]

It was not until 1876 that a new system of "voluntary admission", *placement volontaire,* was introduced in France as a reaction to protests against the existing preference of the system for the criminally insane.[32] "Voluntary" did not mean that the patient could or would bring himself to the attention of a psychiatrist through their own volition; rather, this new system allowed family members, friends or neighbours to place a person in a psychiatric asylum.[33] In France, most patients placed through "voluntary admission" were brought to the asylums by their husbands or wives: Patricia Prestwich's 1994 research showed that almost 40 percent of "voluntary admissions" in France in the late 19th and early 20th century were demanded by spouses.[34]

Even after the introduction of this law, the strong focus of institutional psychiatry on criminal patients remained. The fact that only the dangerous insane were admitted to mental hospitals while all other patients, because they posed less of a danger to society, were sent away, was also the case in the colonies.[35] French colonial psychiatrists complained that this focus on "criminals" left non-threatening cases without treatment, cases that could be more easily cured than the "criminally insane". Antoine Porot, for example, wrote in 1936 that this focus of psychiatric treatment on criminality meant that in Algeria patients with "light psychoses" were left without care or medical help because there was only enough space in the psychiatric institutions for the most dangerous patients.[36]

These laws focusing on the internment of the "criminally insane" brought new legal problems. How could one decide whether somebody was truly insane or merely pretending in order not to be put into prison? How could insanity be defined and deduced, especially in persons who committed truly horrific crimes? The people who took it upon themselves to act as judges of this important subject with absolute authority were psychiatrists. In the 19th century psychiatrists became the specialists in Europe for determining responsibility in criminals. They defined themselves as the only ones capable of drawing the line between the "criminally insane" and the "common criminal", between prisoner and patient, and they were increasingly asked to do so in court. They deplored less developed countries like their colonies, where

---

31   Prestwich, Family Strategies, 800, FN 13.

32   Dowbiggin, Back to the Future, 386, FN 11.

33   A person placed through "voluntary admission" could also be withdrawn from the asylum at any point. Prestwich, Family Strategies, 800.

34   Ibid., 803.

35   The same happened in non-French colonies, for example in Indonesia and India. Ernst, Idioms of Madness, 174; Pols, Development, 363 f.

36   Porot, Services hospitaliers, 796.

"criminally insane people" were still placed in prisons. The psychiatrists Lwoff and Sérieux, for example, disapprovingly described in their 1911 report that in Morocco the criminally insane were often confused with common criminals.[37]

In Muslim colonies, the expertise of psychiatrists was contested due to differing notions of insanity. In Islamic law, nobody could be held responsible while insane and was, therefore, not punishable – a criminally insane person had to be delivered to the care of their families, and only if their families could not take them back were they transferred to Islamic hospitals.[38] The experts responsible for determining whether somebody was sane, insane or in a lucid moment of his insanity were traditionally judges with a completely different set of ideas about the causes, scope and definition of insanity.[39] The Muslim process of admission into "medical care" was purely legal, based on witness testimonials – no medical expert was involved, as recorded by Henry Bouquet in his 1909 dissertation on the "Alienated in Tunisia". Having heard the witnesses brought before him by the family of the potential patient, the judge would decide on whether the accused was sane or insane. If insane, he could either be immediately arrested and brought to a mental asylum or stay in the care of the family responsible for his upkeep.[40]

Another problem psychiatrists were faced with was the separation of the "dangerous insane" from the "harmless insane" within their institutions. While this separation was introduced in most of Europe in the late 19th century as well as in the British colonies in India[41] and Egypt[42], this was not the case in France, which only instituted its first asylum for criminal cases in 1910 with the establishment of the Villejuif *Quartier de Sûreté*.[43] Unsurprisingly, there was no segregation of the "dangerous insane" and the "harmless insane" in the Maghreb either,[44] despite French psychiatrists repeatedly

37   Lwoff/Sérieux, Aliénés au Maroc, 472 f. The same regret – about the traditional confusion of the "criminally insane" with criminals in Muslim societies, caused by the absence of psychiatric expertise – is also stated by Henri Soumeire in his 1932 dissertation on "Murder in the Indigenous Alienated in Algeria". Soumeire, Meurtre, 23.

38   Chaleby, Forensic Psychiatry, 21; Pridmore/Pasha, Psychiatry and Islam, 383.

39   As the Islamic scientist Michael Dols pointed out, the Maliki School of Law is the only one of the four Islamic Schools which does not have the idea of "lucid moments" in insanity. Dols, Insanity in Islamic Law, 84.

40   Bouquet, Aliénés en Tunisie, 75 f.

41   Ernst, Idioms of Madness, 153.

42   Abbasîya and Khanka, 794. In Egypt, this architectural separation only concerned male patients. Warnock, Twenty-Eight Years, 244.

43   Fau-Vincenti, Vers les UMD, 69.

44   French colonial psychiatrists often claimed that this confusion of criminals with the criminally insane was due to pre-colonial Islamic conceptions and treatment of insanity. The colonial administrator Joseph Luccioni, who wrote a report on the situation of traditional Muslim

requesting this in their publications.[45] Consequently, they felt that, in this respect, they were behind other colonial powers in their treatment of the colonial mad.[46] The lack of segregation throughout French colonialism in the Maghreb is partly explained by the aforementioned differences in implementing theories about committing the mentally ill in France and Britain. Further, the first European-built and -run mental hospitals for Muslims in the Maghreb were only founded in the 1930s, while those in India and Egypt were built in the 19th century, a period when France still sent its colonial "mad" to asylums in France.

2.5 The Violent Muslim Man and the Passive Muslim Woman

Another explanation for the lack of segregation of the "criminally insane" concerns a specific, "race-related" quality of North African patients. Frantz Fanon wrote in 1961 that French colonial psychiatry was one of the cornerstones in reinforcing and validating the settler notion of the North African as a "born criminal",[47] a "hereditary" and "congenital criminal".[48] In Fanon's eyes, colonial psychiatry, especially the theories propagated by the *École d'Alger*, was the scientific foundation of these notions.[49] Porot and Arrii, for example, wrote in their 1932 article on "Criminal Impulsivity" that "*the frequency of criminal impulsivity*" was a "phenomenon especially particular to this race";[50] while Charles Bardenat suggested in 1948 that the low intelligence

---

    asylums in Morocco, in 1953, claimed: "Those who have committed detrimental acts or have become dangerous were imprisoned for an indefinite amount of time, or confused with common criminals. Like criminals, they wear iron fetters, riveted to the ankles, and at night they are attached to a chain by an iron collar." Luccioni, Maristanes, 462.

45   For example at the time of the instalment of the first hospital for the criminally insane in France, in 1911. Livet, Aliénés algériens, 42. As late as 1948, Charles Bardenat still demanded institutions for criminally insane Muslim men. Bardenat, Criminalité, 480.

46   This regret was also palpable with respect to other aspects of colonial psychiatry's duties. Bouquet, for example, professed his shame in his 1909 dissertation about the state of French colonial psychiatry, regretting that, unlike Holland and Great Britain, France had not yet developed a psychiatric assistance for the colonial mad. Bouquet, Aliénés en Tunisie, 83.

47   Fanon wrote that colonial psychiatry solidified the idea of the North African as "born slackers, born liars, born thieves, born criminals". Fanon, Damnés, 285.

48   Ibid., 287.

49   Ibid. This idea is taken up by the secondary literature, for example in: Macey, Algerian with the Knife, 162; McCulloch, Empire's New Clothes, 38 f. As noted above, the notion of the criminal North African already existed before the heyday of the *École d'Alger* and Fanon's criticism of it – Lemanski, for example, described male Arabs as a "race of bold and violent men" in 1913. Lemanski, Mœurs arabes, 136.

50   Porot/Arrii, Impulsivité criminelle, 589. Emphasis in the original.

of Muslims, their "mental insufficiency", made them intrinsically more delinquent than Europeans.[51] This psychiatric theory of male North Africans as "born criminals" had wide-reaching implications. It meant that no money needed to be invested in the education or assimilation of North Africans because criminality was too deeply ingrained in their inherited "racial" characteristics, and the money saved on education should instead be invested in the police and psychiatric hospitals to ensure the protection of the settler population against an innate criminality that made Muslims inaccessible to the French ideals of the *mission civilisatrice*.[52]

From the point of view of colonial psychiatrists, criminality was not a sign of insanity – because male North Africans were dangerous and violent even in their normality[53] –, and if this definition held true for normal North African men then, naturally, male North African mental patients who had lost their reason were dangerous and violent as well. Because of this alleged penchant for violence, the separation of the "dangerous insane" from the "harmless insane" in North African hospitals was not necessary since other mechanisms of separation were already operating: a "racial" separation of Muslim patients from European patients as well as gender segregation.[54]

Female wards for the "dangerous insane" were deemed unnecessary because the theories of French psychiatrists mirrored popular conceptions of normal femininity. Female Muslims were not only seen as set apart from the "born criminal" class discussed by Fanon but viewed as almost genetically incapable of being violent and dangerous[55]

---

51   Bardenat, Criminalité, 468 f. Even postcolonial North African writers support this theory. In 1965, the Tunisian sociologist Abdelwahab Bouhdiba wrote: "These data [i. e. repeat offenders] are disturbing, because they seem to question the perfectibility of man, and the reform of criminals proves to be at the very least illusory. Without going as far as to talk about 'professional criminals', it seems that we are dealing with something very deeply rooted in the mentality of the Tunisian Muslim." Bouhdiba, Criminalité, 59.

52   Keller, Colonial Madness, 16.

53   In Fanon's eyes, the danger posed by North Africans was not a purely colonial construct, as violent protest was one of the only forms of dissent open to the colonised. In his interpretation, North Africans were forced, by colonial oppression, into violent reactions. See for example: Fanon, Damnés, 83. Though Fanon used the word "Algerian", which nominally included women, it is clear from his examples and from the quotes of French psychiatrists that he reproduced in his texts that he was actually referring to men. This has been noted by Anne McClintock, for example, in her 1995 book "Imperial Leather". "Potentially generic terms like 'the Negro' or 'the Native' – syntactically unmarked for gender – are almost everywhere immediately contextually marked as male [...]." McClintock, Imperial Leather, 362.

54   For example in: Desruelles/Bersot, Assistance aux aliénés en Algérie, 591. See also: Schwarz, Psychiatrie in Algerien, 88.

55   For example: Lemanski, Mœurs arabes, 117. This notion is still widespread. The aforementioned Tunisian sociologist Bouhdiba wrote in 1965: "Crime in Tunisia remains, as elsewhere in the world, an essentially male manifestation. Women, and Muslim women in particular, remain

and, instead, were traditionally portrayed as the victims of male aggression.[56] Women were seen as being too passive to be the perpetrators of criminality, a notion that fitted in with Muslim concepts of gender segregation and patriarchy, or at least the French interpretations of these concepts.

The reason for the widespread male violence against women was believed to be jealousy, which Kocher defined in 1883 as the moral basis of the Algerian male psyche.[57] In Kocher's opinion, there were multiple causes for this jealousy: "*polygamy, divorce, and marriage*, which is often, with Arabs, only a shameful commerce – the young girl is allocated to the highest bidder, and jealousy and hatred awake between rivals."[58] The basis for Muslim women's suffering was therefore seen to be part of Muslim family law, which, in the eyes of the French, permitted and tolerated excessive sexuality and all the vices that came with it, such as violent jealousy.

The repetition of quotes about the Muslim woman's status as an eternal victim, discussed in Chapter 1, enabled the French to criticise societies in the Maghreb.[59] France did not actively interfere in Muslim civil law and Muslim traditions because they feared uprisings would ensue if they did.[60] Having allegedly no opportunity to change Muslim civil law or traditions, but still wishing to voice their outrage, many colonial authors instead focused on the miserable life Muslim women led, which they attributed to Muslim civil law and Islamic traditions as much as to male Muslim normality, as discussed in the previous chapter. Presenting Muslim women as victims of male Muslim despotism soon became a trope yet never sparked any real urgency

---

the guardians of morality and virtue. If they participate in crimes, they do so ten times less often than men." Bouhdiba, Criminalité, 69. He even postulated that "Tunisian Women stay morally and socially superior to men. But their entry into public life led them to participate more in the building of society. The increase in female imprisonment reflects quite accurately the social evolution in progress. Indeed, it is in the interior and in the South that the percentage of female criminality is the lowest, [and] it is also there that the traditional situation of women is the slowest to change." Ibid., 73. Capitalisation in the original.

56 The psychiatrist Sextius Arène wrote in his 1913 dissertation on "Criminality in Arabs": "The crimes of Muslims are mostly *crimes of passion*, motivated by adultery or jealousy. The lack of loving emotions between men and women should be emphasised here; Arabs are *male* and *female* [animals]: an Arab man cannot see a woman without desiring her and an Arab woman cannot see a man without wanting him for her personal pleasure; from this comes the jealousy of men and the explanation of the confinement of women." Emphasis in the original. Arène, Criminalité, 105 f. See also: Porot/Arrii, Impulsivité criminelle, 589.

57 This notion was taken up by many later psychiatric authors. See for example: Lemanski, Mœurs arabes, 141; Bardenat, Criminalité, 325 f.; Aubin, Indigènes Nord-Africains, 292.

58 Kocher, Criminalité, 98. Emphasis in the original.

59 Clancy-Smith, Islam, Gender, and Identities, 155 f.

60 For a discussion of this "refusal to intervene" in other French colonies, see: Conklin, Mission to Civilize, 87 f., especially FN 43.

to tackle the deplorable – but perceived as unchangeable – misery of female Muslims. Even though Muslim women were depicted as passive victims, they were, due to their exotic sex drive, also seen as responsible for the crimes committed against them. In 1883 Kocher wrote about the presumed sexuality of young Arab girls who were dressed provocatively by their mothers: "An accusation of rape, produced under these conditions, would evidently lose a great part of its gravity."[61]

The theory that indigenous women were incapable of crime was a colonial construct,[62] showing the notable gap between psychiatric theory and practice, as the case studies show numerous examples of female patients being very violent and destructive. However, there was no question of women not being victims of "criminally insane" men. Muslim women were assaulted by confused or demented male family members, just as they were in Europe at that time, and as it still happens to this day. One can find allusions to women suffering from the hereditary criminality of Muslim men, often in the summaries that psychiatrists gave in court when judging whether a murderer was responsible for his crimes. One can also find female victims of male aggression and violence in case studies of female mental patients – the background information, used by colonial psychiatrists to explain the emergence of diseases, often depicted Muslim women as victims. Jean Sutter, for example, studied cases of "Mental Epilepsy in the Native Algerian" for his 1937 dissertation. One female patient, first married at 17 and mother, widow and remarried by the age of 24 when Sutter wrote about her, was so badly mistreated by her second husband that she miscarried and suffered a traumatic brain injury, which seems to have triggered her first epileptic shock.[63] In Sutter's view of the case, she was completely innocent and fulfilled the criteria of ideal Muslim femininity by being brought to a mental asylum as a victim rather than a dangerous or criminal perpetrator.

Female Muslim perpetrators were extremely rare over the entire colonial period, as some psychiatrists tried to prove through numerical evidence. Porot and his student Arrii described in 1932 40 cases of "criminal impulsivity" in Algerian Muslims, only two of them concerning female criminals.[64] In the same year, only one woman in 14 case studies was documented as being criminal in a psychiatric dissertation on "Murder in the Indigenous Algerian Population", which is, according to Henri Soumeire, in "accordance with the conclusions of all psychiatrists".[65] In Suzanne Taïeb's 1939

---

61   Kocher, Criminalité, 185 f.
62   It coincided with Muslim notions that, while women were maybe untrustworthy and immoral, they were not physically dangerous. In Muslim societies, the danger of women was seen to lie in their association with magic.
63   Sutter, Épilepsie mentale, 181 f.
64   Porot/Arrii, Impulsivité criminelle, 607.
65   Soumeire, Meurtre, 78.

dissertation, she found that none of the criminal cases she looked at were committed by women, which led her to the general conclusion that deliriums and psychoses made Muslim men more violent and dangerous[66] but, interestingly, not to the corresponding theory that Muslim women were somehow incapable of criminality. Finally, Assicot et al. stated in 1961 that among 66 Muslim admissions into Blida Psychiatric Hospital for medico-legal reasons in 1958 and 1959 only one concerned a Muslim woman.[67]

In another statistic covering the admission numbers to Blida Psychiatric Hospital in Algeria from 1933 to 1940, the psychiatrist Charles Bardenat found that out of 1,324 female patients (795 European Christians, 412 Muslims, and 117 Jews), only three were condemned criminals – and all three were Muslim women.[68] He argued that Muslim women were indeed very unlikely to commit crimes, but still more likely than their more civilised European or Jewish sisters. Bardenat concluded: "Without wanting to draw definite conclusions from this fact, we have to admit that the indigenous woman – noisier and more destructive in the hospital than her kind in the other ethnic groups – does not reach the harmfulness of the male native, because of her condition as a minor, in which she is kept in her society, living under a narrow and quasi-slavish dependence."[69]

2.6 Mechanisms of Admission

As has been shown, crimes in general and violent crimes in particular were regarded as a male domain by French colonial psychiatrists, regardless of the reality encountered in their daily lives. Even when they were confronted with criminal female Muslim patients, it was argued that the numbers were so small that they could be neglected. The facts therefore seemed congruent with their theories of gendered aggression and criminality in both normality and abnormality.

However, an examination of the ways in which women were admitted to psychiatric care in the Maghreb reveals a strong criminalisation of female patients. As mentioned above, these mechanisms of admission can be roughly divided into three groups: "voluntary placements", "administrative placements" and "judicial placements", each with their own manner of criminalisation. As neither the case studies nor the statistics state how many patients were interned via each of these possible placements, some of the cases mentioned below could be subsumed under more than one category.

---

66 Taïeb, Idées d'influence, 78.
67 During the same period, only six European patients were admitted in that way, among them also one woman. Assicot et al., Causes principales, 263.
68 Bardenat, Criminalité, 318.
69 Ibid., 320.

2.6.1   Voluntary Placement

One might reasonably presume that "voluntary placement" of mentally ill people
by family members and neighbours should have been the most common mode of
admission of Muslim patients to colonial psychiatric hospitals.[70] However, placement
for health reasons seems to have been quite rare,[71] as people with mental illnesses
were traditionally looked after by their families,[72] brought to local healers or placed
in purpose-built Islamic hospitals (*māristāns*) next to the tombs of saints.[73] Only
under extreme circumstances did Muslim families contact colonial psychiatrists. Livet
explained this in 1911 through the distances between Muslim families in rural Algeria
and the general hospitals in Algiers or even the mental institutions in France.[74] He
stated: "As to the families, given that the asylum is two days travel [away], they resolve
with much difficulty to [agree with] the separation from the sufferer who, despite
everything, is dear to them. For this, it is necessary that the insane has shown some
dangerous or offensive symptoms."[75]

---

70   In a 1936 article on the "Psychiatric Hospital Services in North Africa", Antoine Porot quoted
     instructions from the Governor-General of Algeria at the time, Jules Gaston Henri Carde,
     from the 10th of August 1934. Article 5 of these instructions stated that people with "light or
     inoffensive" mental problems could be admitted by either their own request or that of their
     families. Carde, Jules Gaston Henri, Instruction, article 5. As quoted in: Porot, Services hos-
     pitaliers, 798.
71   Frantz Fanon and François Sanchez even mentioned in 1956 that they knew of patients who
     had been interned against the express wishes of their families. Fanon/Sanchez, Attitude, 27.
     This was also observed in postcolonial psychiatric texts. The British psychiatrist John Racy
     wrote in 1970 that female patients in Arab countries were still mostly brought to the atten-
     tion of the authorities by their male family members, or through official forms of placement.
     Racy, Psychiatry in the Arab East, 40.
72   See for example: Lemanski, Mœurs arabes, 122; Desruelles/Bersot, Assistance aux aliénés en
     Algérie, 581; Al-Issa, Mental Illness, 57.
73   Lwoff/Sérieux, Aliénés au Maroc, 473 f. The French colonial administration in Tunisia and
     Morocco tolerated these *māristāns*, as a means of institutionalising the indigenous insane,
     but only when the patient had not committed a crime. In Algeria, the French disbanded all
     traditional hospitals or reorganised them under European rule at the beginning of the French
     conquest. Desruelles/Bersot, Assistance aux aliénés en Algérie, 594. One of these traditional
     māristāns became, for example, the Civil Hospital of Mustapha. Livet, Aliénés algériens, 13 f.
     These traditional asylums will be discussed in detail in Chapters 3 and 4.
74   Ibid., 35.
75   Ibid., 53. See also: Susini, Quelques considérations, 27 f. The Iraqi psychiatrist Ihsan Al-Issa
     and his Finnish wife Brigitta Al-Issa wrote in a 1970 article on psychiatric problems in Iraq that
     Muslims were very tolerant towards people with mental issues, "as long as it is not expressed in
     unprovoked violence, sexually shameful behaviour, or uncontrollable motor overactivity [...]."
     In their opinion "the mental content of a patient is seldom enough to bring him to the healer

Due to a too literal and rigid incorporation of Muslim ideals about gender segregation into their simplistic interpretation of Islam, it was a widespread colonial belief that Muslim families would never voluntarily bring their ill female family members to a male doctor[76] and that this accounted for the reluctance to admit patients to psychiatric care.[77] While Muslim ideals of gender segregation might have hindered some women from contacting male European specialists, and while others might have been stopped by jealous husbands or worried families, just as many might have had completely different reasons for preferring other cures. Many patients, especially at the time when they were still shipped to France, did not survive their placement in colonial care – the death rates were shockingly high.[78] Families that could afford to look after their patients without involving colonial care would do so at almost any cost.[79] While Muslim women who were treated by local healers or in a traditional *māristān* for mental disorders were readily accepted back into society once healed,[80] those who spent time in colonial asylums, and were lucky enough to survive, usually suffered stigmatisation.[81] The reluctance to bring female patients to psychiatric

---

or doctor; it is the behaviour which is decisive." Al-Issa/Al-Issa, Psychiatric Problems, 17. This distinction between "disease" and "behaviour" also seemed to have played a role in Maghrebi conceptions of supportable and insupportable mental diseases, of patients that could be kept at home, and those that were brought to the attention of colonial psychiatrists.

76 For example: Matignon, Art médical, 91. Unsurprisingly, this belief can also be found in the texts of French female doctors, as for example in the 1905 dissertation by Hélène Abadie-Feyguine about "Medical Assistance of Indigenous Women in Algeria". Abadie-Feyguine, Assistance médicale, 65.

77 This explanation, for example, was given in an article published in the journal *Hygiène Mentale* in 1955 – one of the authors was Frantz Fanon. Dequeker et al., Aspects actuels, 1112.

78 See Chapter 3.3.1 "Chances of Death".

79 This tradition of keeping people with mental problems with their families was repeatedly criticised by French psychiatrists. Reboul and Régis, for example, felt in 1912 that the Muslim insane were mistreated by their families, because of their lack of psychiatric knowledge. Reboul/Régis, Assistance, 76.

80 This tolerance was caused by traditional notions of insanity being caused by "Jinn", who might attack anybody, regardless of their actions or behaviour. Especially among women, possession by a "Jinn" was seen as normal and was therefore socially tolerated. Aouattah, Ethnopsychiatrie maghrébine, 242 f.

81 Lemanski, for instance, wrote that because of a stigma connected to all kinds of European hospitals, only the poorest population of North Africa brought their female mental patients to the French doctors and psychiatrists. Lemanski, Mœurs arabes, 122. This stigma attached to former patients of psychiatry in Arab countries is still observed in postcolonial and even contemporary research. See for example: Katchadourian, Survey, 24; Al-Krenawi/Graham, Gender and Biomedical/Traditional Mental Health Utilization, 226; El-Islam, Mental Illness, 133; Okasha, Mental Health Services in the Arab World, 45; Mejda et al., Histoire, 691.

hospitals therefore might have had less to do with Muslim gender segregation and clinging to traditional healing than with negative connotations of colonial care, of which the psychiatrists had little awareness.

Still, some patients were admitted through "voluntary placement" by their families. In his 1907 dissertation "Diet and Treatment of the Indigenous Insane in Algeria", Camille-Charles Gervais mentioned a woman who was brought to psychiatric care and his personal attention by her husband, who seemed to have been earnestly worried about her health. At a time when patients from Algeria were shipped to Aix-en-Provence, this could have easily meant the end of the contact between husband and wife, but the husband, who apparently had eight other wives – so that "one more or less did not really change anything"[82], as Gervais noted patronisingly and clearly against the evidence of his own case study –, was a retired military man with money. Shocked at how much the asylum in Aix-en-Provence made him pay for the upkeep of his wife, he decided to get her back, but on his arrival at the hospital, he was denied permission to see his wife, despite the long journey he had expressly made to meet her. He returned to Algeria, only to turn up again in Aix-en-Provence, this time demanding to talk to someone in authority. He spoke to the director of the asylum and allegedly told him: "Your doctors cannot cure, do you want to try my remedy? Give me back my wife; in Algiers, in my village, I will take charge of her cure."[83] Unsurprisingly, they did not give him the chance to cure his wife with traditional medicine, and Gervais mentioned no more about either husband or wife.

This case seems to have been unique: no similar stories about families worrying about the health of an interned family member and trying to be actively involved in the treatment are to be found in published case studies.[84] However, in her 1941 dissertation Eliane Demassieux mentioned Muslim mothers and wives visiting the psychiatric services in Algeria to inquire about institutionalising a male family member, whose violent reactions they feared.[85] More often, however, voluntary placement took the form of formal complaints by neighbours or family members to local magistrates in order to protect themselves from the violence of a mentally ill person rather than seeking treatment for their mental health problems per se. When these magistrates thought the claim of insanity was justified by the unreasonable actions of the patient

---

82 Gervais, Contribution, 72.

83 Ibid.

84 This is also shown through a passage in a 1954 article, in which the French doctor Pierre Charbonneau explicitly stated that "[...] some requests of voluntary placement are sometimes made by Moroccans to the hospital in Fes [...]." Had voluntary placements of Muslim psychiatric patients occurred regularly, this remark would have been unnecessary. Charbonneau, Assistance, part 2, 792.

85 Demassieux, Service social, 41 f.

and verified by witnesses, they transferred the case to a *māristān*.[86] As already mentioned, in Islamic Law it was the *qāḍī*, the local judge, who determined whether the accused was sane or insane. Under colonial rule, a doctor's statement was added as an extra step between magistrate and asylum, and the final decision about whether a person was deemed sane or insane lay with the "true experts", the colonial psychiatrists.[87]

This more common manifestation of the "voluntary placement" mainly concerned women who were, for some reason, unbearable to their families, who usually looked after their "insane" female relations until their death, although this line of action was only taken under extreme circumstances, most often when patients uttered wild threats or became too violent for the makeshift restraints at home. The psychiatrist Jean Sutter described in his 1937 dissertation cases of "voluntary placement" and the threat that violent "madwomen" posed to their families. One was the aforementioned case of a woman whose mental epilepsy was triggered by the physical abuse she suffered at the hands of her second husband. Her violent epileptic crises disturbed her neighbours, who finally contacted the police.[88] A second case study concerned a 37-year-old Kabyle woman with another heart-breaking life story of young marriage (first wedding at the age of 12), young widowhood (at 18), another marriage, then a divorce, after which the woman was "always sad", "fleeing all society", "often crying", and "speaking to herself in a low voice [...]." Six months before her internment in Algiers, she underwent a "crisis", in which she tried to "hit her mother", whom she later threatened to kill.[89]

Another psychiatrist who described cases of Muslim women becoming a danger to their families was Suzanne Taïeb in 1939. One female epileptic "had quickly become 'malicious', hitting her mother, hitting her brothers", running away into the countryside, and "slapping children she encountered [...]." Her parents reacted to these crises by "locking her up in a room, hoping that she would calm down, but seeing that she became more and more violent, they ultimately had to hospitalise her."[90] In another of her case studies, Taïeb wrote about a schizophrenic, who, in phases of "general over-excitement", threatened "to kill everybody, her mother included, who wants to approach her. In her anger, she breaks everything within her reach. She is furious." After those phases, the patient became calmer, sadder, and refused to speak or let other people look after her.[91] In cases like these, it is probable, though often not specifically mentioned, that either families or neighbours contacted the local magistrates, who

---

86 Bouquet, Aliénés en Tunisie, 75.
87 Bouquet also mentioned that families sometimes sidestepped local magistrates and contacted the asylum directly to get help with their violent family members. Ibid., 75 f.
88 Sutter, Épilepsie mentale, 181 f.
89 Ibid., 156 f.
90 Taïeb, Idées d'influence, 95 f.
91 Ibid., 104 f.

then interned them. It is also important to understand that these patients were taken from their family homes and brought to psychiatric asylums because of the perceived danger they posed due to their violence and threatening manner and not because they were seen as being ill.

There were also women deemed dangerous not to others but to themselves. Jean Sutter, for instance, summarised the danger that Muslim women posed in 1937 as follows: "In women [...] one notes fewer dangerous or criminal reactions, but [instead] a disorderly agitation which leads sometimes to auto-mutilation."[92] French psychiatrists held the theory that suicide, prohibited through Islamic law, had been unknown in North Africa before France started its *mission civilisatrice*.[93] To them, it was only with the civilising project that suicide started in the Maghreb. Kocher wrote in 1883 that, "especially in women", suicide, formerly infrequent, seemed to increase with the contact with France.[94] Kocher went on to say that, unlike in Europeans, where single men and women killed themselves, suicide in the Maghreb concerned married Muslims in two thirds of all cases. In his opinion, "this number should not astonish us, if we think of the cruel suffering which brings with it, for women, the state of abjection in which they are kept by their husbands."[95]

2.6.2 Administrative Placement

"Administrative placement" is the name the French gave to the admission of patients who were picked up by the police because they behaved in a way that was unacceptable to local and French social customs or, often, morals.[96] Antoine Porot, quoting again from the instructions of the general governor of Algeria concerning mental hospitals,

---

92 Sutter, Épilepsie mentale, 215.

93 Kocher, Criminalité, 143 f.

94 Ibid., 233. Suzanne Taïeb also described several cases of Muslim women who tried to commit suicide, often in very violent ways, both prior to their internment and during their psychiatric treatment. These Muslim women often had to be physically restrained in the hospitals in fear of self-harm. Taïeb, Idées d'influence, 89 f.

95 Kocher, Criminalité, 148 f. Apart from the general malaise regarding the low status of Muslim women, Kocher also blamed, in another part of his dissertation, the alcoholism that France's *mission civilisatrice* brought with it for the rise in both suicide rates and "insanity". This reason for the rise of suicides, however, seems to be applied mainly to Muslim men. Ibid., 28.

96 Henri Bouquet described Islamic "administrative placements" in his 1909 dissertation, translating article 629 of the pre-colonial Tunisian Civil Code from the year 1861: "Each individual, in a state of drunkenness or dementia, will be hindered from circulating in the streets... The police will arrest the madman and will bring him to his parents or, in the absence of those, to the house of the alienated." Bouquet, Aliénés en Tunisie, 76, FN 1.

wrote in 1936 that "administrative placements" took place when a subject was disturbing the public order or menacing the security of people.[97] As with "voluntary placements", these cases were brought before a local magistrate who determined whether
the patient should be deemed sane or insane. Next, a local doctor was contacted, who
might again send them on to a psychiatric hospital where psychiatric experts decided
whether the person was merely difficult or truly insane.[98] Porot went on to say that the
normal rules (necessitating an official statement, a medical certificate and personal
papers) could be bypassed "in case of urgency or of imminent danger, at the request
of the patient, or of his family, or of authorities [...]."[99]

In such cases, the manner of admittance itself, reinforced by the involvement of
the police, stressed the potential danger of these patients to society. Police involvement was, surprisingly, almost never mentioned in the published case studies, but
it is reasonable to assume that patients described in ways that pointed to this idea
of "disrupting the public order" were admitted to psychiatric hospitals by "administrative placements". These disruptions could take various forms. Adolphe Kocher,
for example, mentioned in 1883 that many Muslim patients were institutionalised
after having committed "public crimes against decency",[100] while Reboul and Régis
explained almost thirty years later that "only those who reveal publicly their excessive extravagance" came to the attention of colonial psychiatrists.[101] Charles Bardenat
regretted in 1948 that "an act of violence, impossible to hide" was needed "to trigger
the intervention by the authorities" and to initiate psychiatric treatment,[102] while
in 1955 a group of French psychiatrists – among them Frantz Fanon – further elaborated on this unease about "administrative placement" by explaining that Muslim
patients only arrived at Blida Psychiatric Hospital after having passed through "stages
of scandal and public danger [...]."[103]

These disruptions of the public order, with regard to Muslim women, can be
divided into three possible categories: a) women classified as prostitutes, b) women
with alcohol problems, and c) vagrant women, who behaved in a socially, morally
or even legally unacceptable way. However, the lines between these categories were

---

97 Carde, Jules Gaston Henri, Instruction, Article 7. As quoted in: Porot, Services hospitaliers,
    798.
98 Bennani, Psychanalyse, 111; Keller, Colonial Madness, 90.
99 Carde, Jules Gaston Henri, Instruction, Article 8. As quoted in: Porot, Services hospitaliers,
    798.
100 Kocher, Criminalité, 160.
101 Reboul/Régis, Assistance, 11. Similarly, Jude and Assad Hakim stated in 1927 that, in Damas-
    cus, patients were only brought to the psychiatric institutions after they had caused a scandal.
    Jude/Assad Hakim, Troubles mentaux, 126. See also: Bullard, Truth in Madness, 120.
102 Bardenat, Criminalité, 319.
103 Dequeker et al., Aspects actuels, 1112.

blurred, for instance women classed as prostitutes were likely to be described as alcoholics or vagrants as well.

Prostitutes

Police, magistrates and psychiatrists could define women as prostitutes just because they behaved in an unaccepted way,[104] but, while technically legal, prostitution was seen to be closely connected to criminal offences[105] and was, both in France and in the North African colonies, frequently cited as a symptom of insanity, as a lifestyle finally leading to insanity or as only undertaken by women already insane.[106] The psychiatrist Camille-Charles Gervais proposed in his 1907 dissertation that, among Muslim women, "[...] those who come to Aix are mainly those who trade in prostitution."[107] However, colonial observers understood that not all prostitutes were classified as insane and that most of them ended in prison rather than in a psychiatric institution, as a visit to a Moroccan female prison in 1923 showed, where "almost all [the inmates] were thieves or women with light morals".[108]

Meilhon, a doctor at the mental asylum in Aix-en-Provence, wrote in 1896 that one of his case studies concerned a Muslim prostitute, whom he called "une fille galante". This woman had been brought to Aix-en-Provence after having been treated at the Civil Hospital of Mustapha in Algiers for syphilis. She initially showed no signs of mental alienation but became agitated in the hospital. Once transferred to Aix-en-Provence, she was kept in the asylum, even though, interestingly, Meilhon never could confirm that she was suffering from any sort of syphilis-induced mental illness.[109] A second of Meilhon's case studies described the history of a hysterical "fille soumise", who

104 Kocher implied that there was a relationship between female homosexuality and prostitution. He wrote that female homosexuality was only observed in prostitutes and was generally not widespread in Arab societies because "it seems that this vice demands a certain degree of civilisation to flower". Kocher, Criminalité, 168.

105 Lazreg, Eloquence of Silence, 23.

106 Sérieux, Recherches cliniques, 26. Jules Comby even hinted in 1923 that psychiatrically normal Muslim women were brought to traditional Moroccan asylums "by the pasha" because "of their light conduct" – a practice he claimed to have witnessed himself in Meknes. Comby, Voyage médical, 1203. On the other hand, prostitution was imagined to be an acceptable alternative for Muslim women to life in the two "cages" discussed in Chapter 1. See for example: Lazreg, Eloquence of Silence, 56.

107 Gervais, Contribution, 48.

108 Celarié, Un mois au Maroc, 213.

109 Meilhon, Aliénation mentale, part 2, 195 f. Similar to the case study discussed at the beginning of this chapter, the story of this allegedly syphilitic prostitute shows an alternate possibility of psychiatric internment: admission by passing through a prison or, in this case, through the

was brought to the asylum in Aix-en-Provence because she was "alcoholic, addicted to venereal excesses" with both violent and "erotic" tendencies.[110] Based on this vivid description, it is easy to imagine that this patient had been arrested by the police for indecent behaviour, although Meilhon did not think it necessary to explain the reason for his patient's admission.

Interestingly, the only psychiatrist openly classifying patients as "prostitutes" after Meilhon, using the same colourful euphemisms, was one of the few women working in colonial North Africa, Suzanne Taïeb. One might ask whether this was due to a stricter moral high ground that Taïeb took, as was described for many European women living in colonies,[111] or a mechanism of self-defence in a profession still dominated by male authority. A Tunisian Jew,[112] speaking fluent Arabic,[113] and with a Maghrebi surname, she might have felt a stronger need to differentiate between herself and the women she treated. Taïeb mentioned, for example, cases of patients who were "filles soumises" or who had been forced to work in brothels.[114] One case study, for example, concerned a 40-year-old Muslim woman, who came to Blida Psychiatric Hospital suffering from deliriums. This woman told Taïeb that she left her husband, whom she had married at the age of 13, and her three children to be with another man, who treated her very badly. One day, after a violent dispute with her abusive partner, her landlady brought her to the police. "They" – presumably the police – brought her to a "house of tolerance"[115], where she was said to be highly unhappy. This happened years before her admission to Blida, but it was still perceived to have been relevant with regards to her present illness in the eyes of Taïeb.[116]

Both Meilhon and Taïeb, even though they wrote with 40 years of colonial experiences separating them, described their patients using strikingly similar terms – "filles légères", "filles galantes", "filles soumises"[117] –, though it is not always certain whether they really meant to imply that the described patients had been working prostitutes.

---

field of vision of general medicine. In both cases, the initial reason for the internment was, psychiatrically speaking, highly questionable.

110 Ibid., part 4, 40.

111 This theory that European women were the cause of a heightened racism in the colonies has been criticised by the historian Ann Laura Stoler. Stoler, Carnal Knowledge, 56. It is not implied that Taïeb was "more racist" than her male colleagues, but that, as a woman, she was seen to embody French colonial morals and was probably conscious of that. Ibid., 57.

112 Taïeb, Idées d'influence, 15.

113 Keller, Madness and Colonization, 315.

114 Taïeb, Idées d'influence, 85; 92; 105.

115 "Maison de tolérance" is a French euphemism for a brothel, and used in colonial sources quite often. For example: Nicole, Prostitution, 211.

116 Taïeb, Idées d'influence, 120 f.

117 Meilhon, Aliénation mentale, part 2, 195; part 4, 40; Taïeb, Idées d'influence, 85; 92.

Arguably, by that time an automatic connection between the "Oriental woman" and prostitution had already become a colonial trope.[118] It was often stated that, perhaps due to the (one-sided) facility of divorce in Islamic family law,[119] sex work was always a possibility for North African women. This notion had been present from almost the beginning of French colonial medicine in North Africa. In 1855 the doctor Émile-Louis Bertherand, for example, suggested a strong link between the normal life of Muslim women and their will to prostitute themselves. "One can say with reason that the Arab woman willingly trades her body. Habituated from a very early age to see herself lowered to the role of slave or a simple instrument of pleasure, prematurely delivered to despotic men who treat her like a commodity, having no principles of moral education which could support her in this series of distressing tests which could inculcate aversion to vice, she gives in promptly and easily to her whims, to her instincts, to the possibility of fleeing an existence of bad treatment and of having some distractions in compensation. Also prostitution is widespread with Arabs; it [prostitution] is recruited generally from among repudiated women."[120] This quote from 1855 was, in a way, still valid a century later as the colonial medical and psychiatric understanding of how the world of Muslim women worked had not changed much. It was still supposed that normal Muslim women could very easily be forced to become prostitutes by certain circumstances. In 1959, for example, Sutter et al. mirrored Bertherand by stating that "prostitution is essentially the result of girls married too young and repudiated long before they come of age."[121]

This classification of normal women as prostitutes seemed to occur regularly with "vagrant women": Alice Bullard thus wrote in her 2001 article "The Truth in Madness" that only destitute prostitutes, having been repudiated not only by their husbands but also by their extended families, could no longer rely on their care in cases of insanity and therefore had to become insane vagrants.[122] Even if there was no other sign of insanity or prostitution in a vagrant woman, it was often assumed that all three things must go together.

---

118 Lazreg, Eloquence of Silence, 56.
119 Divorced women from the poorer classes were seen to be the most likely to become prostitutes in the eyes of French psychiatrists, as stated in an article in 1959. Sutter et al., Quelques observations, 908.
120 Bertherand, Médecine et hygiène, 198.
121 Sutter et al., Aspects algériens, 895.
122 Bullard, Truth in Madness, 120.

Drug addicts

Addicts were often regarded as potential criminals by colonial psychiatrists, but deciding whether the addiction was also a sign of insanity was more difficult, especially considering the often very large amounts of alcohol the French population of North Africa drank on a daily basis.[123] Most Muslim men were described as suffering from addictions (mainly to alcohol or hashish, and often to both),[124] but it is difficult to tell in these cases whether drug addiction was the cause, a symptom or actually its own form of insanity. With women, this differentiation was easier. Female drug addicts needed no other symptoms of insanity apart from their addiction itself – their obvious breaking of social norms was sign enough. Not only did they break their own religious laws, they also behaved in a way that was distinctly unwomanly to French observers.[125]

French colonial psychiatrists often mentioned that before the start of colonialism in North Africa in 1830, alcohol, alcoholism and alcohol-related mental diseases were unknown. Kocher wrote in 1883 that North African men – Muslim women were mostly seen as abstinent – had managed to "assimilate the vices" of French civilisation and quickly became addicted to alcohol.[126] Many deplored the advent of alcohol in the indigenous population, who seemed unable to control themselves under its influence, and the psychiatric experts blamed alcohol not only for the strong rise in certain specific organic diseases but also for the rise in both mental problems and general violence. In 1926 Military doctor S. Abbatucci, for example, stated about the situation in all French colonies that "the boost of a toxic, such as *alcohol*, on a primitive brain, triggers immediately sudden and violent impulsive crises."[127] Alcoholism was therefore not only a "trigger" for mental disorders but also for the much-feared innate violence of Muslim men.

---

123 See, for example, Armand, Algérie médicale, 474; Lemanski, Hygiène du colon, 80. On this topic, see also: Studer, Green Fairy in the Maghreb.

124 The propensity of Muslim men towards addictions became a colonial trope. Writing about psychiatry and North Africans without mentioning them was soon impossible, as the psychiatrist Raoul Vadon mentioned humorously in his 1935 dissertation "Medical Assistance of Psychopaths in Tunisia": "Not to speak about kiff or mint tea, in an essay about psychoses in Tunisia, would be a gap that I ought not to leave." Vadon, Assistance, 49. See also: Matignon, Art médical, 88; Reboul/Régis, Assistance, 51; Maréschal, Héroïnomanie, 255. This notion persisted during colonial times and is still present today. See for example Al-Issa's chapter on "Culture and Mental Illness" from the year 1990, republished in 2000: Al-Issa, Culture and Mental Illness, 112.

125 See also: Faradj Khan, Hygiène et islamisme, 57.

126 Kocher, Criminalité, 72.

127 Abbatucci, Assistance, 653. Emphasis in the original.

While there were a number of case studies dedicated to female Muslim alcoholics, none specifically dealt with other addictions. Drug addictions were seen to be so closely connected to Muslim men, so inherently unfeminine, that female Muslim patients were normally excluded from the French psychiatric investigations.[128] Those who did remark upon addictions in Muslim women usually emphasised their rarity.[129] In 1955, for example, Manceaux et al. presented a paper on heroin addiction in Algeria at the Congress in Nice. In it, they stated: "All our patients are men. There is, to our knowledge, only a very small number of prostitutes indulging in heroin in Algiers [...]."[130] This automatic equation of a marginalised group of society with a form of socially unacceptable and potentially morbid behaviour occurred regularly. The first case study of a female Muslim alcoholic to be found in the published source material was the aforementioned "fille soumise" in Meilhon's 1896 article.[131] Whether the woman was really both an alcoholic and a prostitute or whether one was assumed because the other was "found" is impossible to say. The same problem occurs when evaluating another, aforementioned, case study by Taïeb: a former vagrant "fille soumise" had been treated at Blida Psychiatric Hospital after suffering terrifying visions, brought on by the patient's alcoholism.[132] Assicot et al.'s research on the patients at Blida Psychiatric Hospital between 1958 and 1959 also only described one case of female Muslim alcoholism – in a prostitute.[133]

Other case studies on addictions were not concerned with women labelled as prostitutes. Chronologically, the next case study about female patients with alcohol problems after Meilhon's was written by the psychiatrist Levet in 1909 and published in the *Annales Médico-Psychologiques*. A 35-year-old woman from Algiers, who had

---

128 For example, in the 1941 article on "Alcoholism and Mental Troubles in the Indigenous Muslim Algerian" by Maurice Porot and J. Gentile, where they wrote: "The extreme rarity of alcoholism in Muslim women (apart from prostitutes) has made us limit this investigation to only men." Porot, M./Gentile, Alcoolisme et troubles mentaux, 126 f. In 1957 the Moroccan psychiatrist Ahmed Benabud analysed the frequency of hashish addiction in Morocco and justified the neglect of female patients by stating that "the number of observations of female hashish addiction – 15 – is negligible". Benabud, Aspects psychopathologiques, 4.

129 The same was described for the Muslim populations in Egypt. In 1903, for instance, John Warnock stressed the rarity of female Muslim hashish addictions in Egypt. Warnock, Insanity from Hasheesh, 109. See also: Parant, Review of Warnock, 455. Gervais, however, claimed in 1907 that many Muslim women at the asylum in Aix-en-Provence suffered from a "passion for tobacco" and the consequences of tobacco withdrawal once interned in French asylums. Gervais, Contribution, 56 f.

130 Manceaux et al., Héroïnomanie, 294.

131 Meilhon, Aliénation mentale, part 4, 40.

132 Taïeb, Idées d'influence, 92.

133 Assicot et al., Causes principales, 272.

been brought to the asylum in Aix-en-Provence in 1905, was described as an "alcoholic" with "excited periods and hallucinations".[134] Louis Livet wrote in his 1911 dissertation on "Algerian Mad and their Hospitalisation" that out of 21 female mental patients at the Civil Hospital of Mustapha in Algiers only one was an alcoholic – but because of the overall low numbers of female patients, this still amounted to 5%.[135]

In his 1940 dissertation on "General Paralysis in Muslim Natives of Tunisia", Jean Olry wrote about his experiences while working at the Manouba Psychiatric Hospital in Tunis. He described a 40-year-old widow, "a proven alcoholic (wine, spirits, eau de Cologne)" also suffering from "eroticism" and "claiming men [...]".[136] A second female patient he described had been moved to the Manouba Psychiatric Hospital from the French Civil Hospital in 1936. Her family said that "in her history, one can find 'teaism', but no alcoholism".[137] In a third case study, Olry described another widow, whom he categorised with one word: "alcoholic". She was brought to Manouba Hospital and her "neighbours were unanimous in asserting her habits of alcoholism".[138]

The connection between alcoholism and prostitution seemed to have been clear to colonial psychiatrists.[139] Quoting Scherb's 1905 article on "The Rarity of Nervous Accidents in the Muslim Indigenous Algerian", the psychiatrist Georges Sicard wrote in his 1907 dissertation that syphilis was widespread among people living in cities, port workers and prostitutes, all of whom were seen as heavy consumers of alcohol.[140] Louis Livet wrote in his 1911 dissertation that "in Arab women, it [alcoholism] is a vice of almost all prostitutes [...]".[141] The same connection was made as late as 1940 by the psychiatrist André Donnadieu, working at the Berrechid Hospital in Morocco.[142]

---

134 Levet, Assistance, 53.

135 Livet, Aliénés algériens, 66 f.

136 Olry, Paralysie générale, 53.

137 Ibid., 54. "Teaism" was one of the specifically North African diseases that French psychiatrists liked to name and describe. It was thought to be a dangerous addiction, as it affected the work force of the North African populations. On the topic of the colonial medical and psychiatric construct of the particularly Tunisian "addiction to tea", see: Studer, 'Was trinkt der zivilisierte Mensch?'.

138 Olry, Paralysie générale, 55.

139 For example: Donnadieu, Alcoolisme mental, 164; Porot, M./Gentile, Alcoolisme et troubles mentaux, 126 f.

140 Sicard, Étude, 12 f. The same quote is mentioned in the 1919 dissertation by Étienne-Paul Laurens about "Nervous Syphilis in Algeria". Laurens, Contribution, 14.

141 Livet, Aliénés algériens, 66.

142 André Donnadieu suspected in his 1940 article "Mental Alcoholism in the Indigenous Population of Morocco" that "contact with French civilisation" was the reason behind the few cases of female Muslim alcoholics that French psychiatrists observed: "Moroccan women also provide their share [in numbers of alcoholics at the Berrechid hospital], but almost exclusively in the category of prostitutes or domestic servants." Donnadieu, Alcoolisme mental, 164.

Even in postcolonial times, this connection between addictions and prostitution was regularly made. The Moroccan psychiatrist Ahmed Benabud, for example, wrote in a 1957 article in the *Annales Médico-Psychologiques* about the Muslim hashish addicts he treated at the Berrechid Hospital in 1956. He concluded that of 15 female Muslim cases – compared to 1,252 male cases in the same period –, five were prostitutes while three came from the middle classes.[143]

Vagrants

Descriptions of "vagrants"[144] took many different forms and it is difficult to determine what kind of women warranted this classification and for what reasons. One explanation for the low numbers of North African patients in colonial hospitals was that North African families traditionally either kept their insane at home or let them roam the streets as harmless vagrants, who did not need to be interned in the opinion of the Muslim population.[145] Those vagrant females selected to be categorised by the expert opinions of the psychiatrists were the aggressive, the demented and those who behaved in a socially unacceptable way. Consequently, an automatic linking of vagrancy with prostitution and drug addiction occurred very often.

One might also ask whether these women were truly vagrants, homeless and begging in order to survive, or whether there was a cultural misunderstanding behind the French concept of Muslim vagrancy. One can easily imagine women on local pilgrimages, or perhaps Sufi women, who might have been viewed as "holy fools" because of their unorthodox lifestyle, being judged to be home- and friendless by the French colonial authorities, taught that all respectable Muslim women were kept from the view of those who did not belong to their families.

In his 1891 article "General Paralysis in Algeria", Meilhon quoted patient records from E. Battarel, which were sent to Aix-en-Provence with a patient, a 50-year-old woman "without profession [...]." She was "found in a state of vagrancy by the police service" in Algeria and brought to the Asylum in Aix-en-Provence because of her "mania", where she was classified as "dangerous to herself and the people around her".[146] Meilhon also described several cases of female vagrancy in his article on "Mental Alienation in Arabs": one woman was placed under his observation after having been sent to Aix-en-Provence from a city in Kabylia, where she had been arrested by the police in a "state of vagrancy [...]." In the asylum, she was violent, destroying everything she laid her hands on and hitting other patients and the religious sisters who looked after

---

143 Benabud, Aspects psychopathologiques, 8.
144 The French terms range from "mendiante" to "vagabonde".
145 Desruelles/Bersot, Assistance aux aliénés en Algérie, 581; 593.
146 Meilhon, Contribution, 391.

them.[147] Another case study was concerned with a woman, described by Meilhon as a 30-year-old "beggar", who was admitted to the asylum in Aix-en-Provence in 1887. Even though he described her as "docile" in her state of vagrancy, he reported that she suffered from aggressive moments in France: "Agitated, she is malicious, angry, hits her neighbours, rips apart and breaks everything she can reach [...]."[148]

Jean Sutter wrote about the case of a 20-year-old vagrant, suffering from epilepsy, who had thrown a stone at a child "without motive" and attacked the passers-by who had wished to intervene. "A policeman arrived at this moment and took her with him to the Commissariat, where they found out that she was a woman who had formerly worked as a domestic servant, but who, without employment for several months, had been begging in the quarter where she had been arrested and where she was considered as simple minded."[149]

Suzanne Taïeb wrote about the case of a 36-year-old vagrant – an "ancienne fille soumise" (former prostitute) – who was arrested in Bel-Abbès, "where she looked for trouble with passers-by in the street, causing a scandal in public; she became menacing and she exposed herself." She also suffered from "terrifying visions" because of her alcohol addiction. Asked about her "mode of existence", she admitted to having lived off begging but denied ever having been an alcoholic.[150] Another vagrancy case Taïeb described concerned a female general paralytic. She was "found on the public street" and brought to a general hospital, where she "became agitated, took her clothes off, scratched her face, and became dangerous to other patients."[151] Taïeb also wrote about a 40-year-old Moroccan woman at Blida Psychiatric Hospital, who seemed to have been a vagrant and was picked up by the police because she tried to dig up bodies, saying "she was happy to see the corpses discovered by digging in the cemeteries [...]."[152]

Demented vagrants were often interned for indecency because they took their clothes off in public. The naked female lunatic, freely roaming the streets of North African cities, seems to have been a colonial anecdote, almost from the very beginning of French colonialism. The military doctor Adolphe Armand, for instance, wrote in his 1854 book "Medical Algeria": "[...] it is not uncommon to find in the cities or in the ksours [settlements in the countryside] the insane in the most absolute poverty, and sometimes without any clothing. At Constantine, 'madmen and idiots met in the streets, among other things, I saw two women, said Mr Deleau, one of sixteen to

---

147 Ibid., Aliénation mentale, part 2, 198 f.
148 Ibid., part 3, 370 f.
149 Sutter, Épilepsie mentale, 151 f. Emphasis in the original.
150 Taïeb, Idées d'influence, 92.
151 Ibid., 122.
152 Ibid., 117 f.

seventeen years, walking absolutely naked.'"[153] Armand further claimed to have personally seen one of these naked madwomen in Taouila, a small town in the Algerian
Sahara.[154] In his 1926 book on "Ritual and Belief in Morocco", the Finnish ethnologist Edward Westermarck also mentioned having personally witnessed a naked mad-
woman: "The saintly lunatic is not held responsible for any absurdity he commits.
During my first stay in Fez there was an insane woman who used to walk about in
a state of perfect nudity; and when I visited the same town again, after an interval
of nearly twelve years, she was still alive and continued her old habit."[155] Other such
cases of Muslim women being brought to the psychiatric attention by their willing-
ness to shed their clothes can be found in the psychiatric texts themselves. Jean Sutter,
for example, writing about the cases brought to the University Hospital in Algiers
in 1937, mentioned a 28-year-old woman, interned for public indecency. The police
"arrested in the street a Moorish woman completely naked, who gesticulated, cried
and hit passers-by". They brought her to the commissariat of police, where it was
decided to have her interned.[156]

This nakedness was shocking to the colonial observers, not only because it hurt
their own social sensibilities but also because it did not correspond to their notions
of how the North African societies worked. One of the most repeated and well-
known facts about Muslim female normality in French texts was the veil; therefore,
these women broke one of the most important rules among the perceived Muslim
customs – the hiding of femininity.

Often mentioned were cases of women not arrested for running naked in the
streets, but who insisted on being naked in the asylums. Meilhon wrote in 1896 that
a female patient "absolutely wanted to stay naked" and "ripped apart all clothing, no
matter whether European or indigenous [...]."[157] Sutter wrote in his 1937 dissertation
about four female epileptic patients, whose nakedness seemed to be part of their disease. In the first case, Sutter described a woman brought to the hospital because she
attacked a passer-by. She was described as "ripping apart her clothing" and sitting
"all naked in her cell [...]."[158] The second patient, openly described as a vagrant, was
"probably found 'ill on a public street'" – and one might ask whether Sutter's term
"voie publique" was a euphemism for a brothel. This woman tried to flee the hospital
"all naked [...]."[159] The third case study concerned a Moorish woman who tried to run

---

153 Armand, Algérie Médicale, 445.
154 Ibid., 446.
155 Westermarck, Ritual and Belief, Vol. 1, 48.
156 Sutter, Épilepsie mentale, 148.
157 Meilhon, Aliénation mentale, part 3, 367.
158 Sutter, Épilepsie mentale, 153 f.
159 Ibid., 155.

away from her parents "entirely naked", and when they tried to bring her back, she tried to scratch and hit everybody, so that they had to tie her down.[160] The fourth case occurred in Oran and was treated by a Dr Camatte – a murder case, in which the perpetrator was a young girl who, for seven months before her crime, had suffered from epileptic crises, in which she stripped naked and ripped her clothes apart.[161]

2.6.3 Judicial Placement

Psychiatrists were, as already mentioned, the officially accepted experts in judging the responsibility of criminals and were mostly asked for their official reports in murder cases. In 1932 Antoine Porot and Don Côme Arrii claimed that murder and attempted murder cases made up 90% of medico-legal reports: "At first sight, the considerable proportion of attacks [...] is striking, in the judicial statistics, and we can say that nine-tenths of [cases of] expertise [on] natives assigned to overseas psychiatrists relate to murders or attempted murders. The native plays with the baton, the knife or with guns with an ease, a quickness and savagery, which most often cause death. These are, very often, close relatives, father, mother, brother, and especially wife, who are beaten and, in a certain number of cases, there are several victims of the impulsive fury of the murderer."[162] In this passage, Porot and Arrii established the frequency of these violent crimes and repeated the clearly gendered imagery belonging to the roles of perpetrator and victim.

Regarding female Muslim perpetrators, their responsibility was usually questioned in cases of the suspected murder of husbands or of illegitimate newborn children.[163] Most often, a verdict of "responsibility", i. e. of psychiatric "normality", was given, but the psychiatrists argued that the hard life Muslim women led, as nothing more than "beasts of burden" and "instruments of pleasure", limited their responsibility, and even normal Muslim women could not be held completely responsible for their actions. One illustration of this can be found in 1883, when Kocher looked at seven cases of murder by poison, all of them committed by women. While the women were all deemed responsible for their actions, i. e. not insane, the sense of them not being completely responsible is tangible in Kocher's dissertation: "All of these poisonings have been committed by women, against a single person, their husband, be it through jealousy,

---

160 Ibid., 198 f.
161 Ibid., 206.
162 Porot/Arrii, Impulsivité criminelle, 589.
163 In Islamic law, there was no place for illegitimate children – they had no status, they did not exist. Unmarried women therefore often felt they had no choice but to take drastic measures in order to prevent repudiation by their families. Bousquet, Morale, 62.

or to save themselves from ill treatment, or through the instigation of a lover."[164] For all three motives, Kocher diagnosed a certain lack of responsibility in female poisoners, arguing that female jealousy was only natural in an environment dominated by polygamy and by the simplicity of getting a divorce; that Muslim women, since they were continually suppressed by their husbands, were prone to take drastic action; and that, though it was morally reprehensible to have a lover, the responsibility for the murder surely rested with the instigator, not with the woman who had been pushed to extremes.

One of the most detailed case studies about a female Muslim patient concerned a woman accused of infanticide, as reported by Don Côme Arrii in his 1926 dissertation, which he based on notes taken by Antoine Porot. He stated that on the 15th of January 1925 "the cadaver of an infant, born at term" was found, "who had been breathing and who carried clear signs of strangulation". The inquest found a 20-year-old woman, living just 200 metres from where the body was found, who had given birth two or three days before. She confessed, but accused a neighbour, "an old man", of having raped her and said that his wife, who had helped her with the birth, had taken the child with her. In prison, she showed signs of "rather tumultuous nervous disorders" and a "mental assessment" was ordered, which Antoine Porot gave in court.[165] Once in prison, overwhelmed by the internment, she had what Porot called a "crisis of maniac excitation", with manifestations of hysteria, where she hit and "even bit" other inmates.[166] "She screamed, sang [...]; she demanded men be brought to her, she took her clothes off, threw herself on the floor, writhed, with haggard eyes, or indulged in obscene gestures [...]. At other times she fell into a lethargic attack, pretended to be dead, threw the people around her into a panic, and, at the moment when they approached her, jumped at the throats of her neighbours."[167]

She only calmed down once her parents had been to see her, bringing Porot to the conclusion: "Still, she does not seem unintelligent to us, she does not have the facial expression of an idiot. There is, in her silence, more reluctance than incapacity to answer and we do not think that her intellectual level is much lower than that of the subjects of her race, her age and her condition."[168] But she was not insane, for Porot concluded that "she was not in a state of dementia at the moment she committed the crime of infanticide, [which] she is accused of. But she presents a light

---

164 Kocher, Criminalité, 126.

165 Arrii, Impulsivité criminelle, 84.

166 Biting people was, as Meilhon assured his readers in his 1896 article, a widespread characteristic of alienated Arabs. Meilhon, Aliénation mentale, part 2, 196.

167 Arrii, Impulsivité criminelle, 85.

168 Ibid., 86.

degree of mental debility and of hysteric imbalance, likely to attenuate her responsibility slightly."[169]

Another medico-legal court report was written by Jean Sutter in 1937, concerning an epileptic woman accused of having murdered another woman by cutting her throat.[170] The victim died in hospital a few days after the attack, having told a judge who had attacked her.[171] Accused of homicide, the woman accused her mother of having been the perpetrator before finally confessing,[172] but she demanded "indulgence" for herself, saying "she did not know what she was doing [...]."[173] The girl was finally brought to the University Hospital in Algiers, where Sutter himself examined her. He concluded that she was an epileptic with strong epileptic impulsions, characterised partly by her violent attacks on people around her. The young woman "did not always fully enjoy her mental faculties; her responsibility is inexistent regarding the crime she is charged with, because, in the absence of witnesses, it [the crime] seems to have been committed after a crisis or the equivalent of an epileptic attack [...]."[174] In his opinion, the murder had been committed while the young woman was in either an epileptic crisis or following a post-epileptic impulsion – which seems bizarre, considering she probably took the murder weapon, a razor, with her while showing the victim around. However, Sutter also said that the accused, "through her violent actions, is capable of compromising public security; she is therefore dangerous. We estimate that it would be best to place her in an establishment for the alienated and to leave her there, locked up until the day her mental state appears sufficiently healed to suppress the dangers which she poses at the moment."[175]

2.6.4 Exceptions

In addition to these three official mechanisms of admission, for which the patients' consent was not needed, there were also other ways and reasons for women to be treated by French psychiatrists. One of them was the aforementioned concept of "voluntary admission" or "free entrances", requested not by the family but by the patient. This only happened from the 1940s onwards and only seems to have occurred with middle

---

169 Ibid., 87.
170 The medico-legal report upon which he based this case study was by a Dr Camatte from the psychiatric service of the Civil Hospital in Oran.
171 Sutter, Épilepsie mentale, 204.
172 Ibid., 205.
173 Ibid., 206.
174 Ibid., 208.
175 Ibid., 208 f.

class women.[176] Another means of entrance entailed some patients being brought to mental hospitals from other hospitals, to which they had previously been admitted for physical problems only. Once in the hospital, doctors sometimes detected mental problems, which made their relegation to a psychiatric asylum necessary. Antoine Porot, quoting article 6 of the instructions from the Governor-General of Algeria at the time, Carde, from the 10th of August 1934, mentioned that all sick people who "accidentally presented mental troubles" should be brought to the psychiatric hospitals.[177]

There were also individual cases which did not fit into any of the sanctioned patterns of admission. One example concerned a young Muslim woman that Antoine Porot had met in 1912 in Tunis, and whom he brought to his hospital, which at that time was reserved for European patients, the French Civil Hospital.[178] This woman was the only Muslim patient there, and would remain the only Muslim patient in a French psychiatric hospital in North Africa until the building of the first asylum on North African soil some 20 years later. In this case, the motive for the impromptu institutionalisation was pity for an individual who was seen as a victim, without any criminalisation implied – if anything, Muslim society was criticised for not offering other possibilities for compassionate care in such cases.

2.7 Criticisms of Admissions

In the processes of institutionalising Muslim psychiatric patients, the focus clearly lay on security and order. Those patients interned were perceived to threaten both the safety and the decorum of the French settler societies in North Africa. This resulted in a selection that, administratively speaking, excluded more easily controlled, more easily "mastered" potential patients, like the allegedly meek Muslim women.[179] L. Couderc, for example, lamented in 1961 that "there is a paradoxical selection of admission: calm patients, women, who are often easier to keep at home, rarely benefit from priority of admission; relatively older patients, who seem less dangerous, are often systematically dismissed from the mental hospitals."[180] Instead of admitting governable and curable

---

176 It seems that this rise coincided with the establishment of asylums on North African soil. The fact that the patients were no longer brought to another country, away from their friends and families, seems to have attracted a certain clientele of voluntary patients. However, among the published case studies, no voluntary admissions of female Muslim patients can be found.

177 Carde, Jules Gaston Henri, Instruction, Article 6. As quoted in: Porot, Services hospitaliers, 798.

178 Ibid., Tunisie, 58.

179 See also: Meilhon, Aliénation mentale, part 1, 25.

180 Couderc, Conséquences, 254.

patients, the mechanisms of admission favoured the most challenging group among the colonised populations – dangerous young men, who were seen to pose difficulties to both the budget and the security of the psychiatric institutions.

While all male North Africans were frequently criminalised in the psychiatric writings of the time, the same theories stressed that Muslim women, with their passive femininity and lack of agency, could not be criminals. Nominally, therefore, nothing pointed to a definition or classification of female Muslim mental patients as criminals, but, as shown, the selection of female patients – which was not based on medical criteria but on those of public order and prevention of crime – caused exactly such a criminalisation, which explains why so few women were voluntarily brought to the attention of French psychiatrists. Paradoxically, French psychiatrists were convinced that Muslim women could not be de facto criminals, but the end result of the patient selection was that most of their institutionalised female patients *were* criminalised to some degree. Through their lack of awareness, colonial psychiatrists failed to notice that this criminalisation deterred Muslim women and their families from contacting them and requesting their help in cases of mental disorders.

However, colonial psychiatrists criticised these different mechanisms of admission on several levels. The most general complaint, voiced by Antoine Porot in 1943 for example, was that voluntary admissions were rare and that "administrative placements" were "applied often with excessive rigour [...]."[181] Others claimed that the neglect of voluntary treatment, in favour of internment by official institutions, falsified their colonial accounts. The abundance of violent Muslim patients, for instance, noticed by so many of the psychiatrists responsible for colonial patients in France, was explained by Abel-Joseph Meilhon in 1896 in terms of this skewed selection mechanism, as the administration was only contacted after potential patients had already committed a violent act. Meilhon concluded that this specific selection, caused by the focus on security, made "the alienated Arab in general seem so dangerous to us [...]."[182] Though emphasised by Meilhon in his important text for French colonial psychiatry, the selection of Muslim patients remained highly problematic during the colonial period. Almost 50 years later, Charles Bardenat still insisted that "in hospital statistics, the proportion of dangerous patients tends to seem stronger, relatively, among the natives."[183]

However, by far the biggest criticism of the admission mechanisms was the question of who possessed the authority to decide on admission into colonial psychiatric care. Meilhon, for instance, claimed in 1896 that Muslim patients could be admitted to a psychiatric institution after "scenes of violence" "on the grounds of a simple

---

181 Porot, Œuvre psychiatrique, 362.
182 Meilhon, Aliénation mentale, part 2, 178.
183 Bardenat, Criminalité, 319.

police report" – without the involvement of a psychiatric expert.[184] This outrage at their profession being sidestepped by other groups endowed with colonial authority can be found in many other texts. Bouquet, for example, wrote in 1909 that "the arbitrariness of the police, the goodwill of a doctor who possessed no special power alone regulated the question of admissions and releases."[185] While Bouquet's concern was generally directed at the wellbeing of patients and the involvement of non-experts in the processes of psychiatric selection, other psychiatrists were more specific in their attacks. In the same year, Levet stressed that the general nature of the terminology of disorders in the patient records, delivered with the patients shipped to Aix-en-Provence from the Civil Hospital of Mustapha in Algiers, proved that the initial diagnosis could not have been conducted by specialists. He smugly stated that "this formulation indicates clearly a doctor foreign to mental pathology."[186] Clearly, in the eyes of many colonial psychiatrists, this involvement of non-experts was to blame for the one-sided selection of patients.

Finally, a third, more general cluster of criticism focused on the idea that the system of admission in North Africa was hopelessly outdated and that French colonial psychiatrists were therefore prevented from working to the best of their abilities by unprofessional regulations. This criticism is expressed in the following quote by Henri Aubin, taken from his paper on the "Native Psychiatric Assistance in the Colonies" at the 1938 Algiers Congress: "Thus, in Algeria, an outdated text demands, for the internment of a patient in Blida [...], a report by the Police Commissioner, supported by the written statements of witnesses; practically, these [witnesses] are the nurses of the Service... who thus control their own head of service."[187] Aubin therefore objected to the "outdated" restriction on psychiatric authority in the mechanisms of institutionalisation by those most directly involved in the everyday treatment of patients.

Psychiatrists strongly disagreed with the system of admission in place in colonial North Africa, mainly because it interfered with their efforts to compile objective statistics and because their professional expertise and authority was seemingly not valued enough. The stigmatisation of institutionalised female Muslim patients, however, remained unnoticed.

If Muslim women were admitted because of complaints from their families or neighbours, they were classified as dangerous. They had usually physically attacked family members or neighbours and often uttered death threats, which the colonial authorities took very seriously, not least because this contrasted so deeply with their picture of normal Muslim femininity. If they were questioned by the police and

---

184 Meilhon, Aliénation mentale, part 1, 28 f. See also: Woytt-Gisclard, Assistance, 165 f.
185 Bouquet, Aliénés en Tunisie, 46.
186 Levet, Assistance, 55.
187 Aubin, Assistance, 174. Capitalisation in the original.

escorted to a hospital, they were almost always defined as vagrants, addicts or prostitutes. This over-zealous reaction to prescribe a criminalising classification to women in asylums compounded the stigma of the involvement of the police, who were often called in because of physical violence committed on the streets. Due to the criminalisation of the "administrative placement" – which meant being arrested for violence or indecency in a public place, picked up by the police and classified as immoral –, the stigmatisation caused by colonial psychiatry could hardly have been greater. Finally, if Muslim women came to the attention of French psychiatrists through court cases, it was mostly as soon-to-be-condemned murderers.

The mechanisms for admission into colonial psychiatric care did not reflect an unaugmented desire to care for patients or to cure a mental disease, but rather official condemnation. Muslim families had realised that only women recognised as too dangerous or immoral for the supervision of their own families would be admitted into colonial care.[188] Indeed, the admission processes seemed to almost eliminate all placements for purely medical reasons, while those women who were admitted were stigmatised for life, even if they had been admitted for other reasons, as shown by the criminalisation of possibly harmless vagrants. No family, if they could help it, would therefore seek to have their female family members admitted to the charge of colonial psychiatry.[189] With male patients, the situation was slightly different; North African men were already criminalised as a whole and could not be stigmatised much further by the additional criminalisation of admission processes. Men also had other ways of being admitted to colonial care, for example because of the complaints of employers.

Arguably, French psychiatrists used this criminalisation of Muslim female patients through the admission processes as a means of determining which of the Muslim women they encountered were sane or insane. As discussed in Chapter 1, it was difficult for French psychiatrists to differentiate between normality and abnormality due to the strangeness that normal Muslim women embodied for them. The conclusions drawn from their experiences with female Muslim patients did not change their picture of female normality – they still maintained the idea that no Muslim woman was violent or criminal. Even without acknowledging it, their experiences with often

---

188 This contrasted not only with colonial notions of femininity but also with Muslim ideals of what women should or should not be.

189 The psychiatrist Pierre Maréschal wrote in 1956, summarising his twenty years of practical experience in Tunisia: "Afraid of what people would say, for fear of the stigma that plagues the insane and prevents girls of the family from marrying [...], the insane are not directed to our consultations at the beginning of their illness." Maréschal, Réflexions, 69. As already mentioned, this stigmatisation by psychiatry has also been noted in Arab countries in postcolonial contexts, especially in ruining marriage prospects for Muslim women. For example: Al-Issa/Al-Issa, Psychiatric Problems, 21; Al-Krenawi et al., Ethnic and Gender Differences, 48.

very violent Muslim women in the psychiatric asylums and institutions reinforced those differences between normality and abnormality. With only the female Muslim "insane" being able to react in an aggressive, immoral or even criminal way, it was much easier to determine who was insane and who was not. "Normal" Muslim women were, as described above, "de-criminalised" as far as possible. Consequently, the contrast between this construct of "normality" and the institutionalised patients must have been overwhelming.

Chapter 3
The Visible Patient: Categorising Deviance

3.1 Case Study on Patient Transit through the Psychiatric System

The psychiatrist Pierre Battarel published three case studies on female Muslim patients in his 1902 dissertation on general paralysis at the Civil Hospital of Mustapha in Algiers, in comparison to 21 case studies on Muslim men. One of these three case studies concerned a 27-year-old Algerian woman, who had been sent to the hospital in Algiers on the 26th of April 1895. According to Battarel, this patient, who had both an Arabic and a French first name, suffered from a combination of general paralysis, megalomania and alcoholism.[1] At the hospital, Battarel described her as follows: "The causes for the disease are unknown; there is no information on [her] heredity. This is the first attack [of her disorders] observed. This patient, orphaned in the famine of 1867, was brought up by Cardinal Lavigerie [Charles Martial Lavigerie; archbishop of Algiers from from 1876 onwards]. Her delusions continued [at the hospital]. She has ideas of grandeur, wealth; she married, she said, the King of Annam; one of her sons is called Jesus Christ, she does not know the [name of the] other, but it is also a 'Great'; she offers rewards in cash to all who may come. The patient had been docile up to that day. Her general condition is good. She has been evacuated to the Asylum for the insane in Aix, on the 15th of May 1895. We should note, with regards to this observation, that almost all indigenous women gathered by the Cardinal Lavigerie are syphilitic or tubercular, often alcoholics. A visit to the Hospital of Saint-Cyprien des Attafs [founded by Lavigerie to care for his orphanages] confirms this suspicion."[2]

The story of this patient's journey from Algeria to France is remarkable for three reasons: first, Battarel's case study conveys an idea of how quickly some patients were shipped to France, which gives context to the general information about patient transfers detailed in this chapter. In the course of only 20 days, this patient travelled from the provinces to Algiers, was psychiatrically examined and finally sent on to Aix-en-Provence. Especially in the light of this being her first "attack", this seems like a swift and also rather drastic measure, considering how unlikely it was for North Africans to ever be released from the asylums in France.[3] Secondly, Battarel must have had a lot

---

1 Battarel, Quelques remarques, 63.
2 Ibid., 64. Capitalisation in the original.
3 See Chapter 3.3.1 on "Chances of Death".

more information about this patient than the colonial psychiatrists usually possessed. Even though her parentage was unknown, as she had been orphaned in 1867, and even though Battarel could not, for that reason, establish whether there had been psychiatric precedents in the family, she still had been in colonial care for practically her whole life.[4] Yet despite this supposed wealth of patient information, Battarel's case study remained very concise, with very little said about both the patient herself and, surprisingly, her myriad of diagnoses. Battarel's brevity can be explained by the third point of interest in this case study: he portrayed a female patient who had very obviously been influenced – negatively – by France's *mission civilisatrice*, as shown by her French first name, the fact that she had been brought up in a Catholic orphanage and her claim of having a son called Jesus Christ. As such, the case study shows an uncertainty as to the moral benefits of this direct contact of France's civilisation with Muslim women. The last paragraph of the case study, Battarel's side remark on the state of Lavigerie's orphanages, seems to show the real reason behind him choosing to publish this particular case study: he claimed that all the orphans under Cardinal Lavigerie's care suffered from syphilis, tuberculosis or alcoholism, at least two of these diseases being firmly connected with (European) vices in the minds of contemporary medical observers. Whether Battarel meant to criticise only the state of the Catholic missions or France's general attempts to civilise Muslim women cannot be determined.

3.2 Counting Muslim Patients

This chapter examines the numbers of female Muslim patients in colonial care, over time and in specific asylums and psychiatric hospitals, and tries to numerically contextualise the claim of French colonial psychiatrists that Muslim women almost never developed mental disorders. This chapter gives a basis for the understanding of both case studies on female Muslim patients and psychiatric theories on normal and abnormal Muslim women by providing the historical context (i.e. patient numbers in France and North Africa, death rates and distribution of diseases) available in the source material. The numbers of female Muslim patients will be compared with the corresponding numbers of Muslim men and European women.[5] More specifically, it

---

4 At the time of her "attack", however, she appears to have been no longer at the orphanage, as her occupation was given as servant.

5 The differentiation between asylums and psychiatric institutions has been adopted from the sources. Antoine Porot argued in 1933 that the old designation of "asylum for the alienated" was outdated, and that it gave the wrong impression with its focus on sequestrating dangerous individuals. He therefore preferred, as did his students, the term "psychiatric hospital". Porot, Assistance psychiatrique, 87.

will be asked whether the neglect of Muslim women in the written sources was justified by the absence of female Muslim patients in the colonial institutions. Was there a correlation between the actual numbers of patients and the relative importance (or unimportance) attributed to them in the colonial writings? What does the statistical evidence say about the prognoses and diagnoses of female Muslim patients and does this data support psychiatric theories?

As a first step, the numbers of Muslim patients in colonial institutions will be analysed, and the ratios of Muslim patients will be compared with those of European patients. Secondly, the percentages of female Muslim patients in both disease categories and death rates will be examined and compared with their overall ratios. Finally, the medium of French colonial statistics, both statistical findings and the way they were used, will be looked at.

It should be added that statistics were not a common tool in French colonial psychiatry. It is therefore rare to find statistical information composed by the author of a psychiatric article. Many sources did not give even the basic numbers one might expect – hospital population, recovery rates, percentages of the individual diseases and the like. Of the statistics that do exist, many lack important information such as gender, age or, in the colonial context, "race". French psychiatrists did not compile official annual reports – unlike their British counterparts in Egypt, for example – about the statistical situation of North African mental patients in France and North Africa. Some articles vaguely refer to the existence of government statistics on asylum populations,[6] which covered the numbers of patients transferred to France from Algeria, but these numbers, provided by the annual reports of the Algerian departments, were not used by colonial psychiatrists, who preferred statistics compiled by themselves or by other, preferably prominent, psychiatrists.[7]

The only official organisation which tried to compile comprehensive statistics was the aforementioned annual *Congrès des Médecins Aliénistes et Neurologistes de France et des Pays de Langue Française*. However, it was only during the 1912 meeting in Tunis, the 1933 meeting in Rabat and the 1938 meeting in Algiers that the participating psychiatrists and neurologists focused their energy on North Africa. Further, only the 1912 Congress collected statistical evidence, and these "eloquent statistics",[8] composed by Henry Reboul and Emmanuel Régis, represent the most complete statistical evidence for the entire period. An analysis of the numerical evidence made available in the published sources reveals that they are too haphazard, too irregular and too infrequent to come

---

6   See for instance: Livet, Aliénés algériens, 34.

7   Furthermore, there are very few statistics on Tunisia or Morocco. The majority of the colonial statistical evidence focuses on Algeria, and was, just like the theoretical evidence, sometimes applied to Tunisia and Morocco.

8   Desruelles/Bersot, Note sur l'histoire, 313.

even remotely close to reflecting reality accurately. Therefore, the statistical evidence is a source material that must be studied carefully as part of the colonial discourse, the scarcity and partiality of this evidence being as significant as the numbers themselves.

3.2.1   Transported to France

Between 1845 and the 1930s several French asylums had contracts for the transfer and care of colonial psychiatric patients. Tunisia had one contract with the Saint-Pierre hospital in Marseille, which covered a total of 13 French patients annually,[9] while Morocco had no such contracts.[10] Antoine Porot, in his paper for the 1912 Congress report, further qualified the number of Tunisian patients in France by saying that, while these places were provided for the French destitute, there were "always two or three Jewish Tunisians" among those patients,[11] but, he added, "in no case" were Muslim Tunisians sent to France.[12] Therefore the Muslim patients from Tunisia and all patients from Morocco were kept either in general hospitals, thus occupying beds needed for physically sick patients, or in traditional Islamic asylums, the so called *mâristâns*, which were, as mentioned in Chapter 2, banished from Algeria.[13]

With Moroccans and Tunisians contractually excluded, only Algerian Muslims were treated in the asylums of the *Métropole*. Several French asylums had unrestricted contracts with the Algerian departments. In 1908, for example, the department of Algiers had contracts with the asylums of Montperrin (in Aix-en-Provence) and Pierrefeu (close

---

9   Porot, Tunisie, 69. Apparently, Italians suffering from mental disorders were shipped to Italy from Tunisia. Mignot, Journées médicales, 162.

10 Naudin, Psychiatrie coloniale, 20. This is something that most colonial sources agreed on, but Jules Colombani, Director of Public Health and Hygiene in Morocco, stated at the 1933 Congress in Rabat that "up to now, it [Berrechid Hospital] sufficed for the most urgent needs; for years now, Morocco has not evacuated the insane to the Establishments of the métropole." Charpentier, Comptes Rendus, 56. Capitalisation in the original. Similarly, Lwoff and Sérieux, in their 1911 report on the psychiatric situation in Morocco, alluded to the fact that French patients had been regularly shipped to Marseille before the beginning of the French protectorate. Lwoff/Sérieux, Aliénés au Maroc, 477.

11 Porot, Tunisie, 69. See also: Mignot, Journées médicales, 162.

12 Porot, Tunisie, 70. In 1935, the French psychiatrist Raoul Vadon wrote in his dissertation on the "Medical Assistance of Psychopaths in Tunisia" that, before the construction of the Manouba Mental Hospital, about 150 Tunisian patients were looked after in the French asylums. It is unclear whether he meant Europeans shipped to France from Tunisia or Muslim Tunisians living in France. Vadon, Assistance, 43.

13 See p. 82, FN 73. Traditional *mâristâns* had existed in Algeria before the French conquest. Linas, Aliénés en Algérie, 492; Bouquet, Aliénés en Tunisie, 88; Livet, Aliénés algériens, 13 f.; Reboul/Régis, Assistance, 35; Desruelles/Bersot, Assistance aux aliénés en Algérie, 580.

to Nice); the department of Oran had contracts with asylums in Limoux (close to Carcassonne) and Saint-Alban (in the department of Lozère); and the department of Constantine had a contract with the asylum of Saint-Pons (close to Nice).[14] Despite this variety of contracts, it was never a question of transporting all Algerian Muslims with mental problems to France, though some psychiatrists assumed just that.[15] Instead, only the most desperate cases,[16] the "bare minimum of internable patients", as the psychiatrists Reboul and Régis regretted in their 1912 Congress report, were shipped to France.[17] The transport of all Muslim patients would have been prohibitively expensive,[18] so colonial psychiatrists focused on deporting the undeniably mad and violent, who would otherwise have been a danger or nuisance to French settlers in Algeria, as discussed in Chapter 2.[19]

In 1939, the psychiatrists Maurice Desruelles and Henri Bersot summarised some of the statistics available in a report entitled "The Assistance of the Alienated in Algeria since the 19th Century". They stated that between 1852 and 1882, 905 transfers were carried out,[20] which amounted to about 30 patients per year. Desruelles and Bersot also quoted from the 1912 collection of articles, edited by the psychiatrist Auguste Marie,[21] who in turn quoted two older texts. Marie's first source was Trolard,[22] who

---

14 Desruelles/Bersot, Assistance aux aliénés en Algérie, 586. The different contracts are also summarised in: Berthelier, Homme maghrébin, 28.

15 Meilhon, for example, thought that his statistical evidence on the rarity of insanity among Muslims, based on an analysis of patients in Aix-en-Provence, represented the whole department of Algiers. Meilhon, Aliénation mentale, part 6, 361.

16 Delasiauve, Review of Collardot, 118; Battarel, Aliénés, 245.

17 Reboul/Régis, Assistance, 49 f. This point was also raised by Richard Keller in his 2007 book, where he mentioned that most of the Muslim patients shipped to France were recidivists, who posed "extreme social danger" to society. Keller, Colonial Madness, 86.

18 Even transporting only a fraction of all cases of Algerian insanity was very expensive and heavily criticised. Lunier, Review of Les aliénés en Algérie, 160; Levet, Assistance, 248.

19 This obviously had an impact on colonial presumptions about North Africans, but also on the statistics of the French asylums: among the Muslim patients in Aix-en-Provence that Meilhon analysed in 1896, 51.22% were aggressive or violent. Meilhon, Aliénation mentale, part 2, 177 f. The role colonial psychiatry played in gathering and controlling dangerous elements of North African society has already been discussed in Chapter 2.

20 Desruelles/Bersot, Assistance aux aliénés en Algérie, 581. This number was also quoted in reports from the 1860s, but regarding transportation for the period of 1852 to 1862 – an average of 90 patients per year. Delasiauve, Review of Collardot, 117 f.; Jobert, Projet, 16. Desruelles and Bersot presumably mistyped the years.

21 Marie, Traité international, 614. The same information, even the same phrasing, can also be found in Marie's 1905 and Margain's 1908 article. Marie, Sur quelques aspects, 766; Margain, Aliénation mentale, 88 f.

22 No references were given, but presumably, Desruelles and Bersot meant Jean Baptiste Paulin Trolard, a prominent professor of anatomy in Algiers. See Loukas et al., Jean Baptiste Paulin

claimed that Algeria, between the years 1884 and 1893, annually sent an average of 139 mental patients to France.[23] The second source was an unspecified text by Moreau,[24] according to which an average of 160 patients were annually shipped from the three Algerian departments to France between 1896 and 1904.[25]

This compilatory effort provided some hard data but also revealed a rather inefficient handling of statistics. The numbers Desruelles and Bersot collected were vague, and they did not quote original sources (i. e. Trolard and Moreau) but relied instead on a more recent and thus accessible psychiatrist quoting them. Moreover, there is no sense of critically looking at the numbers presented, demonstrated through their use of another detail from Marie's "International Treatise", who in turn quoted a paper given by Collardot in 1864.[26] Collardot apparently gave an account of 90 patients, Europeans and Muslims, transferred to France in 1862,[27] when on average, according to Desruelles and Bersot, only 30 patients were shipped to France annually.[28]

These figures for annual patient admissions, vague and contradictory as they are, may seem negligible, but they were important to the French asylums. The numbers of patients forced on the journey across the Mediterranean overwhelmed the French asylums of the Midi. In 1905, for instance, the admission of these colonial patients made up 32.79% of new patients in Aix-en-Provence, and 26.92% in 1906[29] – and many of these patients stayed in French asylums until their deaths. This steady accumulation of patients was another consequence of admitting only grave cases to the general hospitals in Algeria – the chronically ill, the recidivists and the criminally insane –, who stood small hope of ever being released. French asylums became a storeroom – and, ultimately, a cemetery – for the psychiatrically hopeless.

Though there are few concrete numbers, it is clear that the volume of patients shipped from Algeria constantly rose. The 1912 Congress report by Reboul and Régis declared that in 1874 260 and in 1883 500 colonial patients were looked after in French

---

    Trolard (1842–1910).

23 Desruelles/Bersot, Assistance aux aliénés en Algérie, 583.

24 Again, no references were given. It could not have been Jacques-Joseph Moreau de Tours, who died in 1884, but perhaps his son Paul, also a well-respected psychiatrist, who died in 1908. Morel, Dictionnaire, 179 f.

25 Desruelles/Bersot, Assistance aux aliénés en Algérie, 585.

26 This paper, given at the Société Médicale d'Algérie in 1864, has been untraceable, but a review of it was published in the Journal de Médecine Mentale in 1865. See: Delasiauve, Review of Collardot.

27 Desruelles/Bersot, Assistance aux aliénés en Algérie, 583.

28 Ibid., 581. As mentioned, this figure of 30 patients annually relied on a typing mistake. See also p. 109, FN 20.

29 Levet, Assistance, 48. Very few colonial psychiatrists gave the numbers in percentages. To aid comparison, the numbers have been expressed as percentages in this chapter.

asylums. In 1885 there were already 610, in 1895 800, and in 1903 948[30] – an overall increase of 264.62% between 1874 and 1903. The French psychiatrist Livet claimed that in 1909 there were already 1,224 colonial patients in French asylums, 276 more than six years earlier.[31] Compared with the initial number of 260 patients for the year 1874, this amounted to an increase of 370.77%.

After 1909, no precise numbers covering all colonial patients in France could be found in the published source material, which implies it was only of secondary importance to the colonial psychiatrists.[32] Alexandre Lasnet and Antoine Porot stated in 1932 that over 1,400 colonial patients were institutionalised in the French asylums.[33] At the 1933 Congress in Rabat, Sasportas, the official delegate of the Algerian Government, commented that there were 1,500 colonial patients currently in the asylums of the *Métropole*, with an average of 400 new admissions annually.[34] Eliane Demassieux, who wrote her dissertation on "Social Service in Psychiatry" at the University of Algiers in 1941, mentioned that "merely ten years ago [i.e. in the early 1930s], the Algerian mad, after a short stint in the local cells of the Hospitals of the major cities, were evacuated to metropolitan asylums, which housed nearly 2,000 of them."[35] As mentioned in the introduction, "Algerian" could but did not necessarily mean Muslim, as the mix of European settlers identified themselves as *Algériens*. In this context, the category of "Algerian mad" covered Europeans, Jews and Muslims.

3.2.2 Proportion of Muslims

The asylum in Aix-en-Provence contained most of these patients from North Africa, but how many of them were Muslim? The French psychiatrist Abel-Joseph Meilhon identified 482 Muslim patients for the period from 1860 to 1888, or 498 for the period 1860 to 1889, amounting to just 16.62 new Muslim patients (excluding 1889) and 16.6 including 1889, on average per year.[36] His colleague Élie Pascalis gave the

---

30 Reboul/Régis, Assistance, 50.
31 Livet, Aliénés algériens, 34. This development has been put together in a graph in Appendix B, Fig. 1, p. 264.
32 Practically no statistical evidence exists for the years from World War I to the end of patient transfers in the 1930s. During the war the treatment of "civilian" North African mental patients was of only secondary importance, and in the 1920s the focus of psychiatrists was on the absence of psychiatric institutions in North Africa, which urgently needed to be addressed, and collecting evidence to support the emerging theories of the *École d'Alger*.
33 Lasnet/Porot, Organisation, 386.
34 Charpentier, Comptes Rendus, 59.
35 Demassieux, Service social, 33.
36 Counting every year fully. Meilhon, Aliénation mentale, part 1, 19.

number of Muslim patients in Aix-en-Provence between 1860 and 1893 as 541 (an average of 16.39 new Muslim patients per year).[37] Battarel, quoting a table personally given to him by Monestier, a psychiatrist working in Aix-en-Provence, added that between 1890 and 1900 133 Muslim patients were admitted from the department of Algiers, or 13.3 on average per year.[38] Summarising Battarel's own statistical results, Goëau-Brissonnière mentioned in 1926 that between 1860 and 1902 633 insane Muslims (or 14.98 on average per year) were accepted into the asylum in Aix-en-Provence.[39] Finally, Auguste Marie gave the numbers of indigenous patients shipped there from the department of Algiers as 296 between 1890 and 1906 – a slightly higher yearly average of 17.41 new patients.[40]

These averages, though modest, are significant if one considers the numbers for the colonial patients in Aix-en-Provence given by Livet – from 1896 to 1910, an average of 511.6 colonial patients per year were housed in the asylum.[41] The numbers given above for the Muslim patients are those of the yearly newcomers and can therefore not be directly compared, but among the 104 "new" patients shipped there in 1906, only 28 (26.92%) were Muslims and 76 (73.08%) were Europeans, according to Levet.[42] In 1910, according to Reboul and Régis, 59.81% of all patients shipped to Aix-en-Provence were Europeans – a category subdivided into the "races" of Northern Europeans, Southern Europeans and Maltese – 8.08% were Jews and 32.1% were Muslims.[43] The surprising difference in the proportion of European patients between 1906 and 1910 might be partially explained through Livet's choice to not provide numbers for a Jewish category. It is likely that Livet included Jewish patients in the number of Europeans, as Algerian Jews were officially French after the Crémieux-Decree of 1870.[44]

While it is unremarkable that most colonial patients in the asylums of the French Midi were European settlers rather than Muslims, it is surprising to find Muslims equally underrepresented in the general hospitals in Algeria, where mental patients were gathered before being shipped off to France.[45] Louis Delasiauve, for example,

37 Pascalis, Paralysie générale, 15.
38 Again, it is not clear whether he counted 1900 as a full year or not. As a decade would make more sense, it has been read as such here. Battarel, Quelques remarques, 17.
39 Goëau-Brissonnière, Syphilis nerveuse, 30.
40 Marie, Question, 418.
41 Livet gives numbers for every year between 1896 and 1910, with the exception of 1902, for which no statistics were available. Livet, Aliénés algériens, 48.
42 Levet, Assistance, 243.
43 Reboul/Régis, Assistance, 52.
44 For example: Betts, Assimilation and Association, 20.
45 This was a problem that both general medicine and psychiatry faced. In 1907 Georges Sicard, for instance, gave the general patient numbers of the Civil Hospital of Mustapha for the year 1905. Among its patients, only 22.3% were Muslims. Sicard, Étude, 54.

compiled numbers of mental patients destined for France, accommodated in general hospitals from all three Algerian departments between 1853 and 1862. He concluded that 28.03% of all patients in Algiers were Muslims, 16.09% of all patients in Oran, and 47.09% of all patients in Constantine.[46] In total, 31.1% of all patients were Muslims. Adolphe Kocher's statistics for the Civil Hospital of Mustapha in Algiers between 1867 and 1882 listed 72.03% European, 23.35% Muslim and 4.62% Jewish patients.[47] Livet, who collected the numbers of mental patients in the same general hospital between the year 1900 and 1910, gave the numbers of European patients, which he – like Reboul and Régis after him – further divided into Northern Europeans, Southern Europeans and Maltese, as 71.91%, Jews as 7.42% and Muslims as 20.66%.[48]

It is evident that Muslims made up a much smaller percentage of psychiatric patients than the ethnic mix in North Africa would have suggested, especially if directly compared with the numbers of Jewish patients. French psychiatrists thought that Jews, as "the transition between Arab and European", were more developed than Muslims and would naturally have proportionally higher numbers of mental diseases.[49] The demographic development of Algeria during French colonisation was analysed by Dominique Maison in 1973, who examined the National Census results in Algeria from 1856 to 1954.[50] In 1856, 6.45% of the whole population of Algeria were classified as "non-Muslim". This proportion grew over time, peaking in the 1911 census at 14.38%, then slowly declining again to just above 10% in 1954.[51] In 1941 there were about 111,000 Algerian Jews and 6,625 "foreign" Jews in Algeria, which was, compared to the 1936 census, only 1.65% of the total population.[52] The numbers for Jewish psychiatric patients were therefore substantially higher than their proportion in the Algerian population, as shown by the numbers for Aix-en-Provence and the Civil Hospital of Mustapha stated above. This can also be seen in the statistical evidence for other French asylums in the 1912 Congress report – in the asylum of Saint-Alban,

---

46 Delasiauve, Review of Collardot, 117 f. The percentages of Muslim patients from the department of Constantine were significantly higher than in any other sample; this can also be observed in the Saint-Pons Asylum, which accepted patients from the department of Constantine: 39.34% of the colonial patients there between 1909 and 1911 were Muslims. Reboul/Régis, Assistance, 54.

47 Kocher, Criminalité, 71.

48 Livet, Aliénés algériens, 70. Livet's tables were also used by Reboul and Régis in their 1912 report at the Tunis Congress. Reboul/Régis, Assistance, 51.

49 Livet, Aliénés algériens, 73. On this topic, see also Victor Trenga's 1902 dissertation on "Psychoses in Algerian Jews".

50 After the Crémieux-Decree from 1870, Algerian Jews were included in the European category of "non-Muslims". Betts, Assimilation and Association, 20.

51 A graph illustrating this development, taken from Maison's numbers, can be found in Appendix B, Fig. 2, p. 264. Maison, Population de l'Algérie, 1080 ff.

52 Sussman, Jewish Population.

15.18% of colonial patients were Jews (1903 and from 1907 to 1912);[53] in Limoux, 15.13% in 1912;[54] and in Saint-Pons, 12.57% between 1909 and 1911.[55] The clinical reality in the French asylums therefore fitted nicely with psychiatric theories of insanity as a disease of civilisation, with patient numbers representing a "racial" degree of civilisation rather than their proportions within the population.

3.2.3 Numbers in Māristāns

Outside of these colonial establishments, there were traditional local institutions in Tunisia and Morocco, so-called *māristāns*, descriptions of which were not only part of the psychiatric narrative[56] but also of a broader spectrum of art, journalism and tourism.[57] The fascination with these almost romantically "picturesque" institutions was regretted by some psychiatrists,[58] who saw them as symbols of Muslim backwardness[59] and often as "barbaric prisons"[60] rather than places of healing. The psychiatric

---

53 Among the patients from the department of Oran in Saint-Alban, 58.93% were Europeans and 25.89% were Muslims. Reboul/Régis, Assistance, 53.

54 Limoux also accepted patients from the department of Oran, and there were 55.46% European and 29.41% Muslim patients. Ibid.

55 The patients from the department of Constantine were transferred to Saint-Pons. Among them 48.09% were Europeans and 39.34% Muslims. Ibid., 54.

56 French interest in Islamic *māristāns* went further than a purely practical interest in the care of patients outside the French institutions. The often very heated discussion on whether the first mental asylums in the world had in fact been built in the Muslim Middle East was still open in the 1930s. See for example: Desruelles/Bersot, Assistance aux aliénés chez les Arabes, 690.

57 The two most famous descriptions of Islamic *māristāns* in European literature can be found in Henrik Ibsen's novel "Peer Gynt" (first published in 1867) and in Guy de Maupassant's travel description "La vie errante", describing his 1871 visit to Tunisia, first published in 1887. Ibsen, Peer Gynt, 99 ff.; Maupassant, Vie errante, 201–8. While Ibsen's fictional portrayal of an asylum in Egypt was not taken up by French psychiatrists, Maupassant's description of his visit to the lunatic ward at the Sadiki General Hospital in Tunis cropped up in many medical and psychiatric texts. Brunswic-Le Bihan, Hôpital Sadiki, 377; Dupouy, Chronique, 535 f.; Coudray, Considérations, 15 f.; Duplenne, Étude, 54 f.; Maréschal, Réflexions, 73.

58 Discussion du rapport d'assistance psychiatrique, 189.

59 Agitated patients in these *māristāns* were often chained to the wall, which upset colonial psychiatrists greatly. For example: L'hôpital arabe de Tunis, 175.

60 The Tékia in Tunis was regularly described as a "barbaric prison", first in a report by the psychiatrist Perrussel, then repeated by Maréschal and Lamarche in 1937 and by Aubin in 1938. Even postcolonial Tunisian psychiatrists echoed this sentiment, and in 1969 and 1972, Sleïm Ammar described the Tékia with the same phrase. Maréschal/Lamarche, Assistance médicale, 401; Aubin, Assistance, 154; Ammar, Relations, 189; Ammar, Assistance psychiatrique, 650.

reports gave few numbers for Muslim patients looked after in these *māristāns*; numerical information was almost entirely displaced by sentiments of pity and compassion for the "suffering" of the inmates. Consequently, the data in the psychiatric sources cannot be used to construct any development of patient numbers, or gender, ethnic or age distributions. Nonetheless, we know that the Tékia, in Tunis, housed about 45 to 50 men and 24 to 30 women in 1904, "and was insufficient to give asylum to all who solicited their admission."[61] In 1909 and 1912 "about twenty madwomen" were housed there[62] and in 1922, 81 men and 19 women, of whom 54 were insane.[63] In 1911 Lwoff and Sérieux reported on their visit to the *māristān* of Sidi Fredj in Fes, where "no European, we believe, had been admitted up to now", and where 15 insane patients, out of an urban population of 100,000, lived.[64] In 1922 Du Mazel thought the patient numbers in Sidi Fredj, 25 to 30 at the time of his visit,[65] curiously low.[66]

This internment rate of only 0.015% to 0.03% of the total population of Fes was not so much a proof of the rarity of insanity in North Africa than a criticism of the inadequacy of the existing psychiatric care. The lack of patients in the North African *māristāns* was seen as a fault of the traditional Islamic care system and the imprecise numbers given in these reports demonstrated not the infrequency of insanity among Muslims but the absence of any real psychiatric traditions in these North African countries.[67] It was generally assumed that the places available to mental patients in *māristāns* like Sidi Fredj and the Tékia could not possibly cover all psychiatric cases. Raoul Vadon, for example, regretted in 1935 that before the construction of the Manouba Psychiatric Hospital in Tunisia in 1932, "psychopaths" had to be sent away from *māristāns* and general hospitals, because there were no available beds.[68]

Māristāns presented colonial psychiatry with a dilemma. Though beds for Muslim psychiatric patients were badly needed in the absence of French asylums in North Africa, the care provided in these Muslim institutions was highly inadequate, both

---

Other *māristāns*, like Sidi Fredj in Fes, were also described as prisons. Lwoff/Sérieux, Aliénés au Maroc, 474. See also: Lévy-Bram, Assistance médicale, 35.

61 Gomma, Assistance médicale, 157.
62 Bouquet, Aliénés en Tunisie, 57; Porot, Tunisie, 65.
63 Comby, Médecine française, 981. The other patients came from among the chronically ill, the destitute and the senile. Bouquet, Aliénés en Tunisie, 41.
64 Lwoff/Sérieux, Aliénés au Maroc, 474.
65 Comby mentioned the same numbers for his 1923 report. Comby, Voyage médical, 1231.
66 Mazel, Visite, 15.
67 Lwoff and Sérieux, for example, introduced their description of the Moroccan *māristāns* in 1911 by claiming that, because of the "state of decadence" of the whole country, "the assistance and treatment of mental illnesses are, so to speak, non-existent in Morocco". Lwoff/Sérieux, Aliénés au Maroc, 470.
68 Vadon, Assistance, 43.

in quality and quantity, and the disappearance of these *māristāns* was desired and often predicted. On the one hand, French psychiatrists were pragmatic and did not press for the abolition of these institutions while there was no alternative, but on the other hand, these same psychiatrists were highly idealistic and saw themselves, in the tradition of Philippe Pinel, as great liberators,[69] and they lobbied for the construction of modern mental asylums in North Africa – with sufficient beds and modern treatments – which, they argued, would solve the problems posed by the *māristāns*. To their astonishment, however, the *māristāns* endured even when alternatives to them had been constructed. As late as 1938, Henri Aubin still predicted their speedy demise with very much the same vocabulary as psychiatric experts before him: "The ancient moristans such as Sidi Fredj in Fes, though under [French] medical control, are witnesses to inhuman customs and will disappear soon."[70]

3.2.4   The Disproportionate Absence of Muslims

Even without detailed statistical evidence, the disproportionate absence of Muslim insanity – in general hospitals, French asylums and traditional Islamic institutions – was observed by colonial psychiatrists and compared to the situation in France. At first, French experts confronted with numbers on insanity in the Maghreb were sceptical. In 1864 Collardot gave a statistic-heavy presentation on the establishment of a mental asylum in Algeria, and Delasiauve, who reviewed Collardot's paper in 1865, showed his surprise at the low number of indigenous patients, 705 for a period of eleven years. He asked: "Our colleague did not say how he reached that total. Are they only those who have passed through the civil hospital [of Mustapha]? Did his investigation cover every town and village? In this case, which is more likely, it seems difficult

---

69   This was discussed in Keller's 2005 article "Pinel in the Maghreb", where he argued: "Psychiatrists spoke in a common voice of the filth and decay they witnessed in Tunisia's and Morocco's maristans. [...] The maristans quickly became a flashpoint for debates over not only psychiatric reform in the colonies, but also for the role of medicine in the advancement of colonial interest." Keller, Pinel in the Maghreb, 473.

70   Aubin, Assistance, 154. Writing just a few years after Aubin, Antoine Porot seemed to have regarded the existence of the Tékia as a glaring anachronism: "You can still find, in *the Tékia*, a survival of the ancient care [systems] of the native insane, where some old residents vegetate, expected to disappear by extinction." Porot, Œuvre psychiatrique, 368. Emphasis in the original. Moroccan *māristāns* were still described in the late 1940s and early 1950s. Pierson, Editorial, iii; Charbonneau, Assistance, part 6, 312. In 1977, Fatima Mernissi described Moroccan sanctuaries of saints, which had been defined as *māristāns* during colonial times. The *māristāns* were theoretically disbanded, but the sanctuaries still very much fulfilled their functions. Mernissi, Women, Saints and Sanctuaries, 102 ff.

for us [to believe] that the information provided had been accurate. The doctors of these locations [...] have only been able to mention overt madness, [which is] much less numerous. How many dementia sufferers, hypochondriacs, epileptics block up our asylums, who, [out] in the world, would not be regarded as insane?"[71] In addition to providing a number for Muslim patients, Delasiauve's discussion of Collardot's statistical evidence raised important questions about the differences between the general and the expert perception of insanity.

In any case, initial scepticism soon subsided, and the "fact" that insanity was rare among North Africans became a colonial trope. Many took the small number of patients in the general hospitals and of those transferred to France to be the total number of Algerian madmen and commented on this extraordinary absence of insanity, especially compared to the situation in France. One of the earliest comparisons with insanity in Europe can be found in a book on Algeria, written by the French doctor Émile-Louis Bertherand in 1855, but it was, interestingly for a book on Algeria, a comparison between England and Egypt. Bertherand's quote shows on the one hand that the numbers for insanity in Algeria were still completely unknown at this time, and, on the other hand, it highlights the assumption, discussed in the introduction, that information on one North African country was directly applicable to any other. "Thus, the statistics give for London one madman for 200 inhabitants, and in Cairo 1 for 23,570 only!"[72] Muslim insanity was therefore 118 times less frequent than European insanity.[73] Kocher concluded from his own statistical evidence in 1883 that insanity was 37 times higher in France than in Algeria;[74] and Meilhon's numerical research in Aix-en-Provence in 1896 brought him to the conclusion that insanity was 134 times less frequent among Arabs.[75]

Comparisons by other early psychiatrists provided less dramatic numbers. In 1868, the psychiatrist Jobert, lobbying for the construction of an asylum in Algeria, wrote:

---

71 Delasiauve, Review of Collardot, 117.

72 Bertherand, Médecine et hygiène, 297.

73 John Warnock, who was the leading psychiatrist in Egypt between 1895 and 1923, used similar numbers in his 1923 report about the 28 years he spent there, specifying, however, that the extremely low proportion of patients only applied to the countryside and providing very different numbers for Cairo. He wrote: "Much of the disparity in the rates of the two countries is due to the different customs as to interning the insane. But, making allowance for that factor, there is evidently a higher rate in England. Is the low rate of insanity of the Egyptians a racial characteristic? The fact that the insanity-rate for Egyptians generally, 1 per 22,000, alters to 1 per 2,500 in Cairo, makes me think that the low general rate is chiefly due to the simple life of the fellah." Warnock, Twenty-Eight Years, 399.

74 0.01 Muslim and 0.37 French patients per 1,000 inhabitants. Kocher, Criminalité, 72.

75 0.018 Muslim and 2.42 French patients per 1,000 inhabitants. Meilhon, Aliénation mentale, part 1, 19.

"In a population of about 200,000 Europeans and about 2,500,000 natives [...] in ten years – from 1852 to 1862 – 905 lunatics were counted: approximately 1 in 3,000 inhabitants. This is small compared with other countries of the civilised world; Russia and Turkey, for example, which are deemed to have the lowest numbers of insane, have 1 in 1,000 inhabitants. This difference is due to the climate and way of life of the Arabs, causing less disorder in the brains, untormented by thought. Evil and good are often in proportion."[76] This modest estimate, which applied to both the European and the Muslim population in Algeria, made insanity three times less frequent in Algeria than in those countries "of the civilised world" which already had the lowest numbers of patients, and about six times less frequent than in France.[77]

The French psychiatrist Dumolard, in a paper given at a meeting of the French Neurological Society in July 1906, put this relative absence of Muslim psychiatric patients in a wider medical context.[78] He argued that insanity only seemed less frequent among Muslims because there were generally fewer Muslim patients. According to him, the percentage of nervous diseases relative to total patient admissions was more or less the same in North Africans and Europeans.[79] In 1926 Goëau-Brissonnière agreed with Dumolard that the statistical evidence of only three Algerians in every ten patients suffering from nervous diseases was due to there being fewer Muslim patients in the French services: "If the number of nervous natives at first seems to be inferior, this is because the number of hospitalised natives is significantly lower than that of Europeans."[80] The low number of Muslim psychiatric patients was not due to their immunity to mental disorders but rather a fault of the French system, just as low numbers of patients in traditional *māristāns* did not reflect reality but the inherent inadequacy of the Islamic care system.

---

76 Jobert, Projet, 13.
77 European numbers were usually taken to be at about 1:500. France had, according to Meilhon, about one mental patient per 413 inhabitants in 1896. Meilhon, Aliénation mentale, part 1, 19. In 1911, Lwoff and Sérieux wrote that no European country had less than 2,000 madmen per 1,000,000 inhabitants, a ratio of 1:500. Lwoff/Sérieux, Note, 696. In 1935, Vadon still used a French ratio of 1:500 for the calculation of psychopaths in Tunisia. Vadon, Assistance, 40 f.
78 See for example: Fréquence des maladies nerveuses chez les Arabes, 49; Teissier, Report, 459. A number of later psychiatrists referred to this unpublished presentation in their texts. Aboab, Contribution, 15; Goëau-Brissonnière, Syphilis nerveuse, 181; Benkhelil, Contribution, 27 f.
79 Goëau-Brissonnière, Syphilis nerveuse, 181. In his 1940 dissertation, Jean Olry described Dumolard as the only theoretical opponent of Porot's *École d'Alger*. Dumolard's theory that insanity was just as frequent in North Africans as in the French was set within a broader world-view where the psychopathology of North Africans was not inherently different from that of Europeans. Olry, Paralysie générale, 32.
80 Goëau-Brissonnière, Syphilis nerveuse, 181 f.

Over time, it became apparent that the small numbers of Muslim mental patients, in all forms of containment, rose, and so, confronted with this clinical reality, the idea of a Muslim immunity to insanity was finally dropped.[81] Whether due to the realisation that Muslims had not made use of colonial institutions or because of the threat posed by these steadily rising numbers, it became clear that the statistical evidence collected needed to be reinterpreted. The statistics composed by earlier psychiatrists had not been wrong – they had just not realised that it was not the diseases that were rare, but the patients that came to get psychiatric support. There was, therefore, a mass of hidden patients awaiting discovery by colonial psychiatry.

Some psychiatrists took the numbers of inhabitants of the different colonies and tried, using the distribution of insanity in France, to calculate how many madmen were yet to be uncovered. Livet, for example, calculated in 1911 a total that included the institutionalised as well as these hidden Algerian patients. For this, he considered that his own statistical figure of 1,200 patients[82] should be "at least doubled". He went on: "Furthermore, as is clear from reports by general Inspectors of the Assistance to the insane, 'that in our departments in France, the recorded figure of madmen, who are regionally known the moment a special asylum is created there, doubles five years after its opening'. It is very likely that it will be the same in Algeria, and that, therefore, we must estimate the population of the future asylum to be an average of 4,000 patients."[83] But even that was not enough – Livet further suggested that this number was "an average" and that "a maximum of 6,000" should be taken as a possibility: "It is obvious that even this figure of 6,000 does not represent the totality of mad Algerians. According to the latest statistics, the proportion of the interned mad represents one third of the total number of the insane."[84] His calculations of the true numbers of Algerian insanity ended with the following: "Taking into account all of these results, if we were to look for what would be, in Algeria, the total number of insane, both hospitalised and free, we would see that, for a population of 5,000,000 inhabitants, we should count, altogether, 25,000 lunatics."[85] By doubling and doubling again his own statistical findings, then randomly adding another 50% – even though he should have added 66.67%, if the psychiatrically interned equalled only a third of the actual

---

81 As discussed in Chapter 1.2 "Female Muslim Normality in Psychiatric Theories". In 1939, Desruelles and Bersot summarised the situation in Algeria as follows: "These statistics show that the widespread opinion about the rarity of insanity among the natives was an unfounded prejudice and that, from the small number of alienated Arabs once deported to Europe, we should not conclude that mental diseases were rare in the colony." Desruelles/Bersot, Assistance aux aliénés en Algérie, 594.

82 Livet, Aliénés algériens, 34.

83 Ibid., 36. Capitalisation in the original.

84 Ibid., 37.

85 Ibid.

insane – and then quadrupling that number, all nominally in comparison with France, Livet arrived at the grand total of 25,000 Algerian lunatics – that is, 23,776 "hidden" lunatics when compared to his initial findings.[86]

In the same year as Livet, Lwoff and Sérieux calculated the number of potential patients in Morocco by comparison with Egypt – again relying on this supposed sameness of the Muslim North African societies. As Egypt had 30,000 lunatics out of a population of 11,000,000,[87] they estimated that Morocco, with a population of 8–10,000,000, should have between 15–20,000 lunatics.[88] Even though the methods of Lwoff and Sérieux on the one hand, and Livet on the other had been very different, the results were surprisingly similar: the sense of an unimaginable number of Muslim lunatics lurking beyond the perception of colonial psychiatry.

Numbers of potential patients for the smaller colony of Tunisia were noticeably lower. Raoul Vadon quoted an unspecified article by the psychiatrist Georges Perrussel, who had calculated in 1924, by direct comparison with France, that Tunisia had about 700 "psychopaths". In 1935 Vadon thought 700 to be a reasonable number[89] at a time when the only psychiatric hospital in Tunisia interned exactly 100 European and Muslim patients.[90] In 1956 the psychiatrist Pierre Maréschal calculated, by comparison with other countries, that there should be about 3,500 lunatics for the total population of 3,000,000 inhabitants in Tunisia, but the institutions only housed 1,045 patients.[91] These numbers of potential patients were lower because the focus of the experienced psychiatrists Perrussel and Maréschal was on gathering only dangerous – and therefore visible – patients. Neither estimate included all patients with mental problems, unlike those by Livet, and Lwoff and Sérieux: "So, only 1,045 mental patients from the 3,500 which Tunisia must conceal are interned; this means that 2,455 dangerous lunatics are left to themselves, without care and roaming the streets and countryside."[92]

---

86   Livet's random number coincided more or less with later estimates. In his 1961 article, for example, L. Couderc stated that Algeria was in need of 20,000 psychiatric beds. Couderc, Conséquences, 252.

87   Lwoff/Sérieux, Aliénés au Maroc, 475, FN 1.

88   Ibid., 475.

89   Vadon, Assistance, 40 f.

90   Ammar, Hôpital, 663.

91   Maréschal, Réflexions, 70. In 1970, the Tunisian psychiatrist Moncef Loussaief calculated that there were about 4,500 Tunisian patients to intern, many of whom were still at large. Loussaief, Assistance psychiatrique, 78 f.

92   Maréschal, Réflexions, 70.

3.2.5 Psychiatric Hospitals in North Africa

After years of planning psychiatric institutions on North African soil, whose establishment was rejected because of costs or interrupted by World War I,[93] the 1930s finally saw their construction. The Manouba Psychiatric Hospital, south of Tunis, opened in December 1931[94] with a capacity of 180 beds,[95] and a psychiatric hospital in Blida, south of Algiers, was officially opened at the Algiers Congress in 1938, with an impressive capacity of 1,200 beds.[96] Morocco had already established a small psychiatric hospital in Berrechid, south of Casablanca, in 1920, but it underwent major redevelopments in 1926 and again in the early 1930s.[97] The numbers of Muslim patients increased immediately after the construction of these institutions because of a change in the policies of patient selection – it was no longer important to limit the number of patients to the absolute minimum because of exorbitant shipping costs, and the admission, control and cure of all mental problems became the main objective.

All three psychiatric hospitals were instantly overrun,[98] which, for Antoine Porot, writing on Blida in 1936, was proof of the "amount of mental patients, who did not receive care in Algeria [before the construction of Blida], for lack of proper organisation."[99] But it was not merely an increase in numbers: the population of the new hospitals was composed differently and the numbers of Muslims soon equalled and then

---

93 For example: Jobert, Projet, 13; Porot, Assistance psychiatrique, 86; Porot, Services hospitaliers, 796.
94 Maréschal/Chaurand, Paralysie générale, 248.
95 Douki et al., Psychiatrie en Tunisie, 51.
96 Desruelles/Bersot, Assistance aux aliénés en Algérie, 593. In reality, Blida Psychiatric Hospital, or Blida-Joinville as it was officially called, had accepted its first patients in July 1933. Porot, Œuvre psychiatrique, 361.
97 Pierson, Editorial, iii. See also: Potet, Au sujet, 449.
98 These psychiatric hospitals were therefore constantly extended. Berrechid, for instance, had 620 beds in 1949 and 800–1,000 beds in 1953. Ibid.; Thierry, Œuvre, 40. The 180 beds initially provided by the Manouba were increased to 440 in 1951, then to 1,018 in 1957. Möbius, Entwicklung der Psychiatrie, 14; Douki et al., Psychiatrie en Tunisie, 51. The Tunisian psychiatrist Sleïm Ammar has put together a table showing the admissions into the Manouba Psychiatric Hospital between 1931 and 1971, which shows another enormous increase just after Tunisia's independence in 1956. Ammar, Hôpital, 663. An article in the *Information Psychiatrique* from 1969 gave a similar overview of the admissions to Blida Psychiatric Hospital, without, admittedly, the detailed information that Ammar had for the Manouba. Here the increase was more gradual and had already started during the Algerian War of Independence. L'hôpital psychiatrique de Blida, 824. The information from these two statistics has been compiled into a graph in Appendix B, Fig. 3, p. 265.
99 Porot, Services hospitaliers, 796.

overtook the numbers of European patients.[100] It was only with this increase in Muslim patients in these new institutions that a real interest in the numbers of female Muslim patients began. Hoda El-Saadi, who analysed statistical evidence for the ʿAbbāsiyya Asylum in Egypt published by the Ministry of Public Health for the period of 1930 to 1936, established an increase in the numbers of Muslim women admitted to the asylum for this period of the early 1930s, which she interpreted as an indication of deeper changes in Egyptian society.[101] It is certain that the numbers of female patients grew in the Maghreb states, but Muslim women remained the smallest group within colonial psychiatric care until the late 1950s, excluding Jewish patients.[102] In 1951, for example, François-Georges Marill and Abdennour Si Hassen wrote an article on general paralysis in North Africa, in which they concluded that among the patients institutionalised in Blida between 1937 and 1949, 21.6% were European men, 18.99% European women, 3.98% Jewish men, 3.59% Jewish women, 39.25% Muslim men and 12.59% Muslim women.[103] By the late 1950s, however, female Muslim patients

---

100 Maréschal gave slightly different numbers for the "racial" distribution at the Manouba Psychiatric Hospital between 1931 and 1936. In an article with Chaurand in 1937, he claimed that Europeans only amounted to 28.38% of all patients, while Jews made up 16.95% and Muslims 54.67%. In the same year, he wrote another article with Lamarche and, in this, 24% of all patients were Europeans, 17% were Jews and 59% Muslims. Maréschal/Chaurand, Paralysie générale, 248; Maréschal/Lamarche, Assistance médicale, 399. Charles Bardenat analysed the population at Blida Psychiatric Hospital for the years 1933 to 1940, where 43.66% of all patients were European, while 7.1% were Jews and 49.29% were Muslims. Bardenat, Criminalité, 318. In the external consultations, however, the numbers of Muslim patients often stayed below those of European patients. In 1955 Pierson et al. analysed the Pavilion of Neuropsychiatry in Casablanca: In 1952 only 32.49% and in 1953 32.29% of all external consultations involved Muslim patients. Pierson et al., Assistance psychiatrique, 31.

101 El-Saadi, Changing Attitudes, 301. This change in attitudes was only really perceptible in the postcolonial Maghreb – and even then only in Tunisia. Morocco and Algeria had significantly fewer female than male Muslim patients during and after French occupation, and the numbers of female patients today are still below those of Muslim men. Particularités de la pathologie algérienne, 880; Bensmail et al., Considérations, 394; Douki et al., Women's Mental Health, 187. Tunisia, on the other hand, claimed its female patient population had been growing, in comparison to the male population, ever since Independence, which was interpreted as a sign of women's emancipation in Tunisia. More importantly, Tunisian psychiatrists claim that this growth was already noticeable during colonial times. Ammar, Hôpital, 660.

102 Desruelles and Bersot, for example, gave patient numbers for Blida Psychiatric Hospital during 1937 and 1938: "Among the men admitted, 65.4% were natives and 34.6% were Europeans, while among the women, 37.7% were natives and 62% were European women." Desruelles/Bersot, Assistance aux aliénés en Algérie, 592.

103 They also gave the numbers for the small psychiatric service of the general hospital in Constantine for the years of 1935 to 1942, where there were slightly more Muslim women (15.59%) than European women (15.07%). Marill/Si Hassen, Paralysie générale, 453 f.

had overtaken the numbers of both European men and women in Blida. Assicot et al. analysed the admissions to one of the services of Blida for the years 1958 and 1959, and concluded that 49.9% of all patients had been Muslim men, followed by 30.93% Muslim women, 10.8% European men and 8.37% European women.[104]

In the 1930s, therefore, the quantitative hierarchy changed from (in descending order) European men, European women, Muslim men and Muslim women to Muslim men, European men, European women and Muslim women.[105] The question of how much physical space should be given to the relatively low numbers of female Muslim patients had been long debated,[106] but only now was real importance attached to it. According to some psychiatrists, it was not necessary to give female Muslim patients any special room. Levet, for example, wrote in 1909: "It is indisputable that the Algerian asylum should consist of two asylums: the European asylum for the settlers, the civilised natives and women, and the Arab asylum for the native men, Arab in manners and life. [...] Given the small number of indigenous women interned, and given that most of those are Europeanised, the urgency of an Arab building for women does not seem immediate [...]."[107]

For financial reasons, it was clear that the hospitals had to be "mixed", by which they meant accommodating both genders, but division by "race" was obvious to French colonial psychiatrists, too.[108] Therefore, a strict division of patients in these institutions along both gender and "racial" lines was envisaged: sections, varying in size and comfort, for European male, European female, Muslim male and Muslim female patients were proposed.[109]

---

104 Assicot et al., Causes principales, 262. Michèle Chappert's 1962 dissertation described the patient population in one of the services in Blida between 1958 and 1961. Among the female patients, 92.28% had been Muslim. Chappert, Contribution, 20.

105 In both hierarchies, Jewish patients made up the smallest groups, with more male than female patients. Summarising the situation at the Civil Hospital of Mustapha in 1937, Desruelles and Bersot stated that while only 8.35% of men at the Mustapha were Jewish, 14.35% of the female patients were Jews, against only 18.8% Muslim women, which coincided, again, with the notion of Jews being more civilised than Muslims: "Note the very small portion of indigenous women and the high proportion of Jewish women." Desruelles/Bersot, Assistance aux aliénés en Algérie, 589. The few statistical tables showing the distribution of all ethnic groups and genders are found in Appendix B, Fig. 4, p. 266.

106 Jobert, Projet, 61 f.

107 Levet, Assistance, 248.

108 Alexandre Lasnet and Antoine Porot, for example, stated in 1932 that "one could not take the responsibility to let natives and Europeans mingle [...]." Lasnet/Porot, Organisation, 387. The exact same phrase was repeated by Antoine Porot in 1933. Porot, Assistance psychiatrique, 89.

109 Ibid.; Pierson et al., Assistance psychiatrique, 35.

3.2.6   Percentages of Female Muslim Patients

This leaves the question of how many female patients there were among the already underrepresented Muslims and how their numbers were interpreted by the colonial psychiatrists. The comparison to European women is important in this context because in the 19th century, mental illness was understood to be more of a female than male disease.[110] In France, this notion seemed to be supported by statistical evidence,[111] and most French psychiatrists in the 19th century thought insanity was more prevalent among women than among men.[112] Those who did not subscribe to this view at least supposed that mental diseases were equally distributed among the sexes,[113] but in the statistics on the North African colonies, this was not the case. Only a few colonial psychiatrists used statistical evidence in their publications, but among those statistics published, it was apparent that psychiatric disorders were less frequent among European women. Ranging from 30.88% for the years 1898 to 1909[114] to 57.58% in 1912,[115] the average ratio of European women, compared to that of European men, was 47.21% during the period when patients were shipped to France, 47.56% once psychiatric institutions were built in North Africa, and 47.36% altogether.[116] Among Muslim patients, the smallest percentage of Muslim women in the published statistics was a mere 12.05% in 1880[117] whereas the highest was 38.27% from 1958 to 1959.[118] If these statistics are combined, the result is an average female ratio of 23.25% among Muslim

---

110 This has been discussed by Elaine Showalter in her 1987 book "Female Malady", where she claimed that women were more often declared insane than men in the 19th and 20th centuries, and that women were imprisoned in British asylums as a means of gender control. Showalter, Female Malady, 55 f. Showalter has been widely criticised for this theory. See for example: Busfield, Female Malady, 259 f.; Ernst, European Madness, 369.

111 In 1846, for instance, 51.7% of all mental patients in France were women. Prix de la société de médecine, 316. At the end of 1877, this number was 52.8%. Constans et al., Rapport sommaire, 93. In 1853, the asylums of Bicêtre and Salpêtrière even had 62.39% female patients. Statistique de Bicêtre et de la Salpêtrière, 178.

112 There were psychiatrists who disputed this fact. Lunier, Augmentation progressive, 33. Jobert, for example, concluded in 1868, having analysed the frequency of certain diseases in Algeria, that insanity was a disease of civilisation, with more male patients than female and more Europeans than Muslims, which meant that any asylums built in North Africa would need less physical space for Muslim women. Jobert, Projet, 61 f.

113 Meilhon, Aliénation mentale, part 1, 25.

114 Bouquet, Aliénés en Tunisie, 34.

115 Reboul/Régis, Assistance, 53.

116 For a detailed breakdown of the ratios of European women to European men, see Appendix B, Fig. 5, p. 267.

117 Meilhon, Aliénation mentale, part 1, 25.

118 Assicot et al., Causes principales, 262 f.

patients during the time when patients were shipped from North Africa to France; an average ratio of 26.74% in the few statistics which give the numbers for female patients among the population of the new psychiatric institutions; and an overall average of 24.49%,[119] which means that roughly every fourth Muslim patient was a woman.[120] Returning to the question of whether the silence towards Muslim women in the psychiatric theories was due to their absence in colonial institutions, it is useful to compare the ratios of Muslim women in the French colonial asylums and psychiatric institutions with the gender distribution in the published case studies.[121] The logic behind this comparison is that published case studies were selected for two reasons: they were either exemplary cases, giving the possibility to describe, through one case, a behaviour, symptom or problem that was shared by many more; or they were cases of a special disease or pathological behaviour that the psychiatrist wished to examine and diffuse. Case studies were not selected to adequately reflect the hospital popula-tions – they were selected because of their representative or illustrative value.[122] For example, C. A. Pierson stated in his 1955 article that he had chosen twelve cases from among 118 possible patients in order to represent the social and educational differ-ences in Moroccan society.[123] He wrote: "The twelve medico-social situations [...] were selected because they relate to different categories of individuals. They range from the most ignorant fellah, from the most rustic countryman, the most superstitious and

---

119 A graph with the ratios of Muslim women to Muslim men can be found in Appendix B, Fig. 6, p. 268

120 Findings for other African colonies are slightly higher. Carothers' statistics on Kenya gave one new female admission for every two male admissions in 1947. Carothers, Study, 558. Sadowsky's examination of insanity in colonial Nigeria came up with a ratio of about 1:3. Sadowsky, Psy-chiatry and Colonial Ideology, 100.

121 A detailed analysis of these numbers in the case studies can be found in Appendix B, Fig. 7, p. 269.

122 As mentioned in the introduction to Chapter 2, Meilhon analysed all 83 Muslim patients present in Aix-en-Provence in a specific year, 1880, so there was no process of selection, which could have discriminated against Muslim women. Collections with case studies exclusively concerning men or women were not considered for the calculation of these case study ratios, even though many of them dealt with general psychiatric topics, e. g. Laurens' 1919 dissertation, Vadon's 1935 dissertation or Maurice Porot's 1956 article, without mentioning female Muslim cases. Laurens, Contribution, 28–41; Vadon, Assistance, 45–9; Porot, M., Retentissements, 622–36. Other psychiatrists published case studies on exclusively male Muslim topics (such as the mental problems of Muslim soldiers), but only in 1959 was the first collection of case studies with exclusively female Muslim patients published by Henry and Assicot, followed in 1962 by two collections of case studies on puerperal psychoses in Chappert's dissertation and Mares and Barre's article. Manceaux et al., Hystérie; Susini, Aspects cliniques; Henry/ Assicot, Le 7044 RP; Chappert, Contribution; Mares/Barre, Quelques aspects.

123 Pierson, Paléophrénie réactionnelle, 643 f.

distant from any contact with the European milieu, to the Moroccan in the process of evolution, to the soldier who has stayed in the Métropole, to the career sergeant, culminating in the evolved Muslims, students of our schools, readers of our textbooks of literature and morals."[124] Apparently, Muslim women neither represented these different stages of "evolution" nor contributed to this North African diversity, as not even one female case study was chosen by Pierson.

Most of these collections of case studies were published in psychiatric dissertations. All of them had more case studies on Muslim men than Muslim women, apart from Suzanne Taïeb's collection, one of only a handful of female colonial psychiatrists working in North Africa.[125] As a woman, she looked after Muslim women and drew her information from them. Her collection of case studies therefore reveals a North African insanity which seemingly included Muslim women. The average of Muslim women in these published case studies amounted to 16.26% (one in every 6.15), and if one excludes Taïeb's collection, this percentage drops to 12.99% (one in every 7.7).[126] It is evident that Muslim women were, statistically speaking, underrepresented in the case studies, which, in psychiatric academia, form the basis for further theories; or, put differently, the theoretical disinterest in Muslim women, exemplified by their neglect in the collection of case studies (16.26%/12.99%), did not mirror the actual absence of female Muslim patients (24.49%). The motivations behind the selection of case studies therefore actively excluded women. Either female patients were not seen to be exemplary cases of Muslim insanity, or the specific interest behind the psychiatric publications (on "typically Muslim" forms of insanity, like criminal insanity and drug use) automatically omitted Muslim women.

3.3 Diagnoses and Prognoses

Other important factors in contextualising the statistical representation of Muslim women in colonial psychiatric care are their recovery and death rates, and their distribution among the diagnostic categories employed in colonial psychiatric statistics.

---

124 Ibid., 644.
125 As previously mentioned, among the 51 case studies that Suzanne Taïeb chose to print in her 1939 dissertation, 30 were on Muslim women. Taïeb, Idées d'influence, 85–146.
126 Meilhon summarised his work in both statistics and case studies, and while his ratio of 12.05% female Muslim patients is the smallest among the statistical evidence, it represents the average for the case studies, if one excludes Taïeb's collection. Meilhon, Aliénation mentale, part 1, 25.

3.3.1 Chances of Death

The chances of being cured were slim for all patients shipped to France. Transportation usually involved appalling, inhumane conditions, as described by a variety of outraged psychiatrists.[127] Since only the most desperate cases were brought to attention, those transported were usually delivered to the hands of psychiatrists too late.[128] Consequently, many colonial patients died, the majority soon after their arrival, while the rest, the chronically insane, steadily accumulated and filled up the psychiatric institutions of the Midi, as discussed above. Jobert stated in 1868 that two thirds of all colonial patients sent from Algeria died in France, without further specifying the "race" of the victims.[129] Viewed cynically, these deaths were necessary for the transport system to function, because the spaces provided by their deaths were needed for new patients, as stated by Antoine Porot in 1912, describing the situation of the European and Jewish patients in Tunisia: "The shipments are made according to the vacated beds, almost always through death, exceptionally through being cured."[130] The transfer of new patients from Algeria was not directly related to the deaths of their predecessors, but because of the immense overcrowding in the asylums of the Midi, the care of Algerian patients effectively depended on these high rates of mortality.

The situation was bad for all colonial patients but worst for Muslims, for whom the transfer was usually a one-way journey.[131] The reasons presented were manifold: France was cold, the food and customs unfamiliar, and nobody spoke the patients' native languages.[132] Further, for patients to be released, there had to be family pressure on the asylums, and while this pressure was exercised by Muslim Algerian families before the patients were first admitted to colonial care, it effectively stopped once the patients crossed the Mediterranean.[133]

---

127 For example: Lunier, Review of Les aliénés en Algérie, 160; Gervais, Contribution, 6; Livet, Aliénés algériens, 79. Dupouy quoted Levet, speaking at the 1912 Congress in Tunis, who condemned transportation as being worse than the alarming situation in North Africa: "Mr LEVET speaks against the exportation of the colonial insane to France. The situation of those cloistered in the Thékia is better than that of the natives deported to the asylums of the métropole." Dupouy, Chronique, 533. Emphasis in the original.

128 Delasiauve, Review of Collardot, 117 f.

129 Jobert, Projet, 16. Marie seemed to quote Jobert as he stated in 1907 that two thirds of all Arabs transported to the asylums in Pierrefeu or Aix-en-Provence died. Marie, Question, 418.

130 Porot, Tunisie, 69.

131 Dupuoy wrote in 1912: "The percentage, for example, of Algerian Arabs cured in France is minute and reasons abound to explain this fact." Dupouy, Chronique, 528.

132 Delasiauve, Review of Collardot, 116; Meilhon, Aliénation mentale, part 6, 357 f.

133 Reboul/Régis, Assistance, 46.

A number of colonial psychiatrists, aware of the disastrous figures of Muslim patients dying in France, campaigned actively for the building of asylums in Algeria. Dr Constans, head of the asylum in Aix-en-Provence, admitted in an 1873 discussion on "Lunatics in Algeria" that, because of their shocking death rates, Muslims should not be treated in France: "They almost never get well, and their annual mortality goes up to 49%, while that of European lunatics is only 13 to 14%."[134] In 1896 Meilhon published his findings which showed that amongst the Arabs admitted into Aix-en-Provence between 1860 and 1888, 53.52% had died;[135] and Levet's statistics for Aix-en-Provence revealed that in 1906 exactly 50% of all Muslims and 32.89% of Europeans admitted that year had died.[136] During the same year, 40.79% of all European patients were released as cured, while only 14.29% of all Muslims were allowed to leave the asylum in Aix-en-Provence.[137]

Death rates among Muslims were not quite as shocking in all published statistics. Kocher gave the overall death rates for the patients collected in the department of Algiers between 1867 and 1882 as only 4.81% – being a general hospital, it processed psychiatric patients and sent the gravest cases off to die elsewhere. Male patients had lower death rates than women, and Europeans lower ones than Muslims: 3.98% of European men died; 5.68% of European women; 4.76% of Muslim men; and 6.17% of Muslim women. 37.72% of patients in the same general hospital and period were released as cured and not sent to other, deadlier institutions. This amounted to 40.36% of European men; 41.08% of European women; 32.47% of Muslim men; but only 20.99% of

---

134 Linas, Aliénés en Algérie, 492. This was quoted as a still acceptable fact by Reboul and Régis at the 1912 Congress in Tunis. Reboul/Régis, Assistance, 42 f. These shocking numbers could still be seen as an improvement over what happened in the Algerian-controlled hospitals in North Africa. In the same discussion in 1873, Auguste Voisin described his visit to the Civil Hospital of Mustapha in Algiers, where, according to him, up to 90% of the Arab lunatics died. Linas, Aliénés en Algérie, 491. The same number seems to be mentioned in Livet's 1911 article, where he wrote about the year 1852: "The Prefect of Algiers took the plight of the insane into serious consideration; their mortality, at that time, reached the rate of 90%, a rate that it had never, under the ancient Moorish domination, under the detestable conditions reported earlier, reached [before]." Livet, Aliénés algériens, 15 f.

135 Meilhon, Aliénation mentale, part 2, 185 f. Meilhon did not further specify when, in relation to the date of their admission into Aix-en-Provence, these patients died. He went on to quote the aforementioned phrase by Constans. Gervais, in his 1907 dissertation, quoted Meilhon's Constans quote without reference, while Naudin, in 1913, quoted Meilhon's 53.52%, but added Constans' 13% without referring to Constans. Gervais, Contribution, 5; Naudin, Psychiatrie coloniale, 20.

136 50% of all Muslim deaths in Aix-en-Provence that year were due to tuberculosis. Levet, Assistance, 242 f.

137 Ibid., 244.

Muslim women.[138] Even in North Africa, where there was no Mediterranean separating Muslim patients from the lobbying powers of friends and families, Muslim women were half as likely to be released as cured as Europeans. This disadvantage of Muslim women could also be observed in statistics on cases released as cured from the Civil Hospital of Mustapha. According to Gervais, 43.64% of all patients released as cured in 1905 and 1906 were European men; 47.27% were European women; 7.27% were Muslim men; and only 1.82% were Muslim women.[139]

In a direct comparison with Muslim men, the disadvantage of Muslim women was similarly apparent. Auguste Marie assembled the rates of Muslim mental patients who died or were released as cured for the department of Algiers for the years 1890 to 1906. 55.36% of all Muslim women and 48.99% of all Muslim men died, and while 28.48% of the male Muslim patients were released as cured, only 16.07% of the female patients were set free.[140] The scarce statistical evidence shows conclusively that female Muslim patients were, relative to their total number, the most likely to die and least likely to be cured by colonial psychiatrists.[141]

3.3.2 North African Diagnoses

The general consensus among French colonial psychiatrists during most of the colonisation of North Africa was that, technically, all mental disorders could be found in North Africans, although usually digressing slightly from their "normal" European forms.[142] The notable exception to this was the supposedly rarely diagnosed general paralysis of the insane.[143] One of the first advocates of the idea that all categories of mental diseases were prevalent among Muslims had been Adolphe Kocher, whose statistical evidence for the years 1867 to 1882 had shown that "all genres of alienation can

---

138 Kocher, Criminalité, 70.

139 Gervais, Contribution, 58.

140 Marie, Question, 418.

141 The statistical evidence does not show whether this is due to the treatment or the selection of female Muslim patients. As only the worst cases were admitted into colonial care, the high mortality rate must have been due to the selection processes, but as this also applied to Muslim men, who were less likely to die in comparison to Muslim women, the treatment must also have played a role. The treatment of Muslim women in these colonial institutions will be discussed in Chapter 4. See also: Susini, Quelques considérations, 14.

142 Camuset, Review of Kocher, 346 f.; Poitrot, Influences climatiques, 1254; Igert, Introduction, 1310.

143 This discussion will be analysed in Chapter 5.3 "General Paralysis: Alcohol, Syphilis and Civilisation".

be found among the Arabs, from dementia to alcoholism [...]."[144] But what were the diagnoses "usually" given to Muslims in general and to female patients in particular? Among the Muslim patients that Kocher had personally analysed, all diseases had been found. Male Muslim patients had every one of Kocher's eleven categories of disease,[145] with 5.19% even displaying the symptoms of the European disease of general paralysis. However, Europeans and Muslim women had never been diagnosed as hashish addicts, and Muslim women furnished no cases for the categories of senile insanity, manic insanity or general paralysis.[146] A similar picture emerged from the statistical evidence presented by Meilhon and by Reboul and Régis. In Meilhon's sample of male Muslim patients, all categories, apart from general paralysis, had been diagnosed,[147] but in his, admittedly small, sample of ten female Muslim patients, there were no cases of mental degeneration, delirium, hashish addiction, combined alcoholism and hashish addiction, convulsive insanity, general paralysis, or imbecility and idiocy.[148] Similarly, only four different diagnoses (epilepsy, dementia, mania and melancholia) were given to the 32 female Muslim patients in Aix-en-Provence in 1910.[149]

In Kocher's evidence, Muslim women had less variety in their disorders than Europeans or Muslim men, and in both Muslim men and Muslim women one diagnosis, "mania", comprised two fifths of all cases: 41.56% of Muslim men and 41.98% of Muslim women were diagnosed as "manic" – against 21.43% and 31.59% in European men and women respectively.[150] "Mania" or "maniacal states" were the most frequent diagnoses in Muslims, in both statistics and theoretical texts,[151] a propensity explained by

---

144 Camuset, Review of Kocher, 346. A graph composed of Kocher's findings is shown in Appendix B, Fig. 8a, p. 271.

145 Kocher identified twelve categories of diseases, but obviously no men could be diagnosed with "puerperal insanity".

146 Kocher, Criminalité, 70.

147 That is, if one gathers the categories of acute and chronic mania; the categories of acute, stupefied and chronic melancholia; and of imbecility and idiocy. Meilhon, Aliénation mentale, part 2, 191.

148 Ibid. Meilhon's findings are compiled in Appendix B, Fig. 8b, p. 272.

149 Reboul/Régis, Assistance, 52. In some of the other statistics provided by Reboul and Régis at the 1912 Congress, Muslim women had diagnoses as diverse as the other groups, e.g. at the Civil Hospital of Mustapha between 1900 and 1910, or at the Asylum of Saint-Pons, 1909–1911. Livet, Aliénés algériens, 70; Reboul/Régis, Assistance, 51; 54. See Appendix B, Fig. 8c–8g, p. 273.

150 Kocher, Criminalité, 70.

151 Jobert, Projet, 61; Meilhon, Aliénation mentale, part 3, 369; Livet, Aliénés algériens, 69. The same was noted about Muslims in Egypt. Savage, Report of the Government Asylums, 470. "Maniacal" also became a useful adjective to describe other diagnoses. Among Muslims, there were, for instance, maniacal manifestations in other diseases, "acute maniacal deliriums",

a choleric temperament attributed to North Africans.[152] Mania offered such diverse symptoms as grimaces;[153] uninterrupted speech, laughing and dancing;[154] tearing of clothes[155] and a deep agitation.[156]

Among Meilhon's observed patient population in Aix-en-Provence in 1880, mania supplied exactly 50% of diagnoses amongst Muslim women, and 26.03% among Muslim men.[157] The different statistics provided by Reboul and Régis at the Congress of Tunis painted a similar picture – mania amounted to 39.53% of all diagnoses among Muslim women in the patient population at the Civil Hospital of Mustapha between 1900 and 1910;[158] to 50% in Saint-Alban in 1903 and between 1907 and 1911;[159] to 34.78% in Saint-Pons between 1909 and 1911;[160] to 56.25% in Aix-en-Provence in 1910; and to 33.33% in Limoux in 1912.[161] While Muslim women only made up 6.09% of the total hospital population in the statistics presented at the 1912 Congress, they made up 10.75% of all mania cases.[162]

Diagnoses of European-style "manias" finally became unfashionable under the rise of the *École d'Alger*.[163] Definitions of typically Muslim forms of mania started to appear, even though the founder of the *École d'Alger*, Antoine Porot, had written in 1912 that "maniacal accidents seem to me to be rather rare, which may perhaps be explained

---

"maniacal excitation" and maniacal forms of depression. Pascalis, Paralysie générale, 43; Porot, Tunisie, 58; Porot/Arrii, Impulsivité criminelle, 603 f.; Sutter et al., Aspects algériens, 894.

152   This choleric temperament is obviously at odds with the meekness and passivity that allegedly defined female Muslim normality, as described in Chapter 1. However, it seems that these contradictions were not discernible for the colonial psychiatrists. It was therefore possible for both rage and calmness to symbolise different aspects of North African "normality".

153   Aubin et al., Troubles mentaux, 412.

154   Taïeb, Idées d'influence, 86 f.

155   Gervais, Contribution, 54 f.

156   Meilhon, Aliénation mentale, part 4, 40. Taïeb, Idées d'influence, 85–8. These symptoms coincided with traditional North African interpretations of spirit possession. Aouattah, Ethno-psychiatrie maghrébine, 58.

157   Meilhon, Aliénation mentale, part 2, 191.

158   Livet, Aliénés algériens, 70. Livet's statistics were also used in the 1912 Congress report by Reboul and Régis. Reboul/Régis, Assistance, 51.

159   Ibid., 53.

160   Ibid., 54.

161   Ibid., 53.

162   Ibid., 51–4. These different statistics have been compiled into one graph, in Appendix B, Fig. 9a/9b, p. 278.

163   This is difficult to estimate from the source material because after the 1912 Congress, no French colonial psychiatrist composed further tables with all diseases prevalent among their Muslim patients.

through the calm and traditional serenity of Muslim mores."[164] This statement contra‐ dicted his later theories, where the main characteristic of North Africans – the danger Muslims posed to French society – dominated all disorders. The idea of a traditional Muslim "calm and serenity" cannot be found in Porot's later publications. In 1938, for example, in a discussion following a paper given by him and some of his students at the Congress in Algiers, Porot justified a diagnosis he had given to a patient even though one of the main – European – characteristics was missing: "[...] if there is no euphoria [in the patient's behaviour], this is because mania tends to take impulsive, irritable or choleric forms in natives."[165]

Other diagnoses which were, statistically speaking, frequent in Muslim women, were mostly among those diseases that Reboul and Régis summarised as "psychic infirmities" (as opposed to "psychoses") at the 1912 Tunis Congress: idiocy, epilepsy and dementia.[166] In Meilhon's statistics, 20% of all Muslim women suffered from epilepsy;[167] and Jean Sutter, who wrote his dissertation on "Mental Epilepsy among North African Natives" in 1937, summarised in a 1959 article written with Maurice Porot and Yves Pélicier that epilepsy was twice as frequent among Muslims as among Europeans.[168] In Kocher's statistical evidence, idiocy comprised up 12.35% of all diag‐ noses given to Muslim women, epilepsy 6.17% and dementia 20.99%.[169] In the statistics prepared for the 1912 Congress, Muslim women, who made up 6.09% of all patients, had, proportionally, slightly too many diagnoses of idiocy (6.38% of all idiocy diag‐ noses had been given to Muslim women) and almost twice as many cases of epilepsy (11.54%) as would have been proportionally expected, but not of dementia (5.42%).[170]

---

164 Porot, Tunisie, 71.
165 Porot et al., Cas d'échokinésie chez un indigène, 209.
166 The fourth disease among these "psychic infirmities" was general paralysis. Reboul/Régis, Assis‐ tance, 51. While the diagnosis of idiocy could not be found among the case studies of female Muslim patients, descriptions of epileptics were common. Meilhon, Aliénation mentale, part 6, 353 f.; Sutter, Épilepsie mentale, 153–6; Taïeb, Idées d'influence, 94. Dementia, while frequent in the case studies, seemed to be a symptom of other diseases rather than a category in itself. Meilhon, Aliénation mentale, part 2, 205 f.; Levet, Assistance, 53; Olry, Paralysie générale, 54.
167 Unusually, his statistical sample showed no Muslim woman suffering from idiocy or imbecil‐ ity. Meilhon, Aliénation mentale, part 2, 191. In 1911, Livet concluded from his own statistics that "a high proportion" of Muslims were epileptics. Livet, Aliénés algériens, 69.
168 Sutter et al., Aspects algériens, 894. This was highly disputed by postcolonial Algerian psychi‐ atrists. In a 1969 article on "Particularities of Algerian Pathology" in the Journal Information Psychiatrique, the unnamed authors claimed "the mental disorders of epilepsy were not found as often as previous studies made by the former Algerian school [the École d'Alger] suggest." Particularités de la pathologie algérienne, 881.
169 Kocher, Criminalité, 70.
170 See Appendix B, Fig. 9a/9b, p. 278.

Among the diseases classed by Reboul and Régis as "psychoses" in 1912 (mania, melancholia, mental confusion, alcoholism/hashish addiction and delirium)[171], mania was, as shown, the most common diagnosis in Muslim women. There were opposing theories about the distribution of melancholia among Muslims, which were supported by statistical evidence. While no female Muslim patient in the asylum of Saint-Alban in the years 1903 and 1907–1912 showed symptoms of melancholia,[172] 21.88% of all Muslim women in the asylum of Aix-en-Provence in 1910 were diagnosed with it.[173] Meilhon, in 1896, claimed that while melancholia was not as frequent as mania in Algerians, it still existed,[174] and he openly criticised Kocher, whose statistical tables lacked a category for melancholia.[175] Meilhon's own research had shown that 9.59% of all admitted Muslim men and 10% of the admitted Muslim women were suffering from melancholia.[176] Among the evidence presented by Reboul and Régis, Muslim women's representation among the cases of melancholia (6.17%) was almost identical to that of their percentage in the asylum populations (6.09%).[177] The idea that melancholia was, if not common, at least possible in Muslims was disputed by the *École d'Alger*. In their 1939 article on "Primitivism among North African Natives", Porot and Sutter wrote that *"melancholy is also rare* in the native, as it corresponds poorly to the habitual profile of his emotional life".[178] Melancholy, the *École d'Alger* claimed, was not compatible with Muslim primitivity, and in the infrequent cases where it was diagnosed, its symptoms were dominated by the prominent choleric characteristics of the "race".[179]

---

171 Reboul/Régis, Assistance, 51.

172 Ibid., 53.

173 Ibid., 52. This might be due to an individual psychiatrist. Melancholy was often described in case studies on female Muslim patients. Meilhon, Aliénation mentale, part 3, 366 f.; Soumeire, Meurtre, 55 f.; Taïeb, Idées d'influence, 89; Henry/Assicot, Le 7044 RP, 692.

174 In his experience, it was mainly the Kabyles who were melancholic. Meilhon, Aliénation mentale, part 3, 364. Livet claimed in 1911 that "melancholia is quite frequent among the Muslims." Livet, Aliénés algériens, 69.

175 Kocher, Criminalité, 70; Meilhon, Aliénation mentale, part 3, 364.

176 Ibid., part 2, 191.

177 See Appendix B, Fig. 9a/9b, p. 278.

178 Porot/Sutter, 'Primitivisme', 238. Manceaux, Sutter and Pélicier confirmed in an article at the 1954 Congress in Liége on "Melancholic States in the North African Native" that "melancholic states" were "less frequent in the native than in the European [...]." Interestingly, they added that "the distribution in the two genders is reasonably equal with a slight predominance in women", without proving this by statistical evidence. Manceaux et al., États mélancoliques, 270.

179 Sutter, Maurice Porot and Pélicier stated in a 1959 article that the most common form of melancholia in Muslims was its "anxious form", with typically Muslim symptoms like "agitation and theatricality". They also claimed, without offering any statistical evidence, that "true

The other categories under the heading "psychoses" proposed by Reboul and Régis – mental confusion, alcoholism, and hashish addiction and delirium – were rarely diagnosed in Muslim women.[180] As discussed in Chapter 2, it was believed that addictions were almost exclusively a male problem.[181]

Overall, one can say that Muslim women were diagnosed with all diseases common in Europeans and Muslim men, but some diseases only appeared in specific hospitals at specific times. There were also distinct patterns in the diagnoses: Muslim women were diagnosed with the disease of civilisation, general paralysis, and with unwomanly diseases like alcoholism, but only infrequently and in small numbers, while other diseases were "over-diagnosed", statistically speaking. Furthermore, many diagnoses attributed to female Muslim patients involved predominantly physical symptoms – idiocy and epilepsy were diseases of degenerated bodies; mania and melancholia were usually expressed physically, through agitation and stupor respectively.[182]

One reason for the lack of variety in diagnoses was certainly the small number of Muslim female patients, with some diagnoses being unlikely to crop up among small samples.[183] The Muslim women admitted to colonial care often suffered from physically very demanding diseases, which, like epilepsy, were more openly noticeable even by people not admitted to the confidence of a family, which meant that the patient could be interned by sidestepping the usual admission mechanisms via complaints. Another reason for this lack of diagnostic variety was the theory that Muslims had mainly simple psychiatric disorders, which allegedly corresponded to those of the European Middle Ages, while Europeans were victims of more complicated and modern diseases.[184]

---

melancholy is twice as rare in autochthonous subjects as in Europeans; the distribution among the genders is roughly equal in both ethnic groups." Sutter et al., Aspects algériens, 894.

180 See Appendix B, Fig. 9a/9b, p. 278.

181 The statistics show that there were female Muslim addicts, but – in the eyes of the colonial psychiatrists – in negligible quantities. In Kocher's statistics, 6.17% of all female Muslim patients were classified as alcoholics; 10% in Meilhon's evidence; 4.65% in Livet's statistics; and 8.7% in Saint-Pons between 1909 and 1911. Given the propensity of Muslim men towards addictions in the colonial discourse, it is perhaps surprising that only Meilhon's statistics gave addictions as the most frequent diagnosis in Muslim men. Kocher, Criminalité, 70; Meilhon, Aliénation mentale, part 2, 191; Livet, Aliénés algériens, 70; Reboul/Régis, Assistance, 51–4.

182 This coincides with postcolonial psychiatric notions of the prevalence of somatisation among Arabs in general and North Africans in particular. Boucebci, Aspects de la psychiatrie, 179 f.; Bennani, Psychanalyse, 241 f.; Okasha/Karam, Mental Health Services, 407.

183 This explains why Meilhon only had five different diagnoses among his ten female Muslim patients. Meilhon, Aliénation mentale, part 2, 191.

184 Jean Sutter, for instance, described in 1937 that it was possible to observe "expired" European mental disorders "revived" in North Africa. Sutter, Épilepsie mentale, 13. This theory was

Meilhon, writing in 1891 about the prevalence of mania and aggressive behaviour amongst Muslim North African patients, claimed: "[...] manic forms, aggressive tendencies, these are the two main characteristics of the madness of Arabs, among whom we find, as in any little civilised race, the elementary forms of insanity, [which have] almost disappeared from our asylums."[185] A very similar statement was made by Reboul and Régis, summarising their 1912 Congress report: "By analysing and comparing the various observations received and published on this point of view, we come, however, to the conclusion that psychopathy, in natives, presents itself in its simplest types, such as degeneration in all degrees, manic states, melancholic states, rudimentary systematised delusions, and that, almost always, this psychopathy bears the stamp of religious ideas and tribal superstitions and is accompanied by intensive exterior reactions, sometimes even becoming like those grimacing [female] dancing maniacs, screaming, gesticulating and dancing, which characterised certain epidemics of our insanity of the Middle Ages."[186] If these theories of Islamic medievalism formed the basis of the expectations with which colonial psychiatrists approached their Muslim patients, it is understandable that only a small number of non-complex disorders were ever diagnosed.

Some of these "elementary" diagnoses became umbrella terms for a variety of symptoms that French psychiatrists could not otherwise classify. By far the most common diagnosis for Muslim women was the not very clearly defined "mania", with its main symptom "agitation". Once it was established that mania was prevalent in Muslim patients, diagnosing general symptoms as mania became easier, as French colonial psychiatrists depended heavily on precedents set by earlier psychiatrists. This prevalence can be partly explained by the fact that most psychiatrists understood neither Arabic nor the Berber dialects.[187] The same problems were encountered in the treatment of Senegalese patients transported to France, as Paul Borreil described in 1908: "This difficulty in interpreting the actions or gestures of these lunatics can only lead to lamentable errors. A patient arrives with a card bearing the diagnosis of mania. The doctor cannot question him, he would not be understood; the patient cannot show whether he is aware of the new situation he finds himself in [...]. Can he at least make himself understood by gestures? Alas! The facial expressions of these people are often so different from ours that the interpretation may be completely erroneous."[188] For these linguistically and culturally untrained psychiatrists, the North African

---

analysed by Alice Bullard in 2001: Bullard, Truth in Madness, 121.
185 Meilhon, Contribution, 388.
186 Reboul/Régis, Assistance, 14.
187 Gervais, Contribution, 23; Marie, Question, 418; Sutter, Épilepsie mentale, 150; Susini, Aspects cliniques, 124.
188 Borreil, Considérations, 25. See also: Fribourg-Blanc, État mental, 143.

languages and ways of speaking appeared to be violent, and perhaps some of them misinterpreted the energy of the language as a psychiatric problem. Vadon explained in his 1935 dissertation: "Moreover, the violence of language, the hyperactivity natural to Oriental races, make reactions, which would seem to border on maniacal agitation in a Frenchmen or a European, go unnoticed in a Tunisian."[189] While their aggressive – and for the colonial psychiatrists incomprehensible – languages protected North African lunatics from being identified in the first place, they also made the diagnosis of mania more likely in patients interned for other, not as easily detectable and diagnosable, disorders.[190]

The language barrier influenced diagnoses on another level – diagnosing patients with complex symptoms was difficult, as some of the "more civilised" diagnoses relied, to some degree, on communication between doctors and patients. Being unable to communicate their grievances, these patients were reduced to their physical symptoms, which might in turn have facilitated "simple" diagnoses.

3.4 French Colonial Statistics as a Historical Source

As mentioned in the introduction to this chapter, there are several problems when analysing the presence of female Muslim patients in French colonial psychiatric statistics – psychiatrists were not obliged to compile annual statistics; the data was selective, very often actively excluding Muslim women;[191] and both the paucity and recycling of colonial statistics make comparisons between them impossible. Worse, the numerical evidence that was used was often confused with details from other statistics taken out of context and contained many contradictions and elementary

189 Vadon, Assistance, 44. The same has been noted in other African contexts. G. Allen German described in his 1987 article that the "more dramatic presentations [...] were first noted and put forward as peculiar to the continent". German, Mental Health in Africa II, 443.

190 Only a few of the French colonial psychiatrists relied on interpreters in their diagnoses, and those North Africans who served as interpreters were usually patients themselves. This problematic use of North African psychiatric patients as interpreters will be examined in Chapter 4.4.2 "Psychotherapy", p. 170.

191 One important question is whether Muslim women could be included in the general category of men (i.e. human beings) if they were not separately mentioned. It is important to ask whether colonial psychiatrists saw men and women as part of a colonial population that could be described as male, while still including all females. While this is difficult to argue in the theories, where the colonial norm is very clearly male, many statistics were genderless, as, for example: Meilhon, Aliénation mentale, part 2, 190; Livet, Aliénés algériens, 48; Reboul/Régis, Assistance, 50; Maréschal/Chaurand, Paralysie générale, 248.

calculation errors.[192] This lack of context allowed for certain estimates and hypotheses to become "facts". In 1911, for instance, as shown above, the French psychiatrists Lwoff and Sérieux, comparing Morocco with Egypt, concluded that Morocco should have had 15–20,000 madmen – a figure far greater than the actual number interned in the traditional asylums and beyond the capacity of any planned psychiatric hospital.[193] In the same year, Livet calculated that Algeria should really have had about 25,000 Algerian lunatics.[194] Both Lwoff and Sérieux's comparison[195] and Livet's complicated calculations[196] were taken up by psychiatrists at the 1912 Congress – not as the rather fanciful estimates they were, but as "scientific truths".

The way some psychiatrists handled statistical evidence is also highly problematic, such as in Meilhon's statistics, which seem to have served as illustrations of what he already "knew".[197] Other psychiatrists referred to statistical evidence without producing figures or giving references. The psychiatrist Camille-Charles Gervais repeatedly alluded to unspecified statistical evidence in his 1907 dissertation: "When considering the sex of our patients, we can say that women are less frequent: 10%."[198] Whether he took this percentage from an unspecified patient population from his own experience at Aix-en-Provence, quoted some now untraceable statistics, or just repeated a common belief cannot be deduced anymore. Another quote by Gervais suggests his statistical evidence was nothing more than "conventionally" accepted common knowledge. Concerning Arabs and Berbers in French care, he claimed "Berbers, who constitute two thirds [of the Algerian population], are hardly numerous at the asylum in Aix, about a fifth, according to convention."[199] If Gervais' estimate of 10% for

---

192 Livet, for example, miscalculated the total of patients from the three Algerian departments for the year 1907. Livet, Aliénés algériens, 49. This error was corrected by Reboul and Régis, who used Livet's statistical information. Reboul/Régis, Assistance, 42. Other calculation errors can be found in the tables by Reboul and Régis. The totals of dementia and delirium sufferers at the asylum in Saint-Alban derived from the numbers of the different groups simply do not add up, and the total of patients in Saint-Pons does not match the different diseases. Ibid., 53 f.

193 Lwoff/Sérieux, Aliénés au Maroc, 475.

194 Livet, Aliénés algériens, 37.

195 Reboul/Régis, Assistance, 78; Abadie, Report, 379; Naudin, Psychiatrie coloniale, 13.

196 Reboul/Régis, Assistance, 49 f.; Abadie, Report, 379; Dupouy, Chronique, 529.

197 "And indeed, for those who lived among them, there is no need for statistical results to assert their extreme malignity [...]." Meilhon, Aliénation mentale, part 2, 178. See also: Ibid., part 1, 21 f. This seems to have occurred in other aspects of colonial medicine in Algeria: Pierre Montaldo stated that abortions were very frequent in Algeria, but added, "[...] our personal statistics give us for the Arabs and the Kabyles only a very small number of abortions, certainly well below the reality." He demonstrated, therefore, that his statistics could only be trusted as far as they coincided with the things he "knew" to be true. Montaldo, Mortalité infantile, 88 ff.

198 Gervais, Contribution, 48.

199 Ibid., 47.

female Muslim patients therefore stemmed from a pool of speculative knowledge shared by French colonial psychiatrists, it is important to repeat that this perceived percentage was far below the actual ratio of Muslim women to Muslim men in the statistical evidence.[200]

By far the biggest problem for a historical analysis of the numerical evidence in French colonial psychiatric texts are the gaps in the statistics, a fact bitterly felt by many psychiatric and medical experts. Jules Brault admitted in 1905 that "the disorders of these two categories [diseases of the circulatory system and of the nervous system] are rather rare, as far as can be judged outside of firm statistics."[201] Brault did not connect this regrettable lack with his own professional duties – it remained unclear who should have compiled these "firm statistics" if not he himself.[202] It was usually understood that the compiling of evidence, which could in turn be used by psychiatrists in their theoretical writings, could not be left to non-experts with only limited understanding of psychiatric problems, a point taken up by Louis Lauriol in 1938: "However, as we shall see concerning the psychiatric assistance, psychiatrists are still rare at present, and here lies an important point for the veracity of the statistics."[203]

Trustworthy figures could therefore only be compiled by psychiatrists themselves. Those psychiatrists who did, like Kocher, Meilhon or Livet, seem to have mostly done so because of a personal interest in statistics. Kocher, for example, seems to have felt a deep trust in the powers of statistical evidence.[204] Besides their own findings, they used all the data available and gave the best historical overviews of the statistics of their times. But for many French colonial psychiatrists, statistics were just not part of their interpretation of their duties. Collecting numerical evidence was secondary to keeping settlers safe[205] – by determining who should be institutionalised – and

---

200   See Appendix B, Fig. 6, p. 268.

201   Brault, Pathologie et hygiène, 57.

202   This lack of statistical evidence and the confusion about who should compile statistics was also a problem in other French colonies, as Jeanselme stated in 1905: "In the absence of statistics, it is impossible to say whether madness is as frequent in the Far East as in the West. What is certain is that the insane are not uncommon among the yellow races. They seem to be a highly fertile ground for neuroses." Jeanselme, Condition des aliénés, 497. Ibrahim Sow stated in 1978 that the "rarity and the punctual character" of statistical research on mental troubles in Africa made conclusive statements about the frequency of mental morbidity impossible. Sow, Structures anthropologiques, 16.

203   Lauriol, Quelques remarques, 9.

204   Writing on the rarity of insanity in Arabs, Islamic notions of legal responsibility and the consequences of climate on French settlers, Kocher stated that "only a statistic could give us the solution to these diverse questions." Kocher, Criminalité, 69.

205   See Chapter 2 on the admission processes which favoured the criminally insane.

formulating theories.[206] Georges Sicard, for instance, claimed in 1907 that statistical evidence was not as important as gaining a deeper understanding of North African psyches. He had been discussing the fact that nervous diseases had dramatically multiplied recently and asked whether they really were as rare as had been believed: "But if the question arises, the solution is not easy. If it were only to highlight the proportion of nervous disorders among the Arabs and the Europeans, this would be only a question of numbers and it would be sufficient to accumulate statistics; but such a consideration would be only of mediocre interest. The thing that is important to know is the sensitivity of the nervous system of the natives."[207]

Some psychiatrists did see the lack of data as a personal failing. Pierre Maréschal, head of the Manouba Psychiatric Hospital in Tunis, who left Tunisia after its independence in 1956, regretted that he had neglected the collection of statistical source material: "Certainly, the clinical spoils of my 20 years of Tunisian psychiatry may seem meagre; I feel its whole inadequacy. Properly filed documents and precise statistics could have given some substance to this article."[208] During his 20 years of leading the only psychiatric hospital in Tunisia, collecting numerical evidence appears to have been of secondary importance to him, and no administrative office seems to have requested statistical accounts from him or his staff.

Most of the time, however, North African Muslims were blamed for the absence of statistical evidence, as it was believed that both patients and family members did not cooperate with the French officials in the collection of data. It was believed that Islamic fatalism and respect for lunatics stopped North Africans from contacting the colonial experts[209] and that, consequently, this lack of reporting undermined the statistics, as the North African non-scientific understanding of mental problems conducted them towards traditional healers rather than educated scientists. Henry Bouquet, for example, wrote in 1909: "It is very difficult to know the frequency of insanity among Muslims precisely because the insane are ignored. It is impossible for us to give figures for Tunisia."[210] The grievous insistence of North Africans to let patients either roam freely or be looked after by their families obstructed and falsified the colonial

---

206 See Chapter 1 on the theories on the abnormal normality of Muslims and on the influence of civilisation on human psychopathology.
207 Sicard, Étude, 49.
208 Maréschal, Réflexions, 79.
209 Goëau-Brissonnière, for example, exclaimed in 1926: "As seen, fatalism and religion in their dominant note, put their powerful seals on Algerian medical statistics." Goëau-Brissonnière, Syphilis nerveuse, 65. See also: Marie, Sur quelques aspects, 767; Margain, Aliénation mentale, 89; Susini, Quelques considérations, 27 f.; Marill/Si Hassen, Paralysie générale, 435.
210 Bouquet, Aliénés en Tunisie, 25. See also: Mignot, Journées médicales, 160 f.

records.[211] Desruelles and Bersot quoted, in 1939, Meilhon's 1896 article on the rarity of insanity among Arabs, adding: "Obviously, this proportion of alienated Arabs compared to the indigenous population (5 per 100,000 inhabitants) is extremely low, which Meilhon attributes to the fatalistic and resigned character of the natives. We do not think so; as in all countries where the proportion of the insane seems very low compared to the population, the insane in Algeria were very poorly recorded and a great number of them remained at large, in prison or sequestered by their families."[212]

Even though statistics were relatively unimportant in the writings of French colonial psychiatrists, they were interpreted as a metaphor for modernity – the lack of statistical thinking was seen to be a dividing line between the French and the Muslims. In 1889 the French military doctor Lucien Bertholon, working on criminal insanity in Tunisia, addressed the Muslim inability to appreciate statistics: "We are dealing with a society with delayed evolution, compared to ours. Notions of time, distance, numbers, etc., are almost unknown to most of its members. Statistics are a myth for them. Maybe this exotic plant will become acclimatised on Berber ground."[213]

This negligence of the native population, both in their reaction to mental disorders and in their stance towards the gathering of records and statistics, meant the numbers collected by French colonial psychiatry were "wrong" in any case, and therefore not worth compiling. After a presentation given by Maréschal and Chaurand on "General Paralysis in Tunisia" at the Nancy Congress in 1937, Antoine Porot joined the discussion, adding: "*In terms of statistics*, our services have only received patients indirectly, if I may say, because of an anti-social reaction; they [the numbers available] do not reflect the proportional importance of G. P. [general paralysis] as compared to other [forms of] psychopathy."[214] French colonial psychiatrists were aware that Muslims somehow slipped through their statistical net, which worked so well for European populations. The psychiatrist Georges Sicard, for instance, wrote in 1907: "However, while the number of Europeans encompasses almost all cases, there is, on the contrary, no doubt that most of the alienated natives escape confinement and therefore the statistics."[215] These French colonial psychiatrists were thus conscious of their statistical evidence being faulty and consequently distrusted their own information: they knew that their statistics over-represented Europeans and presented an incorrect picture of insanity being a largely European problem, but they did little about it.

---

211 Olry regretted as late as 1940 that "the mass of Arab populations of the countryside remains outside our field of observation." Olry, Paralysie générale, 17.
212 Desruelles/Bersot, Assistance aux aliénés en Algérie, 584.
213 Bertholon, Esquisse, 390.
214 Maréschal/Chaurand, Paralysie générale, 254. Emphasis in the original.
215 Sicard, Étude, 67.

While French psychiatrists were aware of these problems, they failed to spot the contradictions between the statistical evidence they used and their accompanying texts and theories. One example of this contradiction concerns the "mythe berbère", pitting the good Berber against the lazy, dangerous Arab.[216] This was one of the cornerstones of early French colonialism in North Africa, and even though many colonial psychiatric texts singled out the distinctions between Berbers and Arabs in explaining the different behaviour of the patients and non-patients from these "races",[217] this distinction was very rarely reflected in the psychiatric statistics. There were only a few exceptions to this: Abel-Joseph Meilhon, for instance, distinguished between Arabs and Kabyles in his statistics concerning Muslims in the asylum in Aix-en-Provence in 1880, meticulously filling in table after table for Arab men, Arab women, Kabyle men and Kabyle women – even though there were no Kabyle women in the asylum at that time.[218]

Similarly, as discussed in Chapters 1 and 2, theories of Muslim normality claimed that all Muslim women (patients and non-patients alike) were quiet and docile. This was one of the main justifications given as to why there were fewer female patients in an environment that mainly segregated the dangerous insane. As mentioned above, the main diagnosis for Muslim women, however, was mania, and the case studies show that these "manic" women were very often agitated and deeply aggressive. Another colonial pet theory claimed that Muslim women never suffered from addictions because they followed Islamic religious regulations to the letter, yet one finds female alcoholics in the statistical evidence. These contradictions between expectations, based on widespread theories on femininity, and experiences, based on professional contact with agitated female maniacs and alcoholics, did not find their way into the theories or readjust them – instead, these contradictions seem to have simply gone "unnoticed".

Today, psychiatric theories are often firmly based on statistical evidence.[219] For French colonial psychiatrists this was not the case – their statistics on North Africa were useful because they illustrated already formulated theories and reinforced "truths" that could be applied to any situation, period and area, gaining authority with each additional quotation. Covering these snapshot-statistics from such a broad period

---

216 The theories concerning the superiority of the Berbers over the Arabs have been analysed by
      Patricia Lorcin in 1995: Lorcin, Imperial Identities, 248–53.
217 Gervais, Contribution, 47 f.; Levet, Assistance, 60 f.; Arrii, Impulsivité criminelle, 30. Distinc-
      tions were also made between certain diseases among Arabs and Berbers, for example in: Livet,
      Aliénés algériens, 69.
218 Meilhon, Aliénation mentale, part 2, 191.
219 Hand, Role of Statistics, 471; Everitt, Statistics in Psychiatry, 110. See, for example: Chaleby,
      Psychosocial Stresses, 149; Al-Krenawi, Women from Polygamous and Monogamous Mar-
      riages, 192.

is less than ideal for historical analysis, but it was essential in order to recreate the academic discourse. The ease with which colonial psychiatrists took each other's statistics out of context, the lack of critical thinking displayed by their failure to spot not just elementary errors in calculation but outright random numbers in the data, and their disregard for statistics that contradicted their pre-conceived ideas helps to understand how colonial psychiatry functioned and calls into question the validity of their theories.

The purpose of this chapter was to place the neglect of North African women in colonial psychiatric writing into context. To French colonial psychiatrists, the low numbers of female Muslim patients caused and justified this neglect, even though women made up a quarter of all Muslim patients. The interest shown in female Muslim patients had no correlation with the statistical evidence from the colonial institutions – the weight given to Muslim women in colonial theories did not mirror their actual numbers and Muslim women were not as rare in the hospital populations as the general assumptions made them out to be. The idea that the small numbers of female Muslim patients justified the disregard shown towards them in the theories is nonsensical. While there was a pronounced statistical interest in the rarity of insanity among Muslims in general in the 19th century, this did not extend to female Muslim patients, among whom, after all, insanity was rarest of all.

Most of the compelling questions that an analysis of colonial psychiatric statistics raises – the fluctuations in female Muslim patient numbers over time and in different asylums; the over-representation of Muslim women among the patients who died and their under-representation among those cured; the narrow variety of disorders they were diagnosed with; and the fact that the majority of diagnoses consisted of just a handful of diseases – went completely unnoticed by French psychiatrists, who neither explained nor even alluded to them in their theories. Given the tiny amount of statistical evidence and the even smaller interest in female patients that colonial psychiatrists had, it seems that it was enough simply to "know" that there were substantially fewer female Muslim patients – something that was instantly, almost instinctively, understood by colonial psychiatrists, habituated to civilisational explanations of the numbers of the insane.

Chapter 4
Treating Deviance: The Shock of the New

4.1 Case Study on Treatments and the Question of Civilisation

In 1959 the psychiatrists Jean Sutter, Robert Susini, Yves Pélicier and Gérard Pascalis wrote an article on "Nuptial Psychoses in Algerian Muslims", in which they published three case studies on female Muslim patients. One of these case studies concerned a 19-year-old female patient, described as a "brunette girl, with harmonious features and well-groomed". She was admitted to Blida Psychiatric Hospital on the 11th of March 1959 in a "state of atypical agitation", which was, allegedly, improved by "three days of isolation and electroshocks". Sutter and his colleagues described their patient as comparatively civilised, having grown up in the suburbs of Algiers "where the modes of European and Muslim life are most intimately intertwined". Sutter et al. then went on to describe the patient's family in some detail, thereby implying that the degree of civilisation of her family had some influence on the development of her mental disorder. According to them, her father was a small artisan, "her mother [was] veiled and [did] not often leave the house", but her two older brothers had attended school and even attained an elementary certificate. The psychiatrists further explained that their patient did not possess this same level of education, adding that they did not know whether she had tried and failed or whether she had just never tried. However, the additional information in the case study clearly shows that she could not have attended school regularly because of health reasons. As she suffered from coxalgia and apparently tuberculosis, the patient had spent long periods of her childhood, between the ages of six and 14, in French hospitals in and around Algiers. The psychiatrists described the effect of these formative years spent in French medical care as follows: "She enjoys the comfort [in these hospitals], the cleanliness, which contrasts with the state of the family home. She gets very spoiled there by her aunt, [who was] hospitalised in a neighbouring house, and by the nuns [who work at these hospitals]. Above all, and this is the most important fact, for several years [she] lived in close contact with the European hospital staff." At the age of 14, she returned to her parents "where she was veiled and became more or less a servant of her brothers", to which the psychiatrists remarked: "The years at the hospital have clearly left her ill-prepared for this fate."[1]

Her psychiatric problems fully developed once her family decided that it was time for her to get married, which the psychiatrists explained as follows: "Her previous

---

1 Sutter et al., Quelques observations, 909.

illness allowed her to escape for some time from the all too inevitable, traditional marriage. Then a serious suitor presented himself, who was approved by her parents. She has never seen him, her whole family being opposed to such a break with traditions. Between [her] and her parents, arguments are frequent, the tone rises. After a discussion [which was] more violent than others – we hear that she was again beaten – [she] became so agitated that she tried to kill herself; she was [then] taken to the hospital. The clinical diagnosis is that of a reactive psycho-neurosis; discrete mental confusion, accompanied by dreams: two women, one white and one black, call [her], while she, to escape them, wants to throw herself off a wall. This highly significant nightmare is interspersed with complaints: 'Let me die! I have suffered too much, my parents do not understand me.'" Despite this serious diagnosis, however, the psychiatrists managed to cure her by the psychoanalytic treatment of abreaction, and she was released – back to her family – after a short period of time.[2]

This case study of a Muslim woman, who was described as at least partly civilised, is extraordinarily extensive and many of its details conform to the general hypotheses of female Muslim normality discussed in Chapter 1: the young patient was primarily portrayed as a victim – a victim of her family, traditions and, at least potentially, her future husband. Through her physical diseases, she came into contact with French hospital staff – a contact which civilised her to a degree that made it impossible for her to be reintegrated into the caged "normality" of Muslim women. Sutter et al. saw her partial civilisation and her subsequent detachment from "Muslim culture" as the ultimate reason for her psychiatric breakdown. If she had not been partly civilised, it is implied, she would have accepted the marriage her parents had decided upon, just as she would not have minded being her elder brothers' "servant". The reasons for her unrest and agitation would therefore simply not have arisen.

In the context of this chapter on treatments, however, this case study is illustrative because it shows both the traditional, aggressive, physical treatments – used in the first period of her institutionalisation to calm her down – and the modern therapies, as shown by her being cured by abreaction. This shows that both forms of therapies, which will be discussed in detail in this chapter, could be used on the same patients, depending on the patient's behaviour. A patient could be subjected to electroshocks and neuroleptics,[3] when aggressive or agitated, or receive forms of psychotherapy if he/she exhibited "civilised" behaviour.

---

2   Ibid.

3   Neuroleptics, such as Largactil, are antipsychotic drugs, usually applied in cases of psychoses. Hakkou, Traitements, 244 f.

4.2 Treating Muslim Patients

This chapter analyses the treatment of patients, particularly female Muslim patients, in colonial psychiatric institutions in France and North Africa. It examines the psychiatric theories behind those treatments, and the case studies accompanying those theories, over the colonial period. Treating patients with innovative methods and according to a "civilised" humanitarianism was an integral part of the self-understanding of colonial psychiatry.[4] Especially in the 20th century, colonial psychiatry was defined, or, rather, defined itself, by the experimental and progressive treatments implemented in the colonies. Even though some French colonial psychiatrists were critical of certain treatments, the majority saw the history of psychiatry in North Africa as an accelerated narrative of progress, developing before their very eyes, under their guidance, so to speak, from the medieval barbarism in the traditional Islamic *māristāns* to the enlightenment of modern science. This chapter traces the development of treatments available to Muslims in general, and Muslim women in particular, in theory and in practice. French colonial psychiatry implemented a variety of new approaches to curing mental illness in North Africa: from early, deeply ideological therapies to the advent of psychosurgery, the medicalisation of psychiatry, and finally the restrained introduction of psychotherapy and other social treatments. These treatments will be analysed chronologically. First, the early institutionalisation of patients as a form of treatment will be examined, followed by the treatments during the heyday of psychiatric innovation, the 1930s to 1950s, which have been further divided in order of patient involvement. Finally, problems in the implementation of treatments, their effectiveness and the criticisms voiced against them will be contrasted with psychiatry's self-representation as a contributor to human progress.

4.3 Morals and Degeneration

The 19th century was an important period for French psychiatry, as it endeavoured both to become an independent science of medical experts and to develop a variety of new theoretical frameworks to cement its own budding authority.[5] But it was also

---

4   This combination of humanitarianism and scientific progress was, according to Eugene Rogan in 2002, one of the main components of colonial psychiatry: "the introduction of European norms in the treatment of the mentally ill in a colonial situation gave rise to a 'distinctly colonial psychiatry' that could be justified in terms of modern science". Rogan, Madness and Marginality, 105.

5   Psychiatry in the 19th century had to fight its first battle of legitimacy against the Catholic Church, which also claimed patronage over the insane. This process has been described by

a time in which first the collection and then – because of the resulting overcrowding – the curing of patients became more important. Summarising two classics of the history of psychiatry, Michel Foucault's "Madness and Civilisation"[6] and Andrew Scull's "Decarceration", Ludmilla Jordanova outlined in 1981 four distinct phases in the treatment of insanity in Europe. The first phase, which she called "toleration and integration of the insane", lasted until the mid-17th century. The second phase, one of incarceration of all undesirables, called by Foucault "le grand renfermement", "the Great Confinement",[7] persisted until the end of the 18th century. During the third phase, the 19th and early 20th century, only those undesirables labelled "insane" by the medical establishment were incarcerated and this coincided with the development of the new treatments discussed in this chapter. The last phase started with World War II, called "decarceration" by Scull, which started to give patients more physical freedom.[8]

For this chapter, only the third phase of Jordanova's periodisation is of relevance, beginning at the start of the 19th century and made legally binding in 1838 when France, as mentioned in Chapter 2, passed a law that required all lunatics to be looked after in asylums, which were to be under the exclusive authority of doctors.[9] The fourth phase, the process of "decarceration" did start tentatively in the 1930s in North Africa with the introduction of social work[10] and later with some open services,[11] but the policy of giving patients more physical freedom was only really implemented once independence was gained.[12] During the 19th century, the psychiatric treatment of Muslim patients was mainly influenced by the opposing theories of "moral therapy" and "degeneration" as well as by the aforementioned general ideology of incarcerating all mentally ill, which underpinned both theories. Under both sets of theories, French psychiatry was characterised by the absence of any conventional "medical" treatment – the

---

the historian Jan Goldstein in her 2001 book. Goldstein, Console and Classify, 5.

6   "Histoire de la folie à l'âge classique".

7   Foucault, Histoire de la folie, 67.

8   Jordanova, Mental Illness, 110.

9   See p. 74. Goldstein, Hysteria Diagnosis, 221; Dowbiggin, Inheriting Madness, 4; Harsin, Gender, Class, and Madness, 1050 f.

10   Demassieux, Service social, 18

11   Bennani, Psychanalyse, 165.

12   Psychiatry in the postcolonial Maghreb states remained classic and often conservative, relying mainly on aggressive medical forms of therapies, especially electroshocks and the so-called chemotherapies – i.e. therapies with chemical drugs. See for example: L'activité des services de santé mentale dans l'ouest algérien, 820; Douki et al., Psychiatrie en Tunisie, 51. The same tendency towards "somatic methods, neuroleptics and electro-convulsive therapy" was observed in the psychiatric services of the "Arab East" by John Racy in 1970 and confirmed by others. Racy, Psychiatry in the Arab East, 41; 49 f.; Al-Issa/Al-Issa, Psychiatric Problems, 21; Salem-Pickartz, Mental Health, 268.

therapeutic zeitgeist of the 19th century recommended therapies which were not based on drugs or operations. Sometimes, as in the case of prophylactic measures stemming from the theory of degeneration, the proposed treatments were not even aimed at the patients themselves. In the colonial context of the Maghreb, Muslim patients shipped to France did not benefit from any specific therapies – at least no comments on treatments could be found in the case studies or in the accompanying texts.[13] Being institutionalised in an asylum became a medical treatment in itself.[14]

Towards the end of the 18th century, the French psychiatrist Philippe Pinel had started to develop what is now called the "moral therapy" or "moral treatment" of psychiatric patients, based on the idea that, while suffering from essentially organic disorders, external factors also had an influence on the development of mental illness. This revolutionised the asylum system in France. Patients were no longer restrained by physical chains,[15] but by what Foucault called "moral chains",[16] the capacity to be cured being contingent on the individual will and determination of the patients.[17] The institutions caring for patients were intended to correspond with humanitarian ideas of modernity,[18] and the treatment of patients in these reformed institutions was fundamentally social, and therefore non-medical,[19] focusing on tight control of inmates instead. Cleanliness, serenity, order and a moral surrounding were the main pillars of this new therapy.[20] Michel Foucault put the humanitarianism of this theory into perspective, focusing on the punitive aspects of Pinel's moral therapy, used at once to "infantilise" and "blame" the mad:[21] if insanity was the result of social and especially moral factors, then a mental disorder had to be due to individual misconduct.[22] In

---

13   Abel-Joseph Meilhon's 1896 case studies of Muslim women, for example, did not mention their treatments. Meilhon, Aliénation mentale, part 2, 195–205; part 3, 366–71; part 4, 40; part 6, 353 f.

14   This was also true for contemporary French patients, as proposed by Foucault. Foucault, Maladie mentale, 84.

15   However, straitjackets were still used as a form of "treatment". Jill Harsin analysed this in her 1992 article: Harsin, Gender, Class, and Madness, 1050, especially FN 7. In North Africa, straitjackets were used until the 1950s. Gervais, Contribution, 8; Taïeb, Idées d'influence, 89; Bennani, Psychanalyse, 165; Douki et al., Psychiatrie en Tunisie, 51.

16   Foucault, Maladie mentale, 84 f.

17   Skultans, Introduction, 1 f.

18   Dowbiggin, Inheriting Madness, 4.

19   Goldstein, Console and Classify, 200.

20   Scull, Museum of Madness Revisited, 10. The medical historian Roy Porter fittingly wrote in 1981: "If Freudian psycho-analysis is the talking cure, moral therapy hoped to be cure by silence." Porter, Being Mad, 46.

21   Foucault, Maladie mentale, 85 f.

22   Dowbiggin, Inheriting Madness, 1.

this explanation, mental patients had committed socially and morally reprehensible wrongs, which had caused the disorder in them and could be cured by learning to control themselves. This "infantilisation" of the patients coincided with psychiatric institutions becoming increasingly patriarchal, with the psychiatrist taking on the role of *pater familias* within the asylums.[23] According to the feminist writer Elaine Showalter, whose controversial theses on women and psychiatry were mentioned in Chapter 3,[24] this patriarchal structure had an influence on female patients, as – in this gendered environment – they were expected to behave in a decidedly feminine manner. Those who did not comply with these notions of femininity were deemed "more insane".[25]

Support for the theory of moral therapy declined towards the end of the 19th century, caused mainly by the chronic overcrowding of the existing asylums, which was not only a result of the incarceration of all mental patients but a clear indicator that moral treatment was unsuccessful. By the middle of the 19th century, a new theory had started to gain attention among French psychiatrist: the theory of degeneration,[26] which explained the rising numbers of patients in the asylum system through an evolutionary worldview. The miserable lives led by the lower classes and, importantly, by their parents and grandparents before them, assigned them to an inferior state of evolution, of which mental problems were just one symptom. In this disillusioned interpretation of mental illness, the treatment of patients affected by degenerative diseases was seen to be in vain: psychiatrists could never hope to cure degenerates.

One of the two psychiatrists who formed the theory of psychiatric degeneration was Jacques-Joseph Moreau de Tours, who had written the first account of insanity in the Orient, published in the *Annales Médico-Psychologiques* in 1843. During his travels he witnessed, among other things, the dangers of heredity,[27] and in 1859 he published a treatise on these problems entitled "Morbid Psychology". The other psychiatrist was Bénédict-Augustin Morel, who wrote a book entitled "Treatise of Physical, Intellectual and Moral Degeneration in the Human Species" in 1857. According to Morel, degeneration was a departure from an ideal form of humanity[28] and could be caused by alcoholism and other drug addictions, malnutrition, and unhygienic

---

23 Foucault, Histoire de la folie, 626 f.; Showalter, Female Malady, 50.
24 See p. 124, FN 110.
25 Showalter analysed the preoccupation of psychiatrists with the idea that female patients should make themselves look presentable. Showalter, Female Malady, 84.
26 Dowbiggin, Degeneration, 188.
27 The dangers of heredity were "shown" through the tolerance towards mad Arab saints, who were allegedly allowed to have sexual intercourse in public with any woman they chose and spread their insanity in this way. Moreau, Recherches, 119. For a discussion of this myth in French colonial psychiatry, see: Studer, 'Pregnant with Madness'.
28 See for example: Walter, What Became of the Degenerate, 423.

housing. However, the main reason was heredity.[29] The aim of psychiatry was to protect society from these potentially dangerous degenerates.[30]

The idea that insanity was caused by hereditary problems was common among colonial psychiatrists, who, like Bouquet in 1909, writing about the situation in Tunisia, suspected that, in the colonies, "a large majority of mental troubles is the consequence of phenomena of degeneration, of heredity."[31] In the North African context, this mental degeneration was linked with "race" and consequently questions of heredity dovetailed with racial stereotypes, as seen, for example, in the following quote by Abel-Joseph Meilhon from 1896: "Early marriages further increase the chances of insanity in the offspring; married at ten years, Arab women, although already nubile, often cannot create more than a product destined for moral and physical decay."[32] Meilhon imagined the alleged precocious nubility of Muslim girls[33] to be purely sensual and therefore doubly reprehensible. The colonial psychiatrists agreed that excessive sexuality, especially of and with children, was morally wrong, but even aside from that moral judgement, this form of sexuality could not fulfil, in these young girls, its only justification – the healthy propagation of the "race". Although capable of sexual intercourse, Muslim girls could not yet bear undamaged, non-degenerate children. The decadent lifestyle of the North African masses, already degenerate purely because of their "race",[34] could not lead to psychiatrically healthy offspring – even though, as shown in previous chapters, Meilhon himself was acutely aware of the "rarity" of insanity among Muslims.

In this theory, heredity had doomed those patients suffering from psychiatric degeneration to physical and moral ruin. Since these current patient populations were incurable, prophylaxis against insanity in future generations became a cornerstone of psychiatric concern. As late as 1938, Henri Aubin reminded psychiatrists at the Congress in Algiers of the duties of psychiatric assistance: "[…] our conceptions have profoundly changed: we certainly did not abandon the maintenance of chronic cases, the palliative treatments which are provided for them, the defence of property, the protection of Society against dangerous lunatics, the guarantees of individual freedom, etc.; but the progress of Mental Pathology showed us that we

---

29 Baruk, Psychiatrie française, 87 f.; Dowbiggin, Inheriting Madness, 2.
30 For example: Pick, Faces of Degeneration, 73.
31 Bouquet, Aliénés en Tunisie, 27. See also: Reboul/Régis, Assistance, 14.
32 Meilhon, Aliénation mentale, part 1, 29.
33 Discussed in Chapter 1 under the heading "Sexualité Précoce".
34 While the psychiatric theory of degeneration was separate from theories of "racial" or gender degeneration prevalent in the 19th century, it cannot be seen isolated from them. Regarding concepts of "racial" degeneration, see for instance: Pick, Faces of Degeneration, 21; 37; 73; McClintock, Imperial Leather, 43 f.; 254.

could do more fruitful work by attaching ourselves to the prevention of mental disorders, to the treatment of the initial stages and pre-psychotic states."[35] Aubin advocated a broadening of psychiatric duties in order to save future generations from the degeneration observable in psychiatric patients – for example, by prohibiting drugs, eradicating venereal diseases and implementing consultations for children.[36] He went on to state that, in the colonies, questions of psychiatric prophylaxis and of the control they entailed were important, particularly with regard to the "natives": "We have to prove to the administrative authorities *that psychiatric assistance has become a socially essential work and* [one] *of economic interest*, as it effectively contributes to the conservation, to the enhancement, to the physical and intellectual improvement of the population."[37] Thus, rather than treat and cure them, it was more economical to prevent "natives" from overcrowding the newly constructed psychiatric hospitals by hindering their eventual degeneration and by helping them to become "physically and intellectually improved".

By the time the first French psychiatrists wrote about their personal experiences with North African patients (Kocher in 1883 and Meilhon in 1891), both sets of theories had profoundly influenced not only psychiatry and medicine but also wider society. In the therapeutic context, the advent of new theories – for example the emergence and decline of the hypothesis of insanity depending on the climate[38] – did not supplant the very general treatments that had been implemented by moral therapy, at least not in the colonies. The treatments were no longer seen to be, strictly speaking, beneficial as therapies, but they were common sense, part of how a civilised asylum should work, fighting against the overcrowding in the asylums. In the following pages, three of these early common sense treatments and their implementation will be analysed (labour, food and spatial orderliness), even though there are very few allusions in the sources to either these or other treatments in relation to Muslim patients.

One of the key factors of moral treatment had been the assumption that the patients needed to be appropriately occupied in order to heal.[39] Tightly scheduled work was described as being of therapeutic value for certain patients, while the labour

---

35 Aubin, Assistance, 149. Capitalisation in the original.
36 Aubin saw these measures as a way in which psychiatrists could help the *"increase of the population* and especially the *improvement of the race"*. Ibid. Emphasis in the original.
37 Ibid. Emphasis in the original.
38 This theory had been advocated by, among others, Jacques-Joseph Moreau de Tours in 1843, who emphasised the influence of the changing seasons on mental illness. Moreau, Recherches, 120. Though soon dismissed as a general psychiatric theory, many psychiatrists supported the idea that the climate had some influence on the psychopathology of both North Africans and Europeans: Kocher, Criminalité, 11; Bouquet, Aliénés en Tunisie, 32; Sutter, Épilepsie mentale, 73; Poitrot, Influences climatiques, 1254.
39 For an example of the English version of moral therapy, see: Showalter, Female Malady, 40.

provided by them was useful for the upkeep of the institutions themselves. This form of therapy could involve recreational distractions for patients of the higher classes in European asylums and for European patients in any institutions looking after colonial patients but usually amounted to hard manual work for the European poor and the colonised.[40] Patients were expected to do unpaid chores for their own good. A French military doctor, André Pichon, working in New Caledonia, wrote for the 1912 Congress in Tunis that "we have observed that work is the best treatment for certain [cases of] insanity. It is a distraction to the individual; it is an occupation that allows him to appreciate his usefulness and to tear himself from his delusions."[41]

Farming, with its romanticised associations of fresh air and general healthiness, was believed to be of particular therapeutic benefit to psychiatric patients. The military doctor Vital Robert, one of Emmanuel Régis' students in Bordeaux, wrote a report for the same Congress about the situation in Madagascar, where he stated: "However, an asylum should not be a simple storage facility. It is a place to treat this chronic [patient], calm his agitation, to improve him, if not to cure him. The work of the fields is the best sedative and the best treatment for the insane."[42] In their summary of the 1912 Tunis Congress, Henri Reboul and Emmanuel Régis mentioned the same ideas of labour being beneficial to patients, before admitting that it also had advantages for the psychiatric institutions themselves: "It goes without saying that asylums should include an agricultural facility and various occupations appropriate to the region; work is a valuable treatment for the curable insane, a beneficial distraction for the incurable insane, aside from the relief of the expenses which can result [from it] for the always tight budget of the establishment."[43]

In the North African context, it seems to have been self-evident that manual labour could be obtained from the patients of any planned asylum. Jobert's 1868 suggestion on how a potential asylum in Algeria should function naturally included the exploitation of the patients' efforts: "To this end, we will farm arable land, [...] where the insane will be co-partners in the exploitation. [... This] will provide the best treatment for mental alienation. The asylum, soon becoming a hamlet, then a

---

40 Ibid.; Ernst, Idioms of Madness, 158. In the 1950s other distractions for the patients were introduced to the colonial hospitals, such as games and sporting facilities. See for instance: Fanon/Azoulay, Socialthérapie, 1095–1106; Pierson et al., Assistance psychiatrique, 35. However, the Tunisian psychiatrist Sleïm Ammar stated in his 1955 article about the situation in the Manouba that while these distractions were available to Muslim men, Muslim women only had the possibility to "engage in sewing or laundry" – which was only taken up by a minority among them. Ammar, Assistance aux aliénés, 26.

41 Reboul/Régis, Assistance, 151.

42 Ibid., 133.

43 Ibid., 198.

village, will turn into a rich centre of colonisation."[44] Not only should the labour of
the patients be used in order to turn the asylum into a success, but the theory of moral
therapy gave psychiatrists the possibility to frame this economic advantage as being
beneficial to the patients.[45]

However, Muslim labour was seen to be of doubtful value. Many patients were unable to do "good work" because of their physical symptoms; others were not expected
to undertake "good work" because of their "race" or gender. While Berbers[46] and
Muslim women[47] were seen to be hard-working, Arab men were decried as inherently
lazy,[48] almost enthusiastically so.[49] Yet even the labour of those North Africans both
physically and "racially" able to work was that of untrained brutes, while delicate work
associated with leisurely femininity was, according to Gervais in 1907, essentially too
civilised for Muslim women: "Arab women in general do not know how to sew; they
are sometimes taught knitting [...]. But these works demand too much patience and
meticulousness from these new [i. e. primitive] natures, coarse [and] little formed.
We are thus reduced to take advantage of them for the work of cleaning [...], wash-
ing the dishes from the kitchen, peeling vegetables, shelling peas. It is correct to say
that none of the occupations is rigorously useful or essentially productive for the
common good; their work is intermittent and often, most often, they destroy more
than they produce. As for the men, there is very little work for which one can rely on
their goodwill. The Arab does not like manual labour; the Kabyle sometimes knows
how to till the soil, but tires easily, revolts and knows very well how to turn his spade
into a terrible weapon..."[50] From Gervais' description, it seems that the small number
of Muslim female patients did most of the unskilled chores needed for the upkeep
of the asylum in Aix-en-Provence, even though Gervais himself does not recognise
the value of this work, while Muslim men remained unused because of their "racial
characteristics" of laziness and aggression.

Once asylums were built in North Africa, it went unchallenged that the work of
the patients should remain an important part of their organisation – even though

---

44 Jobert, Projet, 62.
45 The idea of using North African patients to farm the colonial possessions of the asylums was
    still valid 40 years later in 1912, when Porot described the proposed asylum in Tunisia as need-
    ing "an agricultural holding", which "would use the patients likely to work." Porot, Tunisie, 75.
46 Dilhan, Ethnographie, 196; Lafitte, Contribution, 23; Meilhon, Aliénation mentale, part 4,
    35; Porot/Sutter, 'Primitivisme', 226.
47 There was no discernible distinction between the labour provided by Berber and Arab women
    in the source material. Gomma, Assistance médicale, 107; Abadie-Feyguine, Assistance médi-
    cale, 18; Bugéja, Sœurs musulmanes, 84.
48 Lafitte, Contribution, 23; Meilhon, Aliénation mentale, part 1, 23 f.; Duplenne, Étude, 19.
49 Dilhan, Ethnographie, 198.
50 Gervais, Contribution, 53.

the idea of its therapeutic benefit was quietly dropped.[51] The work undertaken by the patients was usually no longer that of performing chores within the asylum itself, but producing marketable objects. In 1943, for example, Antoine Porot could look back on a decade of experience of psychiatric institutions in North Africa and state: "The *work of the patients* has been pushed up to the maximum in recent years: general services, an important farm, workshops for the weaving of palmettos, [workshops] for baskets for the men, for sewing and spinning wool for the women. It is estimated that, for men, work absorbs nearly a quarter of those hospitalised."[52]

Summarising, one can say that patient labour was seen as helpful both from a therapeutic and budgetary point of view, and that Muslim patients performed a significant amount of manual work in both the asylums in France and in the psychiatric hospitals in North Africa. Even those labelled "incurable", who could not hope to be cured by therapeutic labour, profited from working as a form of "diversion". The division of labour within the asylums was guided by racial and gender prejudices, with Muslim women being more often employed than Muslim men. Allegedly, psychiatrists did not want to hurt existing North African traditions,[53] but it is reasonable to suggest that supervision of "dangerous" male patients would have required too many paid staff for the labour to be of economic value.

The patients interned in these 19th century asylums had to receive, it was generally agreed, "adequate food" – being part of the treatment itself in moral therapy while malnourishment was seen as both a cause and a symptom of degeneration[54] and therefore needed to be eradicated. French colonial psychiatrists contrasted the food served in French asylums with that found in traditional *māristāns* and concluded that both the quality and quantity in the *māristāns* was far below that found in the former.[55] As Solomon Lwoff and Paul Sérieux remarked in 1911, the patients of the Moroccan

---

51 The only reference to the therapeutic benefit of work found after the construction of psychiatric hospitals in North Africa was in Pierre Maréschal's account of his twenty years of experience at the Manouba Psychiatric Hospital. Maréschal, Réflexions, 71.

52 Porot, Œuvre psychiatrique, 364. Emphasis in the original.

53 It is indisputable that such a division of labour existed within the Muslim societies of North Africa. Frantz Fanon and Jacques Azoulay addressed this idea of gender-related work distribution among the Muslims in 1954: "He [the Algerian man] practices sometimes a quite rudimentary craft outside the major urban centres, but he is reluctant to work with wool or raffia, because this is a feminine work: it is the women who make baskets or mats. In a psychiatric hospital, we can try to organise workshops for raffia, weaving or pottery. But it would be better, we think, to entrust these works to sick women." Fanon/Azoulay, Socialthérapie, 1106.

54 The conviction that malnutrition caused mental problems was also proposed by later psychiatrists. See for example: Porot, Œuvre psychiatrique, 377; Assicot et al., Causes principales, 276; Chappert, Contribution, 45.

55 Variot, Visite, 538; Bouquet, Aliénés en Tunisie, 58; Mazel, Visite, 17, FN 1.

māristāns were "poorly dressed and poorly fed".[56] However, the culinary situation in the French-controlled asylums was not always better for Muslims – apart from being confronted with food they were not accustomed to, Islamic food regulations were not observed even though French colonial psychiatrists were certainly aware of them.[57] Alcohol and pork were regularly served, and fasting during Ramadan was disregarded. This neglect and disrespect was criticised by many colonial psychiatrists, who wanted Muslim food for Muslim patients in the planned psychiatric institutions in North Africa as part of their general treatment.[58] The problem of how to best feed the North African patients in France had been long recognised: Meilhon, for instance, wrote in 1896 that Muslim patients faced a variety of "disappointments" in the French asylums, which exacerbated their pre-existing conditions, one of them being the lack of adequate food. Here the adequacy was not related to quality or quantity, but to ethnicity: "[...] it will take him several days to get used to the food presented to him; here no more couscous, no more coffee, but immediately, and without transition, soup and the invariable stew."[59]

In theory, the observation of Islamic food regulations was expected to have a positive effect on the health of Muslim patients as part of a broader "common sense" therapy and, in practice, it positively influenced the budget of the psychiatric institutions in a manner comparable to the financial advantages of patient labour. These two advantages of introducing Islamic food went hand in hand and did not exclude one another. Criticism of un-Islamic food for Muslim patients, however, usually focused on the economic, not the religious, aspects. The psychiatrist Louis Livet, for example, stated in 1911, "in our opinion, the native and European quarters have to be distinct, in the plans of the future asylum, just like the diet, the furniture and clothing as well. A simple mat suffices for the rest of the Arab. That he is left, in addition, his cap and his cloak, as clothing; as to his food, it is easy to make it as consistent as possible with his habits. In complying with the customs of the Natives, the Administration will realise, we are persuaded, considerable savings, on equipment, on clothing and on food."[60]

---

56 Lwoff/Sérieux, Aliénés au Maroc, 474.

57 Porot and Arrii, for instance, wrote in 1932: "the wise commandments of the Qur'an about fermented beverages are hardly respected anymore, apart from in the countryside [...]." Porot/ Arrii, Impulsivité criminelle, 599. Other examples are: Duchêne-Marullaz, Hygiène, 61; Levet, Assistance, 241; Trenga, Âme arabo-berbère, 203.

58 Meilhon, Aliénation mentale, part 6, 359; Gervais, Contribution, 28; Bouquet, Aliénés en Tunisie, 58; Levet, Assistance, 241 f.; Livet, Aliénés algériens, 55; Reboul/Régis, Assistance, 201.

59 Meilhon, Aliénation mentale, part 6, 358. See also: Marie/Godin, Malades musulmans à Paris, 43.

60 Livet, Aliénés algériens, 71. Capitalisation in the original.

While it was commonly accepted that food influenced the well-being of patients and that lack of adequate food was a source of mental unease, Islamic food regulations were merely recognised before the construction of hospitals in North Africa but not institutionalised.[61] Refusal of food in the French asylums was not usually explained through religious reservations. In the late 1890s and the first decade of the 20th century some female Muslim patients were reported to have refused the food served in the asylum of Aix-en-Provence.[62] While this may have been a symptom of their diseases or an expression of anguish, it may also have been a rejection of foreign, non-Islamic food,[63] but it was never considered as such by the psychiatrists responsible for them.

Order, hygiene and cleanliness – markers of civilisation in the colonial worldview[64] – were other aspects of these early "cures", and they found their way into the architecture of the model psychiatric institutions of the time. Symmetrical, airy and spotless, they were seen by some to be therapeutic and by others as merely easier to manage – both important during a period when institutionalisation was the only possibility for the mentally ill. As with the food given to colonial patients, the cleanliness of French institutions was favourably compared with the squalor of those in North Africa,[65] and the case studies describing female Muslim patients often focused on their "unfeminine" dirtiness.[66] Additionally, the North African hospitals and *māristāns*, which were usually housed in old buildings with rooms around a central courtyard, were deemed unhealthy because of their lack of windows. In 1881 the French doctor Gaston Variot reported indignantly on his visit to the Arab Hospital in Tunis that the cells had no windows,

---

61 This led to unfortunate cultural misunderstandings between Muslim patients and French hospital staff. Camille-Charles Gervais reported in his 1907 dissertation the heart-breaking case of a male Muslim patient in Aix-en-Provence who had been force-fed, even though he was only observing Ramadan. Gervais, Contribution, 122. This case study was already discussed by Jean-Michel Bégué in 1996. Bégué, French Psychiatry in Algeria, 535.

62 Pascalis, Paralysie générale, 29; Meilhon, Aliénation mentale, part 3, 367; 371; Battarel, Quelques remarques, 65. Similarly, Lemanski reported in 1913 that Tunisian women refused to consume medicines because they suspected alcohol in them. Lemanski, Mœurs arabes, 111.

63 The only other collection of case studies which reported a group of female patients refusing food was Paul Borreil's 1908 dissertation on the "Internment of Senegalese Lunatics in France", on the Saint-Pierre asylum in Marseille. Here the proportion was stark – out of the five case studies on Muslim women, four were reported to have refused food and showed signs of dramatic weight loss. Borreil, Considérations, 39; 42; 44; 47.

64 Lorcin, Imperialism, 657.

65 See, for instance; Bertherand, Médecine et hygiène, 22. The ethnologist Aug. Dilhan wrote in 1873 that Arabs were "of a proverbial dirtiness [...]." Dilhan, Ethnographie, 176. Others also commented on this alleged characteristic: Brault, Pathologie et hygiène, 179 f.; Mansouri, Contribution, 19. There were also some reports which insisted on the cleanliness in the *māristāns*: Bouquet, Aliénés en Tunisie, 57.

66 Pascalis, Paralysie générale, 29; Meilhon, Aliénation mentale, part 2, 199; 201; 206; part 4, 40.

"only receiving air and light through the door opening on the court."[67] Traditional North African architecture, while exotic and picturesque, was seen to be a very unwholesome environment for patients, with its combined absence of air and light.[68]

A bizarre adjunct to the theory that the correct environment could be helpful to psychiatric patients was proposed in the 19th century, illustrating that this was indeed a time when all manner of ideas were voiced in the desperate search for valid remedies. Abel-Joseph Meilhon noticed in 1896 that patients were measurably calmer when they arrived at Aix-en-Provence, compared to their departure from Algiers: "The calmness of the patients we have always attributed to the crossing. The change in milieu, the fatigue of the voyage, and especially seasickness and vomiting, which are inseparable from it, could immediately produce a beneficial effect on the agitated patient; through the revulsion which seasickness operates on the digestive organs, and the plundering of the nervous forces which accompany it, the patient [who was] most agitated at the departure of the boat, arrives often in a state of calm, which contrasts sharply with the information provided [on him]."[69] This alleged benign effect of seasickness on a lunatic mind had been noticed by others before: Dr Barbier from Algiers suggested in 1884 that an asylum should be built on a boat in the Mediterranean, so that patients could benefit from therapeutic nausea.[70] Unsurprisingly, nothing came of these suggestions of institutionalised seasickness.

When it came to the long-postponed establishment of psychiatric hospitals, the ideals of therapeutic architecture were not the most influential ones. By the time the first psychiatric institutions were built in North Africa, these ideas, while still respected, were no longer as important as other factors. The psychiatric institutions

---

67 Variot, Visite, 538. Other psychiatric and medical reports on traditional North African ideals of architecture, which was what the *māristāns* were based on, however, included the descriptions of spacious gardens with fountains. Bouquet, Aliénés en Tunisie, 57; Livet, Aliénés algériens, 25; Mazel, Visite, 11; Comby, Voyage médical, 1231; Duplenne, Étude, 54 f.; Woytt-Gisclard, Assistance, 163 f.

68 The *māristān* of Sidi Ben Achir in Salé, for instance, was described, due to this absence of air, as "dark and damp" in 1934, and in 1953 as dark and sticky. Périale, Maristane, 389 f.; Luccioni, Maristanes, 464. Roger Mignot described his visit to the Tékia in Tunis in 1926 as follows: "I visited this establishment, if indeed one can use such a term to describe an Arab house, very picturesque, which would have delighted the romantic painters, but which is devoid of any of the characteristics of a hospital." Mignot, Journées médicales, 162.

69 Meilhon, Aliénation mentale, part 2, 181.

70 Barbier, Fous et le mal de mer, 229. This has already been discussed by Richard Keller: Keller, Pinel in the Maghreb, 478. In 1913, Naudin reported that the journey from Algiers to France took 30 hours; in 1925, Antoine Porot spoke of 26 to 30 hours. Naudin, Psychiatrie coloniale, 19 f.; Porot, Chronique algérienne, 270, FN 2.

on North African soil, designed to be models of their type,[71] needed, foremost, to be "racially" segregated, as discussed in Chapter 3.[72] The nominal reason for this was that it was healthier for each patient group to be housed exclusively with its own ethnicity. Boigey, for example, wrote in 1907 that hospitals for Muslims had to be "exclusively *native*",[73] and that North Africans would only accept European treatment and care in a "native" setting.[74]

Raoul Vadon printed the photograph shown on the title page of this book, showing the male Muslim "Dormitory of the Serious Ward" at the newly opened Manouba Psychiatric Hospital, in his 1935 dissertation on the "Medical Assistance of Psychopaths in Tunisia".[75] It is one of the rare depictions of the interior of colonial psychiatric hospitals in North Africa and shows the sparseness, order and cleanliness of the "native wards" of these new institutions.

These spatial divisions within the hospitals influenced the treatment of the different patient groups, with the European services receiving both more space and modern equipment than those reserved for Muslim patients.[76] At the 1938 Congress in Algiers, the participating psychiatrists were invited to visit the newly opened psychiatric hospital at Blida, and a description of this visit was published in the reports of the Congress. It described the European pavilion as follows, hinting at the preferential treatment settlers received: "A certain luxury, which is not unsuitable for the pavilions reserved for Europeans accustomed to comfort, also distinguishes this Algerian psychiatric creation, which can compare favourably with the best European establishments."[77] The therapeutic ideals associated with clean, open spaces were not discarded but lost the initial egalitarianism present in early suggestions – the newly constructed psychiatric buildings still took them into consideration, but modern problems, like overcrowding, "racial" segregation and financial difficulties, overshadowed the idea of therapeutic space. While European patients still received the practical benefits based

---

71 For instance, C. A. Pierson, head of the Neuropsychiatric Services of Berrechid, proclaimed at the 1938 Congress in Algiers: "For the *Europeans* [...], the Neuropsychiatric Service in Casablanca, expanded by a new wing, and the modern pavilions of Ber-Rechid offer satisfactory equipment, for which more than one department of the Métropole would envy us." Discussion du rapport d'assistance psychiatrique, 187. Emphasis in the original. See also: Desruelles/Bersot, Assistance aux aliénés en Algérie, 591; Boucebci, Aspects actuels, 953.

72 See p. 123 The idea that "racial" segregation was beneficial for the mental health of all patients was upheld in: Levet, Assistance, 248; Porot, Assistance psychiatrique, 89; Desruelles/Bersot, Assistance aux aliénés en Algérie, 591; Porot, Œuvre psychiatrique, 363.

73 Boigey, Assistance hospitalière, 610. Emphasis in the original.

74 Ibid., 611. See also: Duplenne, Étude, 66.

75 Vadon, Assistance, between pages 42 and 43.

76 Discussion du rapport d'assistance psychiatrique, 187.

77 Réceptions et excursions, 383.

on the initial ideology, with their services even verging on the "luxurious", Muslim pavilions were more basic, if still clean, orderly, and tightly controlled.

Overall, the common sense therapeutics mentioned in early sources became ever more urgent in the overcrowded and understaffed environment of the psychiatric hospitals in North Africa. These "treatments" survived, even though their implementation no longer made therapeutic sense, strictly speaking, because of entirely practical reasons – maintaining patient labour, cheap indigenous food and order through spatial separation was now of economic and administrative interest in the new North African psychiatric hospitals.

4.4 Drugs, Operations and the Absence of Communication

Both of these 19th century theories failed in their attempts to resolve the problems posed by insanity – moral treatment could not cure patients, and the degenerationists could not prevent mental disorders in new generations. Instead, patient numbers both in France and in the colonies rose steadily. Therefore, new therapies were needed and promptly developed, which revolutionised psychiatry from the 1930s onwards. Colonial psychiatry, under the *École d'Alger,* was at the forefront of testing and implementing them,[78] so much so that French psychiatrists working in the Maghreb influenced the *Métropole* with their progressive findings.[79] As discussed in the previous chapter, North African (male) patient numbers started to overtake the numbers of European patients soon after the construction of psychiatric hospitals in North Africa in the 1930s, and therefore the rise of these innovative treatments coincided with a more or less rapid increase in Muslim patient numbers.

---

78   In his 2007 book "Colonial Madness", Richard Keller argued that because French colonial psychiatrists saw North Africa as both a psychiatrically empty place and as a "space of experimentation", they could be more innovative and pioneering than their colleagues in France. Keller described how French colonial psychiatrists "also saw their North African Muslim patients as a data set for testing the efficacy and safety of increasingly invasive treatments in the hope of complementing institutional progressivism with new technologies for healing. French psychiatrists understood the Maghreb and its subjects as a space of experimentation." Keller, Colonial Madness, 84. The same can be observed in other African colonies, as detailed by Jock McCulloch in 1993. McCulloch, Empire's New Clothes, 48 f.

79   Keller, Colonial Madness, 84 f. Also in: Vaughan, Introduction, 7.

4.4.1   Physical Treatments

These new treatments ranged from shock therapies introduced in the 1930s and 1940s (insulin, electro[80] and Cardiazol shocks[81]), to the so-called psychosurgeries in the 1940s (mainly lobotomies), to a variety of drugs in the 1950s.[82] The effect of their introduction was tremendous. In 1956 Pierre Maréschal reminisced about the enormous changes during the twenty years he had been director of the Manouba Psychiatric Hospital, which, in his eyes, were garlanded with success: "In addition, new therapeutic techniques: electroshock, insulin therapy, sleep therapy and also rehabilitation of the patient through work and occupationalism[83] have brought about many cures. The Manouba has lost her reputation as a storage facility for incurables, as a dungeon for lunatics."[84] The vocabulary used by Maréschal to describe the early situation in the Manouba echoes the reports on Islamic *māristāns*, discussed in Chapter 3,[85] even though the Manouba was only opened in 1932 and Maréschal became its second director from 1935 to 1956. However, while Maréschal took the credit for innovating the therapeutic system in Tunisia, he apparently did not think that the former reputation of the Manouba as a "dungeon" was in any way his responsibility.

Once introduced, these treatments became increasingly popular, especially among the psychiatrists of the *École d'Alger*. In 1943 Antoine Porot summarised what he called the "therapeutic activity" of just a single year (1940) as involving "4,510 insulin shocks, 2,482 Cardiazol shocks, 383 lumbar punctures and 5,805 laboratory tests". Electroshock, introduced recently, was also "practiced on a large scale", so that "at the recent Congress in Montpellier [in 1942], we were able to report more than 2,000 electric shocks realised in one year in Blida."[86]

---

80   Electroshocks are nowadays called electro-convulsive therapy (ECT), but in the French colonial sources, the terms used were "éléctrochocs" or "sismothérapie", and this terminology has been adopted for this chapter.

81   Cardiazol, a registered trademark for pentylenetetrazol, a stimulant used to provoke convulsions, was administered from 1934 onward.

82   The different drugs are discussed later in the chapter. Among the biochemical and surgical treatments experimented with from the 1930s onwards, only lobotomies, electroshock and drugs will be examined in this chapter.

83   I have translated Maréschal's neologism "occupationisme" as "occupationalism", meaning the act of being occupied.

84   Maréschal, Réflexions, 71.

85   See p. 114. The term "storage facility" was used, for example, as a description of the Tékia in 1943, but also of outdated asylums in France. Porot, Assistance psychiatrique, 87; Demassieux, Service social, 18; Porot, Œuvre psychiatrique, 368.

86   Ibid., 364. In reality, the paper presented at the 1942 Congress in Montpellier reported on over 3,000 electroshocks administered within one year. Porot et al., Réflexions, 331.

Given the importance placed upon the "racial" segregation of patients as part of their treatment, it is remarkable that Porot failed to state how many of these early "therapeutic activities" had been conducted on Muslims. The theoretical source material published by the *École d'Alger* was mostly silent on the distribution of both "races" and genders among these "therapeutic activities", and on the variations in success in treating different patient groups. Apart from the evidence in the case studies, these texts on medical innovations were usually "neutral", pretending to treat a "race-less", non-gendered patient and to produce universally applicable experiences. The only sources acknowledging that there could be differences in outcomes were Sutter et al., mentioning in 1959, in passing, that "biological methods and drug therapies work in the same way in native patients" as in Europeans;[87] and an article, published the same year, about the treatment of chronic psychoses. In it, the authors, J. Henry and Michel Assicot, stated that no "significant differences" had been noted in the effects of the various treatments on Europeans and Muslims.[88]

The first major new treatment introduced in North Africa had been electroshock therapy, designed in 1938 by the Italian psychiatrist Ugo Cerletti for the treatment of depressed patients. Richard Keller constructed a chronological analysis of electroshock treatment in France, pointing out how cautious and sceptical psychiatrists in France had initially been.[89] French colonial psychiatrists, by contrast, lacked this healthy scepticism – in 1942 2,868 electroshocks were administered to 220 patients at Blida Psychiatric Hospital, the Civil Hospital of Mustapha, and an unnamed private practice.[90] Between May 1941 and the Congress in Montpellier in October 1942, 340 patients had been subjected to the treatment at the Manouba Psychiatric Hospital in Tunisia.[91] Although no further qualifications about the ethnicity or gender of the patients were given, a significant portion must have been Muslim. An article published in 1955 in the *Annales Médico-Psychologiques* on "Tuberculosis and Psychiatric Shock-Treatments", by Maurice Porot and A. Cohen-Tenoudji, hinted at this religious or "racial" prevalence among the patients: discussing the effects of combined electroshock and insulin shock treatments, they mentioned that they were unable to give insights into "racial" differences, as with "the vast majority of our patients being Muslim, we were unable to establish meaningful comparisons."[92]

The high numbers of electroshocks carried out in these early years suggests that these psychiatrists believed they had found a solution to a variety of serious problems.

---

87   Sutter et al., Aspects algériens, 895.
88   Henry/Assicot, Le 7044 RP, 691.
89   Keller, Colonial Madness, 104.
90   Porot et al., Réflexions, 331.
91   Maréschal et al., Résultats, 341.
92   Porot, M./Cohen-Tenoudji, Tuberculose, 395.

They did not yet know exactly which disorders or symptoms could be cured by it, but they were willing to experiment. Pierre Maréschal et al., for instance, wrote in their paper given at the 1942 Congress in Montpellier: "Since May 1941, treatment through electroshock has been applied regularly and systematically at the Hospital of the Manouba to all patients able to bear it."[93] Neither youth nor old age excused patients from these experimental electroshocks.[94] In many cases, it was claimed that the treatments noticeably improved the conditions of patients.

Despite the scarceness of colonial statistics addressed in Chapter 3, these successes were compiled into statistical evidence. Writing for the 1942 Montpellier Congress, Porot et al. summarised that 42.6% of all patients in the acute services had been healed by electroshock, 32.4% improved and 25% were unchanged. Among the chronic patients, 8% were cured, 38% improved and 54% were unchanged.[95] Maréschal et al. presented similar results at the same Congress for Tunisia. Their experiments showed that of the people interned for more than a year, only 17% had been cured by electroshock, while among the patients interned for less than a year, it had been 33.79% and among the outpatients an impressive 66.25%.[96] While electroshocks "worked" better on the recently interned, the statistical evidence gained from experiments on a variety of North African patients showed that they also cured many chronic patients. This was a tangible success, especially as these patients, prior to the advent of electroshock, would probably have remained among the stock of incurables at the "storage facilities" that many asylums had become.[97]

While these individual statistics of psychiatric triumph lacked essential categories like ethnicity and gender, it is clear that many of the patients treated by electroshocks had been women.[98] Even extenuating circumstances such as fragility caused by

---

93   Maréschal et al., Résultats, 341.
94   Ibid.
95   Porot et al., Réflexions, 331.
96   Maréschal et al., Résultats, 343.
97   Colonial psychiatrists were convinced that electroshock therapy was not only efficacious, but also achieved results very rapidly. See for example: Chappert, Contribution, 49. However, this success was put into context by Richard Keller, who reminded readers in his 2007 book that in the 1940s, during those mass experimentations on North Africans, no "paralytic agents and general anesthesia" were administered in combination with electroshocks. Keller, Colonial Madness, 106. It is therefore probable that some patients claimed to be cured in order not to undergo further treatments and to escape the pain.
98   Elaine Showalter claimed that in Britain and the United States, women were more likely to be administered electro-convulsive therapy than men. Showalter, Female Malady, 207. Other research has shown that in the 1980s, black patients in Britain were more often subjected to electro-convulsive therapy than white patients. Littlewood/Cross, Ethnic Minorities and Psychiatric Services, 199.

advanced years[99] or pregnancies did not exclude women from being subjects in this quest for innovation. In 1942, for instance, Maréschal et al. conducted electroshock treatments on a 25-year-old pregnant patient, who suffered "from the mental point of view from a confused and frenzied agitation and from the obstetrical point of view from a transverse position with normal pelvis". A first session of electroshock caused contractions and turned the obstetrical problem into an acceptable breech position. "Three days later, a second session triggered contractions of the same nature, which led to labour and to the expulsion, a month before term, of a viable child."[100] Similar cases were reported by Maurice Porot, both alone and in collaboration with A. Cohen-Tenoudji. In 1949 Maurice Porot described the effects of electroshocks on a young Muslim woman suffering from apathy, whose pregnancy was only noticed in the middle of a 10-session electroshock treatment. The treatment did not improve her situation, but neither did it harm the child, who was born normally after the patient was released unhealed.[101] In the aforementioned article from 1955, Porot and Cohen-Tenoudji referred to one patient, suffering from tuberculosis, who was three months pregnant and depressed, but "a series of electroshocks led to a physical and mental improvement. Later, she gave birth normally and at term."[102] Neither Maréschal et al. nor Porot and Cohen-Tenoudji specified whether their patients were European or Muslim.

Electroshocks were a popular treatment among colonial psychiatrists and remained so until the end of the colonial period. Even though Jean Sutter stated in 1962 that "the year 1957 saw the end not, of course, of electroshocks, but of their almost exclusive reign,"[103] electroshock treatments remained one of the treatments of choice in the North African colonies. In her 1962 dissertation on puerperal psychoses, Michèle Chappert described what she entitled the "basic treatment" in Blida Psychiatric

---

99 Demonstrated by a remark by Porot et al. at the 1942 Montpellier Congress about "a melancholic woman of 60 whose condition lasted for nearly a year and whom we did not dare to treat because of her age, suddenly cured by the third shock." Porot et al., Réflexions, 334. Nonetheless, electroshock could be dangerous: Aubin et al., for example, presented in 1947 the case of a 56-year-old Algerian Jewish woman, whose electroshock treatment had to be "interrupted" because she had difficulties waking up after the treatments and fainted repeatedly. Aubin et al., Troubles mentaux, 412.
100 Maréschal et al., Résultats, 345.
101 Porot, M., Traitements psychiatriques, 1119.
102 Porot, M./Cohen-Tenoudji, Tuberculose, 395. In 1956 Maurice Porot also reported, together with H. Jouanneau, on the case of a 30-year-old pregnant French patient, who had been treated with Largactil, an early antipsychotic. Porot, M./Jouanneau, Traitement par la chlorpromazine, 395 ff.
103 Sutter, Nouvelles médications anti-dépressives, 391.

Hospital as a combination of neuroleptics and electroshocks.[104] She went on to say that "70% of our patients were treated by the addition of electroshocks to neuroleptics".[105]

There are a number of published case studies on female Muslim patients treated by electroshock.[106] In 1959 Jean Sutter and his colleagues at the University of Algiers published two case studies of agitated young Algerian women subjected to electroshock treatments in their article on "Nuptial Psychoses in Algerian Muslims". One of these case studies was discussed in the introduction of this chapter;[107] the other patient had been admitted only eight days after her wedding, having refused to have sexual intercourse with her husband.[108] Within days both cases were cured. The first was initially calmed by a combination of isolation and electroshocks and then healed by a form of psychotherapy;[109] the second was cured by electroshocks and neuroleptics.[110] The social problems which led to the development of their mental problems had been noticed and documented, described as part of the general suppression of Muslim women, but the treatment itself had been mostly medical – and, apparently, effective. Both young women were released back into the hands of their families – and the unsuitable suitor and unloved husband. In 1955, Manceaux at al. wrote about a 15-year-old Tunisian girl who had come to their attention because of a month long retention of urine, "without organic cause", thereby falling into their field of expertise. Her affliction was improved by electroshock, "all prior attempts at psychotherapy having been met with absence of confidence from the patient."[111] In this case study, the French psychiatrists were successful despite the refusal of the patient – new methods gave the psychiatrists the possibility to act without requiring the cooperation or even the consent of their patients. Even though this was portrayed by Manceaux et al. as a positive development – they had, after all, improved the condition of the girl – electroshock treatments plainly had the potential to be used as punitive measures for uncooperative patients.[112]

---

104 Chappert, Contribution, 48.
105 Ibid., 49.
106 Michèle Chappert gave seven examples among her collection of case studies in her 1962 dissertation, and J. Mares and R. Barre four in their 1962 article. Chappert, Contribution, 32 ff.; 40; 42; 44; Mares/Barre, Quelques aspects, 35; 38 ff.
107 Sutter et al., Quelques observations, 909.
108 Ibid., 910.
109 Ibid., 909.
110 Ibid., 910.
111 Manceaux et al., Intérêt diagnostique, 305.
112 However, even with these intrusive treatments, the psychiatrists complained about the lack of cooperation from Muslim patients. The psychiatrists Maurice Igert and L. Viaud explained in a 1949 article concerning their experiences with electroshock in Morocco that the "psychological

All three cases illustrated the victory of French theories over the allegedly widespread "nuptial psychoses" on the one hand and the patient's refusal to cooperate on the other. Once the patients felt better, or claimed they felt better to escape further treatment, they were sent back to their unhappy homes and the psychological pressures that had caused their afflictions. Nevertheless, these were fortunate cases, leaving psychiatric care after only a short period of treatments. Other North African women were permanently harmed by these waves of medicalised psychiatric treatments. In 1935 the Portuguese neurologist Egas Moniz performed the first lobotomy (or leucotomy),[113] and it was soon established as a therapy to heal patients with different neuroses and depressions.[114]

In North Africa, psychosurgery was taken up by a number of psychiatrists, including Antoine Porot's son, Maurice Porot. In 1947 he published an article on "Prefrontal Leucotomy in Psychiatry" in the *Annales Médico-Psychologiques*, in which he expressed some scepticism towards lobotomies: "Prefrontal leucotomy remains an empirical method and will certainly not yet be the 'magna therapia' that all psychiatrists wish for. [...] It has, compared to other modern psychiatric therapies, one big disadvantage: the operative mortality, which cannot be neglected, although it has already been greatly reduced and one can, reasonably, hope to expect it to further decrease with technical progress."[115] Though sceptical, his conclusions were nevertheless in favour of psychosurgical treatment: "If one considers that, up to now, almost all lobotomised patients fulfilled the conditions for severe symptoms – long duration of illness, and especially incurability by modern psychiatric techniques, such as convulsive and insulin shocks –, we can assume that the risk was worth taking. Can we deny certain patients this last chance of cure or, at least, of seeing their symptoms subside, [which] make their lives impossible and themselves often unbearable, even if this sedation is achieved at the cost of an apparently irrevocable lesion?"[116] Psychosurgery was, as Maurice Porot claimed, employed in hopeless cases, where all other treatments – namely electroshock and insulin shock therapy, drugs and even forms of psychoanalysis – had been unsuccessful, as specified in another article on the "Current State of Psychosurgery" that Maurice Porot co-authored with Pierre Descuns in 1955.[117]

---

opposition" of patients constituted one of the "most difficult and troublesome complications of electrical treatment [...]." Igert/Viaud, Bilan, 218.

113 Porot, M., Leucotomie préfrontale, 121. Psychosurgery was usually undertaken on patients who had been put in a coma through electroshocks, as discussed by Maurice Porot and Pierre Descuns in 1955. Porot, M./Descuns, État actuel, 527.

114 Showalter, Female Malady, 208.

115 Porot, M., Leucotomie préfrontale, 139.

116 Ibid., 139 f.

117 Porot, M./Descuns, État actuel, 535 f.

Maurice Porot's appreciation of psychosurgery as a therapeutic tool for "often unbearable" patients was also shown by the fact that he prescribed a significant number of these operations. Between the publication of his 1947 article, which marked the beginning of lobotomies in North Africa, and 1955, he had, according to Richard Keller, "performed psychosurgeries on over two hundred patients" at Blida Psychiatric Hospital.[118] Keller compared this to hospitals in America where, in the same period, only marginally more operations had been carried out, even though there were twice as many patients as in Blida.[119]

As with electroshocks, there are no known statistical details about the patients who underwent psychosurgeries – both the ethnic and the gender distribution remain hidden in the published sources.[120] However, colonial psychiatric theories likened the brains of Africans in general[121] and North Africans in particular[122] to those of lobotomised Europeans, which might point to an assumption that lobotomies posed fewer risks on the already "genetically lobotomised" North Africans. In addition to this general assumption, Alice Cherki, herself an intern at Blida Psychiatric Hospital at that time, described in 2002 the situation encountered by Frantz Fanon in 1953. The neurosurgeons who carried out these psychosurgeries came from Algiers to Blida on fixed dates, whereupon the psychiatrists "chose patients they wanted to submit to [the operation of] lobotomy and organised a convoy of 'selected ones' on the arranged day".[123] The lack of patient consent presented in this description, with psychiatrists deciding whom to lobotomise – possibly Maurice Porot's "unbearable"

---

118 Ibid., 532. As quoted in: Keller, Colonial Madness, 108.

119 Ibid., 106.

120 The only two published case studies on lobotomised Muslim women could be found in the aforementioned article by J. Henry and Michel Assicot from 1959. Both had been subjected to a combination of treatments before being lobotomised – something discussed later in this chapter. In general, however, according to Elaine Showalter, more women were lobotomised than men. Showalter, Female Malady, 209 f.

121 The British psychiatrist John Carothers proposed in 1951 that the brains of "primitive" Africans were similar to those of lobotomised Europeans. Carothers, Frontal Lobe Function, 12; 37. Frantz Fanon and Thomas Lambo attacked him for this. Lambo, Role of Cultural Factors, 244; Fanon, Racisme et culture, 40; ibid., Damnés, 291.

122 The theory about North Africans was slightly different. It was believed by some that North Africans used their diencephalon (the posterior part of the forebrain) instead of their cortex (forebrain). Jean Sutter, for instance, wrote in his 1937 dissertation: "The activity of the Native, whose life is essentially vegetative and instinctive, is primarily regulated by the diencephalon." Sutter, Épilepsie mentale, 215. Capitalisation in the original. In 1939, Antoine Porot and Jean Sutter repeated: "We have, elsewhere, speculated that there might be a certain fragility of cortical integration, giving free play to the predominance of the diencephalic functions." Porot/Sutter, 'Primitivisme', 241. Frantz Fanon attacked them for these statements. Fanon, Damnés, 290.

123 Cherki, Frantz Fanon, 108.

patients[124] – suggests those patients were Muslim, as it is harder to imagine vocal set-tler families, whose consent could have been sought for such an invasive treatment, meekly accepting post facto that psychosurgery had been performed on their family members.[125] It is however questionable, whether any form of consent was needed: in the aforementioned 1955 article, Maurice Porot and Pierre Descuns discussed the problem of patient consent to any therapeutic treatment. They concluded, essentially, that patient consent – or the consent of the families concerned – was rarely needed and even commented that seeking consent from ill-informed patients and their fam-ilies often hindered the effectiveness of possible cures.[126]

The medicalisation of psychiatry in the 1950s brought forth new drugs, which were freely administered to North African patients in an attempt to stem overcrowding in colonial hospitals. Previously, according to the published sources, psychiatry had only rarely used drugs in the treatment of North Africans – apart from the drugs used to induce convulsions in early shock therapies and certain sedatives. Drugs had been successfully used before the 1950s in the sedative treatment of epileptic patients, shown in two of Jean Sutter's case studies from his 1937 dissertation, where two Alge-rian women, both "mental epileptics", had been admitted into psychiatric care by the police after attacking children in the street.[127] In the hospital, they were agitated and suffered epileptic crises, which were alleviated by the administration of the drug Gardenal.[128] These case studies were early success stories of French colonial psychia-try, demonstrating that epilepsy – both the seizures and the unacceptable behaviour resulting from it – could be effectively controlled by modern sedatives.

In the 1950s articles began to be published on specific drugs, tested in the psychi-atric hospitals in North Africa.[129] In 1950, for example, Maurice Porot and Fernand Destaing wrote about the effects of streptomycin, an antibiotic, on people suffering from mental problems and concluded that, far from being helpful, "streptomycin is capable of causing mental disorders".[130] Most of the drugs, however, were "successes" and proudly presented as such. In the aforementioned article on "Nuptial Psychoses

---

124 Porot, M., Leucotomie préfrontale, 140.
125 No complaints from settler families about psychiatrists performing lobotomies on their family members have been found in either the psychiatric source material or the colonial press.
126 Porot, M./Descuns, État actuel, 536.
127 Sutter, Épilepsie mentale, 151; 153.
128 Ibid., 153; 155. Gardenal, a sedative and anticonvulsant, is a registered trademark for pheno-barbital.
129 The following articles are just a sample of those published between 1952 and 1956 alone: Porot, M./Duboucher, Guérison; Porot, M./Bisquerra, Note préliminaire; Porot, M./Duboucher, Quatre ans après; Manceaux et al., Intérêt diagnostique; Porot, M./Jouanneau, Traitement par la chlorpromazine; Ramée et al., Effets favorables; Sutter/Pascalis, Effets psychologiques.
130 Porot, M./Destaing, Streptomycine et troubles mentaux, 525.

in Algerian Muslims" from 1959, Sutter et al. mentioned the case of a 20-year-old patient who had been married to a man she had not known before her wedding. On the wedding night, she refused sexual intercourse and developed hallucinations, believing her family-in-law wanted to kill her. She eventually tried to commit suicide by jumping off a building, but survived, albeit in a catatonic state: "[...] placed in a cast, she at first accepted care with great passivity, then sank into silence, immobility and refusal of food. The catatonic syndrome was very characteristic. After a brief period of delirium, it [the catatonic syndrome] was greatly improved by treatment with reserpine, continued for seven months."[131] Not only were these drugs able to shock the young woman out of her catatonic state, but they also cured her hallucinations and, apparently, even the repulsion she had felt for both her husband and sexual intercourse, as the last sentence of the case study proclaimed that the patient was "currently pregnant..."[132] The rather self-satisfied ellipsis after that statement – hinting at the obstacle of sexual refusal that had been successfully overcome – was part of Sutter et al.'s published case study.

As previously stated, it is not possible to gauge whether the patients who were administered these invasive treatments were Muslim or European, as it is usually not mentioned in the published source material. Nonetheless, from the case studies, it is clear that Muslims in general, and Muslim women in particular, were among those who underwent these experimental treatments.[133] In 1959 J. Henry and Michel Assicot published an article in which they described five case studies with different combinations of modern treatments, observed at Blida Psychiatric Hospital – and they all described chronic female Muslim patients, detailing how they were administered treatment after treatment during their long years in psychiatric care. The article, however, was not exclusively about female patients or Muslims, so the choice of only female Muslim cases is striking. While this selection might be explained by the departments that Henry and Assicot worked in at Blida Psychiatric Hospital,[134] it might also suggest that this group – chronically ill Muslim women – were the patients most likely to end up as testing grounds for new treatments. Among these case studies, four were tentative success stories, with the patients eventually being released.[135] One

---

131 Sutter et al., Quelques observations, 911. Reserpine is used as an antipsychotic.
132 Ibid.
133 For other case studies involving Muslim women treated with these new drugs, see: Assicot et al., Causes principales, 275; 278; 284; Chappert, Contribution, 33 f.; 40 ff.; 44; Mares/Barre, Quelques aspects, 35 f.; 39 f.
134 The article did not specify in which of the departments of Blida Psychiatric Hospital these two psychiatrists worked.
135 A woman suffering from post-puerperal schizophrenia could not be healed. Her treatment, during the seven years of her internment in Blida, was similar to the successful ones and involved "repeated" electroshocks, and insulin and Nozinan treatments, which did not improve her

of them, a mute melancholic with "anxious seizures", had, over the course of seven years, been administered a wide variety of treatments in significant numbers: electro-Coramine shocks[136], 79 insulin-induced comas, two series of electroshocks, and 300 mg of Largactil[137] per day. These treatments "improved" her, but she was only cured by the administration of Nozinan, which prompted her release in August 1958.[138]

Two of Henry and Assicot's cases concerned schizophrenics interned for seven and nine years respectively.[139] Having been unsuccessfully treated with electroshock and insulin therapy, they were both lobotomised in 1954, without improvement to their conditions.[140] In one of the case notes, it was admitted that the lobotomy had been conducted "out of desperation" – "with no better results".[141] After their lobotomies, these women were given other drug treatments – equally unsuccessful – before the administration of Nozinan resulted in them finally being released as "healed",[142] though one can only speculate what condition they were in after they had been, effectively, testing grounds for such a long period.

These case studies show that new treatments were tested on Muslim patients, and that when the psychiatrists responsible did not know which ones would work, they just tried them out. In the absence of statistical evidence, it is difficult to judge whether these very aggressive treatments were applied equally to North Africans and Europeans, but it is clear that Muslim women were a patient group that presented to colonial psychiatrists the possibility of acquiring experiential biomedical knowledge.

---

condition. Henry/Assicot, Le 7044 RP, 694. Nozinan, a trademark name for levomeprom-azine or "7044 RP", is an antipsychotic drug, part of the group of neuroleptics. Hakkou, Traitements, 253.

136 Coramine is a stimulant and a trademark name for nikethamide.
137 Largactil, a trademark for chlorpromazine, is an antipsychotic drug, part of the group of neu-roleptics. Hakkou, Traitements, 253.
138 Henry/Assicot, Le 7044 RP, 692. The last of the five case studies given by Henry and Assicot was very similar. It concerned a schizophrenic woman who was given Largactil treatments, without success, before a "fairly low dosage" of Nozinan cured her, allowing her to be released. Ibid., 694.
139 Ibid., 693; 694.
140 Ibid., 693.
141 Ibid., 694.
142 Ibid., 693; 694.

4.4.2 Psychotherapy

Treatments which demanded the active cooperation of psychiatric patients, such as psychotherapy, were only partially implemented in colonial French North Africa. To this day, the only one of the three Maghrebi countries with a psychoanalytical tradition and praxis is Morocco.[143] This was due to a major French psychoanalyst and Freud student, René Laforgue, travelling regularly to Morocco from 1947 to 1959,[144] where he formed a psychoanalytic circle, influencing other psychiatrists such as Maurice Igert.[145]

At first sight, the ideas of the *École d'Alger* were not really compatible with psycho-analytic theories. The *École d'Alger* upheld that mental problems had organic origins and could be successfully treated with physical treatments such as operations and drugs.[146] Others thought that while psychoanalysis was relevant in Europe, it was not applicable to the "primitive minds" of North Africans. Experience showed that when it was attempted, Muslim patients often refused to cooperate in psychotherapy. For example, as mentioned above, Manceaux et al. reported in 1955 the case of a 15-year-old Tunisian girl, on whom electroshocks were successfully used, "all prior attempts at psychotherapy having been met with absence of confidence from the patient".[147]

Even advocates of psychoanalysis were sceptical about whether psychotherapy could be adapted to the Maghreb. René Laforgue, for instance, wrote an article in

---

143 Bennani, Psychanalyse, 16 f. Psychoanalysis is also not widespread in the Arab world. Salem-Pickartz, Mental Health, 268. The reasons given for this prevalence of physical treatments seem very colonial in both Orientalist ideology and vocabulary. The Iraqi-born psychiatrist Ihsan Al-Issa and his Finnish-born wife and fellow psychiatrist Brigitta Al-Issa, for example, wrote in 1970 that ECT and drugs were more popular in Iraq than other forms of treatments, and that "psychotherapy has little appeal to the patients. This is partly due to the fact that psychotherapy usually takes a long time, unlike the quick magical effect expected from the traditional treatment. People seem to have transferred to some extent their belief in magical power from the healers' treatment to ECT." Al-Issa/Al-Issa, Psychiatric Problems, 21.

144 Laforgue actually moved to Casablanca in either 1947 or 1948 before moving back to France at Morocco's independence.

145 Bennani, Psychanalyse, 132.

146 Jean Sutter, a key figure of the *École d'Alger*, recognised idealistic similarities between his own field of neuropsychiatry and psychoanalysis when he suggested, in an article published in 1949, that psychiatry could learn from psychoanalysis. He stated that psychoanalysts had shown that pathogenic processes worked in an identical way in individuals from the same background, an insight which he judged to be especially relevant in the North African context. He claimed that it had already been established by the *École d'Alger* that the minds of North Africans, whether normal or abnormal, worked in a similar way, and if psychoanalysis helped in understanding their mysterious, pathogenic ways, it should be used for that purpose. Sutter, Quelques aspects, 215.

147 Manceaux et al., Intérêt diagnostique, 305. However, the case study analysed in the introduction highlights a psychoanalytical success. Sutter et al., Quelques observations, 909.

Maroc Médical in 1953 explaining that in North Africa "psychoanalysis can only serve as a means of treatment in cases where the patient's ego remains strong enough to face the grave conflict from which he has become accustomed to flee into the disease. In cases where the patient's ego is too weak to support the cure, psychoanalysis can be inappropriate. It [psychoanalysis] is always [inappropriate] when the disease is too deeply rooted or when the psychoanalyst is imperfectly armed to analyse in detail the family situation or the social environment [...], which created in these patients the traumatising super-ego in question."[148] Laforgue's conclusion was familiar to any French colonial psychiatrist of the period after the construction of institutions in North Africa: the normality of North Africans was too different from European normality to be analysable by French-trained, and therefore "imperfectly armed", experts, or to be treatable by therapies intended for European minds. In 1959 Sutter et al. addressed the same problem: "In practical terms, [...] biological methods and drug therapies work the same way in native patients: it is entirely different when it comes to the various forms of psychotherapy. The first difficulty is that of verbal contact [...]. Beyond the questions of language, there are more challenging obstacles to overcome. The processes and methods of psychotherapy, as varied as they are, have been developed from a psychological knowledge of man, which does not correspond to the particularities of the 'native mentality' [...]."[149] While the main languages of North Africa could be learnt by any medical expert, the "particularities of the 'native mentality'" needed to be meticulously examined and explained first – by psychiatrists, naturally – before psychotherapy could "appropriately" work in the North African context.

Even though Sutter et al. dismissed it as being of only secondary importance, the language barrier alone posed enormous problems for the implementation of these forms of therapy. Due to it, many psychiatrists did not even know the most basic facts about their North African patients,[150] and it is difficult to find evidence of French colonial psychiatrists even attempting to talk directly with their Muslim patients. One of only two female clinical psychiatrists in the colonial Maghreb, Suzanne Taïeb, born and raised in Tunisia, understood North African women, both linguistically and culturally, far better than her male colleagues, and in her collection of case studies there is a variety of instances in which she talked extensively with her patients about their disorders and North African interpretations of insanity.[151] While there were certainly other French psychiatrists who spoke Arabic well enough to communicate

---

148 Laforgue, Aspect psychosomatique, 475.
149 Sutter et al., Aspects algériens, 895.
150 As amply demonstrated by the paucity of information given in the case studies. See for example: Pascalis, Paralysie générale, 29 f.; Meilhon, Aliénation mentale, part 6, 353; Battarel, Quelques remarques, 64; Levet, Assistance, 53; Benkhelil, Contribution, 74.
151 For instance: Taïeb, Idées d'influence, 85 f.; 91 f.; 100 ff.

with patients,[152] Taïeb's case studies were the only published colonial psychiatric source where female North African voices could be found – although obviously coloured through Taïeb's transcription and interpretation of them.

Other colonial psychiatrists relied on interpreters, for example Frantz Fanon and Jacques Azoulay in 1954, but they admitted "this need for the interpreter fundamentally invalidates the patient-psychotherapist relationship".[153] This complaint was not uncommon. In 1907 Camille-Charles Gervais had already highlighted the problems posed by the language barrier and the unusual solution that was forced upon psychiatrists in Aix-en-Provence, far away from the services of trained interpreters. Gervais regretted that "[...] we are often almost completely unaware of the important pathological antecedents: despite our best efforts to try through accidental interpreters, who are themselves insane, to make the patient speak their language."[154] If obtaining relatively simple information, like a patient's medical history, was almost impossible even with an interpreter, how much more difficult would it have been to conduct psychotherapy, especially if the interpreter was himself a psychiatric patient?

Confronted with this range of problems, only a few attempts were made to introduce "softer" treatments, two of them by Frantz Fanon. When he arrived at Blida Psychiatric Hospital in 1953, he was responsible for separate services for European women and Muslim men.[155] Fanon wrote an article with one of his interns, Jacques Azoulay, in 1954, explaining how successful their innovation, which they called "social therapy",[156] had been in the service of European women, where they had organised Christmas and other celebrations, cinema evenings, newspapers etc.: "This fast and relatively easy success only highlights the complete failure of the same methods [when] employed in our service of Muslim men."[157] Realising that Muslim forms of entertain-

---

152 Jean Sutter, for instance, spoke Arabic. Sutter, Épilepsie mentale, 150.

153 Fanon/Azoulay, Socialthérapie, 1104. This issue was also raised by others, such as Michèle Chappert in 1962. Chappert, Contribution, 18. On Fanon's inability to speak (North) African languages, see also: Bullard, Critical Impact, 233; Gates, Critical Fanonism, 468. Other examples of psychiatrists who admitted to needing help from interpreters were Abel-Joseph Meilhon in 1896, A. Fribourg-Blanc in 1927 and François-Georges Marill and Abdennour Si Hassen in 1952. Meilhon, Aliénation mentale, part 4, 40; Fribourg-Blanc, État mental, 143; Marill/Si Hassen, Paralysie générale, 446 f.

154 Gervais, Contribution, 23.

155 Fanon/Azoulay, Socialthérapie, 1095.

156 This form of social therapy was taken up in postcolonial Tunisia by the psychiatrists Tahar Ben Soltane and Sleïm Ammar, who supported journals as well as musical, sportive and recreational activities for the patients at the Razi Psychiatric Hospital, formerly known as the Manouba. Douki et al., Psychiatrie en Tunisie, 51.

157 Fanon/Azoulay, Socialthérapie, 1096.

ment helped Muslim patients better, they established a Moorish café in the hospital, celebrated traditional Muslim holidays and had a professional storyteller come round.[158]

Fanon and Azoulay believed they had committed a mistake in introducing European forms of entertainment to North African patients, and to show that patients were more at ease in their own cultural setting, they described an experience with female Muslim patients: "For six months, the Muslim women regularly attended the parties given in the European pavilions. For six months, they applauded in the European way. And then, one day, a Muslim orchestra came to the hospital, played and sang, and our astonishment was great [when we] heard the applause of the Muslim women: short, acute and repeated modulations (called yous-yous). They reacted therefore to the configurational setting according to specific requirements of this setting. It became obvious that we should look for settings that would facilitate already inscribed reactions in a fully developed personality."[159]

The second innovation introduced by Fanon and inspired by psychoanalysis was the so-called Thematic Apperception Test (TAT), in which patients were given black and white pictures of everyday events, which they had to interpret. While not strictly speaking a form of treatment, it was nonetheless an attempt to understand patient behaviour better and to help in their treatment, while at the same time giving them an active role to play in their own therapy. Frantz Fanon and Charles Géronimi wrote a paper for the 1956 Congress in Bordeaux on the "TAT in Muslim Women", in which they processed information gathered in the treatment of twelve female Muslim patients suffering from hypochondria or anxiety at Blida Psychiatric Hospital. Fanon and Géronimi compared the different approaches of Muslim and European patients, and the difficulties Muslim women had in relating to the pictures. The Muslim patients described what was on the pictures, without telling the story of what happened in them.[160] Fanon and Géronimi concluded that their own approach was wrong,[161] and admitted that their French method was not working in the North African context, refusing to pathologise all Muslim women in order to defend the theory.

Both of Fanon's more social therapies initially failed because of what Laforgue and Sutter et al. had described in their respective articles as the "social environment"[162] or the "particularities"[163] of North Africans. The European forms of entertainment had not appealed to the North African mentality, and the TAT had been unsuccessful because North Africans did not "think" in the same way as Europeans. While

---

158 Ibid., 1106.
159 Ibid., 1102.
160 Fanon/Géronimi, T. A. T., 365 f.
161 Ibid., 367.
162 Laforgue, Aspect psychosomatique, 475.
163 Sutter et al., Aspects algériens, 895.

Fanon and his colleagues accepted the fundamental principle of cultural difference, they rejected both the idea of a pathologised North African "primitivism"[164] and the finality of European treatments. Fanon tried to implement adapted forms of treatment at Blida Psychiatric Hospital, for example the installation of a Moorish Café, but his treatments were interrupted as he had to leave Algeria in 1956 because of his political activities.[165]

4.5 Contextualising Progress

As mentioned in Chapter 3, it became a colonial trope to contrast the traditional psychiatric treatments available in North Africa with those newly developed in Europe.[166] French colonial psychiatry saw itself as a key player in the history of progress – of humanity, of civilisation, of modernity –, which could be demonstrated through the advances made by psychiatry in North Africa, measured in both humanitarian and technical terms. In addition to a real philanthropic outrage felt by many of them, colonial psychiatrists used the treatments available to Muslim patients outside of French controlled psychiatric institutions as an opportunity for negative comparisons to demonstrate the progress made by colonial psychiatry.

In the colonial imagination, North African treatments were represented by the absence of medicine on the one hand and the misinterpretation of magic as medicine on the other.[167] Solomon Lwoff and Paul Sérieux, for example, in the report on their 1911 mission to Morocco, described the decayed state of psychiatry there,[168] regretting the disappearance of the medieval "grand schools of the Muslim world", which had possessed far greater knowledge than their 20th century successors. In the present state of decadence, "the field remained free for the superstitions of the primitives."[169]

---

164 In their article on the TAT, Fanon and Géronimi attacked the theory of "primitivism" of the *École d'Alger*: "To say that the Muslim woman is incapable of inventing, in reference to a particular genetic constitution, which would fall into the overall frame of primitivism, seems to us to be a difficult position to defend." Fanon/Géronimi, T.A.T., 367.

165 Berthelier, Homme maghrébin, 111.

166 See p. 114.

167 This was not only observed in psychiatry, but also in other areas of medicine: Perrin, Essai, 15; Thierry, Étude, 11; Pasqualini, Contribution, 30.

168 Lwoff/Sérieux, Aliénés au Maroc, 470. See also: Mazel, Visite, 18; Desruelles/Bersot, Note sur les origines arabes, 308. It is disconcerting to find the same discourse of decline and a century-long decay in the North African countries in texts by postcolonial Maghrebi psychiatrists. See for example: Ammar, Histoire, 11 f.; Mejda et al., Histoire, 691.

169 Lwoff/Sérieux, Aliénés au Maroc, 471. But this decay of Muslim intellectualism was not the only obstacle to the introduction of medical treatments in the eyes of many psychiatrists.

Apart from the traditional Islamic *māristāns*, these "superstitions of the primitives" included a variety of cures. Among the options available, North Africans suffering from mental problems had the possibility to join one of the exorcism ceremonies performed by a brotherhood[170] or to consult a traditional healer.[171] This diversity was summarised in 1911 by Lwoff and Sérieux: "Before ending up in the moristans, the insane are often subjected to treatments which are little more than rites of sympathetic, demonic or Koranic magic, or magico-medical practices, all aimed at the expulsion of demons. [...] One consults not the doctor (*toubîb*) who heals through drugs, but a *taleb* (scholar, student, teacher) who recommends incantations, fumigations, gives a talisman, etc. The Negroes (*gnaouïa*) are brought in, specialising in the exorcism of madness-producing demons. One leads the patients – as happens still with us – on a pilgrimage to the tomb of a renowned saint, whose *baraka* (divine grace, supernatural power) makes miraculous cures and gives [back] reason by expelling the *jinn*."[172] Colonial psychiatric treatments were therefore only one of a number of therapeutic choices available to North Africans, and, considering the unpleasant mechanisms of admission described in Chapter 2, they might well have

---

Livet, for instance, explained in his 1911 dissertation "Algerian Mad and their Hospitalisation" that "the dominant idea that lunatics were inspired [by God] meant that the Arabs never regarded insanity as a disease, and, therefore, never had the idea of using medical treatment." Livet, Aliénés algériens, 11. This widespread notion was lamented by Lwoff and Sérieux, who vehemently denied that Muslim lunatics were always seen as saints. Lwoff/Sérieux, Aliénés au Maroc, 472; ibid., Note, 695.

170 Woytt-Gisclard, Assistance, 158. As described, for example, by Vincent Crapanzano for Morocco in 1973. Crapanzano, Ḥamadsha, 133 f. A similar kind of ceremony, zar dances, still exists in other parts of the Muslim world and has been discussed by psychiatric experts. The discussion led by the Egyptian psychiatrist Ahmed Okasha from 1966 shows the contempt North African psychiatrists felt for these traditional (and often traditionally female) practices: "With the advent of modern therapies it [zar] has lost much of its former popularity and is only resorted to by very emotive, bigoted women of the lower and middle classes." Okasha, Cultural Psychiatric Study, 1217.

171 The colonial sources usually described three different types of North African healers, here called *marabout*, *faqīh*, and *ṭālib*. Marabouts were portrayed as North African "saints", who North Africans thought were able to heal specific physical afflictions, with some of them specialising in mental problems. Armand, Algérie médicale, 431 f.; Thierry, Étude, 73; Taïeb, Idées d'influence, 45, El-Khayat, Tradition et modernité, 71. Faqīh was one of the names given to religious experts who studied Islamic law and healed through recitation of qur'anic verses. Ifrah, Maghreb déchiré, 23, FN 1; Aouattah, Ethnopsychiatrie maghrébine, 76; Bennani, Psychanalyse, 44; Bullard, Truth in Madness, 117. The *ṭālib*, on the other hand, was thought to be a true "sorcerer", who used magical treatments to heal his patients. Legey, Essai, 140; Pasqualini, Contribution, 69.

172 Lwoff/Sérieux, Aliénés au Maroc, 473 f. Emphasis in the original.

been a last resort.[173] These alternatives, without exception decried as superstitions, were not taken seriously by colonial psychiatrists, who were confident that only their therapies could cure mental problems. In the colonial worldview, it was obvious that Muslims consulting a saint, for example, would eventually end up in psychiatric care.

The only North African treatment that was recognisable as vaguely medical in the eyes of French psychiatrists was that provided by the *māristāns*, because they were analogous to French asylums in the "Middle Ages". Most colonial psychiatrists denied that any medical principles were involved in the organisation of the *māristāns*,[174] but, during the bygone heyday of Islamic medicine, a variety of physical treatments had in fact been available, summarised by the Iraqi-born psychiatrist Ihsan Al-Issa in 2000 as "including baths, fermentations, compresses, bandaging, massage, bloodletting, cupping, and cautery. Medications included sedatives and stimulants."[175] If such medical treatments still existed in the 19th and 20th century, they were never witnessed and described by colonial psychiatrists – the picture painted of the *māristāns* was uniformly one of barbarity, where treatment consisted mainly of iron chains,[176] cages[177] and the occasional outbursts of violence from the semi-nursing, semi-guarding staff.[178]

---

173 Psychiatrists might be consulted either before or after traditional treatments had been tried, or even simultaneously. Michael Dols has described this plurality of treatments, which still exists today, for the Islamic Middle Ages. Dols, Majnūn, 8. See also: Douki et al., Introduction, XI; Aouattah, Ethnopsychiatrie maghrébine, 7; Salem-Pickartz, Mental Health, 268.

174 In 1922 Du Mazel, for example, wrote about the *māristān* of Sidi Fredj that "no medical service is involved, in fact, in the running of the establishment, while it is provided with [...] an administrative service. The certificate issued by the doctor of the indigenous hospital for the admission of the lunatic and for his release has only an administrative value and bears no consequence in terms of treatment, which exists to no degree." Mazel, Visite, 17. The same sentiment was voiced by Joseph Luccioni in 1953, also about the situation in Sidi Fredj: "Of course, there was no question of either care or of medical treatment, or even of control by the authorities on the admissions and releases." Luccioni, Maristanes, 463.

175 Al-Issa, Mental Illness, 56.

176 Moreau, Recherches, 110 f.; Review of Furnari, 150; Variot, Visite, 538; Bouquet, Aliénés en Tunisie, 24; Lwoff/Sérieux, Aliénés au Maroc, 474; Reboul/Régis, Assistance, 35; Mazel, Visite, 8; 17; Comby, Voyage médical, 1230; Arrii, Impulsivité criminelle, 39; Legey, Essai, 156; Woytt-Gisclard, Assistance, 162; Desruelles/Bersot, Assistance aux aliénés chez les Arabes, 705; Luccioni, Maristanes, 463.

177 Moreau, Recherches, 112; Variot, Visite, 538; Lwoff/Sérieux, Aliénés au Maroc, 474; Mazel, Visite, 15; Périale, Maristane, 390; Maréchal/Lamarche, Assistance médicale, 393; Luccioni, Maristanes, 464; Maréchal, Réflexions, 69.

178 Livet, Aliénés algériens, 11; 64; Legey, Essai, 156; Cloarec, Bîmâristâns, 60 f. In the descriptions of traditional asylums in Egypt, the use of the "courbash", the whip, was usually mentioned. For example in: Sandwith, Cairo Lunatic Asylum, 475; Burdett, Hospitals and Asylums of the World, 498.

Only non-psychiatrically trained authors mentioned other treatments available in the *māristāns* in their reports. The journalist Marise Périale, for instance, recounted in a 1934 article about a journey through Morocco the following concerning therapies at the Sidi Ben Achir *māristān* in Salé: "In the past, the madman once chained [...] was whipped with a fennel rod ([with a] flexible and light stem, not able to hurt) dipped in a red liquid. The intended goal is to scare him, because in his dementia the patient believed he saw blood dripping from his body; this fear started to calm him."[179] After this description of effectively an early form of shock therapy, Périale went on to quote other progressive forms of treatments in traditional Islamic institutions: "Not far from him [the patient who was whipped with a fennel rod] an orchestra played soft and nostalgic songs, which had the power to maintain this calm. Finally, the place was constructed in a way that he [the patient] always had a flower plantation before his eyes. This amalgamation of sounds and colour was considered to be the only effective remedy. After a period of this treatment, the patient was cured. But this treatment is not applied [anymore] in Salé. Only the chain around the neck remained and it is the only remedy that is given to these unfortunates."[180] In her account, Périale claimed that, in an unspecified past, North Africans had used forms of treatments which were progressive even in 1934 – but that progress was irrefutably lost, and Périale's refreshingly different account ends on a note of Muslim barbarity, matching the standard psychiatric accounts on the conditions in the *māristāns*.

These barbaric conditions reminded colonial psychiatrists of the situation in French asylums before Philippe Pinel, the founder of "moral therapy" mentioned at the beginning of this chapter, unchained the patients in the hospitals of Bicêtre and the Salpêtrière in Paris in 1793.[181] This iconic founding moment of modern French psychiatry accompanied French psychiatrists to North Africa, where they imagined themselves confronted with those treatments which had driven Pinel to action.[182] By

---

179 Périale, Maristane, 390. This story was also told by the French doctor Françoise Legey in 1926. Legey, Essai, 156.

180 Périale, Maristane, 390. Mustapha Akhmisse repeated Périale's report without acknowledging her in 2005: Akhmisse, Médecine, 57. Accounts of these therapies combining sound, smell and vision can be found in Michael Dol's book. Dols, Majnūn, 124. See also: El-Khayat, Tradition et modernité, 69; Kogelmann, Sidi Fredj, 73; Keller, Pinel in the Maghreb, 472.

181 Foucault, Maladie mentale, 84; ibid., Histoire de la folie, 530 f.; 584 ff.; Porter, Being Mad, 45. Discussions on whether this had actually happened or whether it was just a myth have been led by William Bynum in his 1974 article "Rationales for Therapy", Gladys Swain in her 1977 book "Subject of Insanity" and Jill Harsin in her 1992 article on "Gender, Class and Madness". Bynum, Rationales for Therapy, 318; Swain, Sujet, 41–7; Harsin, Gender, Class, and Madness, 1049 f.

182 Comparisons of North African institutions with "Bicêtre before Pinel" can be found in many psychiatric texts. In 1872, Auguste Voisin was reminded of Bicêtre during his visit to the Civil

denouncing, and eventually changing, the conditions in the *māristāns*, they had the chance of following Pinel's humanitarian lead not just metaphorically but physically. Ironically, this wish of emulating Pinel, combined with the obsession of settler security, resulted in colonial psychiatry's paradoxical aims of both freeing and imprisoning the patients, as shown in a summary of the 1912 Tunis Congress: "The colonial doctor will also need to educate the native, to rid him of his prejudices against madness in order to bring him to entrust the delusional into psychiatric care, instead of allowing them to roam, to chain them or to cage them."[183] For the psychiatric experts, the tolerance that Muslims allegedly showed towards certain cases of insanity was just as objectionable as their assumed barbarity towards those incarcerated in the *māristāns*.

French colonial psychiatrists were united in denouncing the barbarity in the *māristāns*, but this humanitarian outcry was not only restricted to North African treatments. They criticised aspects of the psychiatric system implemented in North Africa on the same grounds: that treatments were inhumane, futile or outdated, imagined either as steps back in psychiatry's history of progress or as obstacles in its way. Outdated treatments were regretted by those who wanted to implement changes[184] and used by others who wanted to demonstrate the unstoppable evolution of psychiatry, where the landscape could dramatically change in a couple of decades. Even criticism could, if applied correctly, be used to highlight progress. In her 1941 dissertation on "Social Service in Psychiatry", for example, Elaine Demassieux described the period before psychiatric services in Algeria were supplemented by social work as a period of despair. She reminded her readers of psychiatric ideologies now deemed barbarous, which, not long ago, were used by mainstream French psychiatry: "Until recently, the Insane were considered as social waste, often dangerous, who could be cut off from Society and who, through a procedure of interment, drawing more from social security than from therapy, could be collected in an Asylum, where the regime was more that of a storage facility than of active therapy."[185] The modern treatments in use in the early 1940s, she explained, both prevented and cured insanity. Where "old" psychiatry had been passive and neglectful of its duties, "new" psychiatry was proactive:

Hospital of Mustapha; in 1935, Raoul Vadon thought of it "despite himself" in describing the Tékia in Tunis, just like Sleïm Ammar in 1955 and Pierre Maréchal in 1956. Linas, Aliénés en Algérie, 491; Vadon, Assistance, 28; Ammar, Assistance aux aliénés, 24 f.; Maréchal, Réflexions, 73. This preoccupation with Pinel as a symbol of modernity in the North African context was analysed by Richard Keller in his 2005 article on "Pinel in the Maghreb".

183 Abadie, Report, 381.
184 Levet, for instance, wrote in 1909, as a summary of his report on the "Assistance of the Algerian Mad in a Metropolitan Asylum": "The foregoing gives the right to conclude that the treatment of the colonial insane, especially the natives, in a metropolitan asylum is a medical and humanitarian mistake." Levet, Assistance, 245.
185 Demassieux, Service social, 18. Capitalisation in the original.

"Instead of waiting in an ancient Asylum for administrative or police authorities to bring the patient to it, Mental Medicine these days will track him [the patient] and find him in his milieu, offering him more welcoming facilities and lending a helping hand to his often distraught entourage."[186]

In trying to contextualise this narrative of humanitarian progress further, it is instructive to look at female Muslim patients. Did this progress have the same impact on the different patient groups within the psychiatric institutions? Were Muslim women given the same treatment as other patient groups within this succession of ever more innovative therapies, considering they were initially the smallest (and consequently least important?) of them? This is difficult to answer due to the almost complete absence of references to Muslim women in descriptions of practical, everyday experiences in the writings of French colonial psychiatrists. As seen in Chapter 3, numerical data simply does not exist. The few statistics published in French sources can neither prove nor refute the psychiatric self-representation as a narrative of progress, much less help in placing Muslim women within this narrative. Female Muslim patients were also absent from most theoretical sources. While early theoretical texts did not focus on any forms of practical treatments – neglecting, as it were, all patient groups equally –, descriptions of therapies were of immense importance in those articles published after 1930, although female Muslim patients remained, apparently, uninteresting. Evidence of the concrete treatment of Muslim women can therefore only be gained from case studies.

During the 19th century, when patients were being shipped to France, both Muslim men and Muslim women suffered the same lack of treatment. Moreover, instead of being medically treated, female Muslim patients were used to undertaking menial chores, but as patient labour was justified as being "beneficial" for the wellbeing of patients, one could say, cynically, that Muslim women received preferential treatment over Muslim men. Despite the enormous changes introduced by the *École d'Alger*, Muslim women seem to have received more or less the same range of treatments as Muslim men with the advent of new therapies in the 1930s – apart from the previously described imbalance in the introduction of new entertainment facilities in the Muslim services in the 1950s.[187] Muslim women certainly participated less in "social" therapies because they were even less likely to speak French than Muslim men, the

---

186 Ibid., 20. Capitalisation in the original. Demassieux further qualified that this task of actively looking for potential mental patients in their own environment was distinctly feminine. Ibid., 42. Most of the patients attended to in this way by female social workers were European women, and Richard Keller points out that all the "success stories" in Demassieux's dissertation involved European patients, which he attributes to a greater efficiency of the therapy in treating patients within the same language and culture. Keller, Colonial Madness, 98–102.

187 Compare p. 151, FN 40.

prerequisite of psychoanalytic treatment in the colonial context. As mentioned in the introduction to this chapter, those few Muslim women who successfully received forms of psychotherapy were explicitly described as different from the masses of "normal" Muslim women because of their class, education or contact with French civilisation.

All of the strictly medical innovations – electroshocks, lobotomies and drugs – were tested on Muslims, and case studies on female Muslim patients were chosen to represent these new treatments triumphing over formerly incurable disorders. All the case studies described above, but particularly those involving multiple aggressive therapies, show that new medicalised treatments were used on Muslim women, even though communication between psychiatrist and patient was difficult and even though, generally speaking, psychiatrists recognised that many of the disorders in Muslim women were caused by mainly social problems.

Finding the right treatment for female Muslim patients was a "hard road" for French colonial psychiatrists, as they tirelessly applied therapy after therapy to their non-consenting patients, as seen in Henry and Assicot's 1959 case studies. The introduction of ever-newer medications and techniques meant that, far from there being an established treatment for each disorder or each set of symptoms, therapies were simply administered in turn in order to find out which worked on which patients. Under the *École d'Alger*, the question, therefore, should not be whether Muslim women received treatments, but whether North African patients in general, and female North Africans in particular, received new, aggressive treatments excessively, which would have been impossible to try out on a European patient population.[188]

There is proof, as demonstrated by some historians, that certain therapeutic techniques were knowingly over-used on North Africans, even if the exact details were not transmitted in the colonial sources. René Collignon, for example, recounted how Salem b. Ahmed Eschadely, the first Tunisian psychiatrist, accused Pierre Maréschal of "gratuitous experimentation" at the Manouba Psychiatric Hospital.[189] Richard Keller mentioned colonial sources hinting at "an abusive approach to ECT" and reported that electroshocks were used in Algeria to intimidate simulators who tried to avoid military service by feigning mental disorders.[190] Simulators, subjected to electroshock, it was argued, would give up all pretence. Porot et al. explained in a paper at the 1942

---

188 Descriptions of the persistence of these aggressive treatments in North African psychiatric institutions – as a colonial legacy – by postcolonial authors support this theory. See for example: Labidi, Rita El-Khayat on Moroccan Psychiatry and Sexuality, 641; Salem-Pickartz, Mental Health, 268.

189 Collignon, Psychiatrie coloniale, 538, FN 37. Richard Keller also mentions that Eschadely witnessed abuses when he worked at the Manouba in the 1930s and 1940s. Keller, Colonial Madness, 172.

190 Keller, Colonial Madness, 105.

Montpellier Congress why electroshocks helped in "unmasking" simulations, a mental fault encountered, allegedly, in many North Africans:[191] Electroshocks worked because, at the moment of waking up, "[...] authoritarian suggestion and re-education no longer found resistance at the moment of semi-consciousness which follows the coma."[192]

Overall, it can be said that colonial psychiatric treatments of North African patients, particularly women, described, in a way, an arc of progress, and, from a purely technical perspective, French colonial psychiatry, under the *École d'Alger*, was a true example of colonies being "laboratories of modernity".[193] French colonial psychiatry could be interpreted as an example of colonies not just being steered by the *Métropole*, not just suppressing the "natives", but as influencing the motherland and trying to save the colonised. This is precisely how many psychiatrists of the *École d'Alger* saw themselves: powering the engine of progress, fighting for notions of civilisation and humanity.[194] In conclusion, however, it must be stressed that if one accepts the self-representation of French colonial psychiatry as a laboratory of modernity, pursuing progress by continually testing and discarding theories, the role accorded to North Africans was that of providing the steady supply of guinea pigs.

191 Simulation, exaggeration and general insincerity, often summarised as "mythomania", were some of the main problems encountered in the treatment of North African patients according to many psychiatrists of the *École d'Alger*. Sutter, Épilepsie mentale, 85; Porot/Sutter, 'Primitivisme', 237; Susini, Aspects cliniques, 115 f.; Manceaux et al., Hystérie, 23.

192 Porot et al., Réflexions, 330.

193 The term "laboratory of modernity" is taken from Ann Stoler: Stoler, Race and the Education of Desire, 15. This point has also been made in: Pelis, Prophet for Profit, 621; Keller, Colonial Madness, 6.

194 For example: Goëau-Brissonnière, Syphilis nerveuse, 77; Aubin, Assistance, 170; Sutter, Quelques aspects, 216; Luccioni, Maristanes, 464 f. Pride in this progress in treatments can also be found in texts by the few North African psychiatrists who worked during the French colonisation of North Africa. See for instance: Ammar, Assistance aux aliénés, 26.

Chapter 5
Making Sense of Absence:
The Curious Case of the Missing Diagnoses

5.1 Case Study on Diagnostic Variety and Hallucinations

Suzanne Taïeb's 30 case studies on Muslim women covered an extensive range of diagnoses. The evidence in her dissertation described a clinical reality in which Muslim women suffered from, among others things, such diverse disorders as mania,[1] melancholia,[2] megalomania,[3] alcoholism,[4] epilepsy,[5] schizophrenia[6] and paranoia.[7] Thus, Taïeb presented a far wider spectrum of diagnoses than previously discussed in Chapter 3. The established consensus that some disorders were frequent among female Muslim patients while others were usually missing could therefore be broken by certain diligent clinical practitioners, without, however, this break being commented on by the network of colonial psychiatrists.

One of Taïeb's case studies concerned a 38-year-old Algerian woman, divorced from her third husband, who was admitted to Blida Psychiatric Hospital on the 27th of October 1938. Her diseases ranged from malaria to "chronic hallucinatory delirium, [with] initial hypochondriac manifestations, [and] an element of mental automatism (verbal hallucinations, ordered acts)", but the patient "also seems to present a weakening of the mental faculties, [as she] gives implausible details about her life." Taïeb sometimes contrasted her own scientific diagnoses with the traditional interpretations given by the patients and their families. According to her, this specific patient suffered from "*liliputian and coenesthetic* [i. e. body-focused] *visual hallucinations*". Taïeb followed this professional statement directly with the explanation proposed by the patient: "[...] *several thousand 'moulouks'* [angels], *very small, but very different in appearance and condition, invade her body and commit numerous depredations,* destroying sometimes an arm, sometimes part of her abdomen, *and they are all connected to each other by safety pins.*"[8]

---

1 Taïeb, Idées d'influence, 85.
2 Ibid., 89.
3 Ibid., 91f.
4 Ibid., 92.
5 Ibid., 94.
6 Ibid., 100ff.
7 Ibid., 105f.
8 Ibid., 119. Emphasis in the original.

These very picturesque visual hallucinations are described in some detail in the case study. As mentioned in Chapter 4.4.2, even Taïeb's notes on her patients were the result of a process of translation and interpretation – and very often also a rather condescending judgement – but as she chose to give the patients' own descriptions and explanations in her case studies, the voices of her female Muslim patients can almost be heard. The rest of this case study described the hallucinations and the aforementioned implausibility in the patient's view of things,[9] starting with the admission process to Blida, with the patient "claiming that she went to the Mustapha hospital to have her teeth done, demands to return there." The hallucinatory delirium had appeared six months before the patient's institutionalisation in Blida Psychiatric Hospital, which the patient explained through the following cause and effect: "[She] admits to having 'lost her head' the previous winter *after seeing the sky reddening, from Algiers to Tunis and even to Constantinople. That day 'the sun faded'*, she felt very overwhelmed by this; her brothers thought it best to call a *taleb*[10]*, who wrote on her left thumb and made her inhale incense.* Unfortunately, this practice burned the moulouks (angels), who had lived in her since her childhood. 'When I fell asleep, she said, I slept with my eyes, but not with my heart, and *I heard angels speak in my stomach and whisper in my ears'.* The angels, furious at having been burnt, tormented her, but now they do not harm her anymore, they tell her what is happening in the world, they announce to her marriages and deaths."[11] The initial and rather alarming delirium with the red sky and the fading sun was deemed unimportant both by the patient – as only the ṭālib's incense started the irritation of the angels – and by Taïeb, whose case study clearly focused on the subsequent hallucinatory development of the angels.

Even though the angels no longer "tormented" or "harmed" her at the moment of Taïeb's consultation, her behaviour was still dictated by the angels' orders, who ordered her to stop eating and to get married again. While at Mustapha and Blida, the patient began seeing a devil and then a number of jinn, but she refused to discuss them with Taïeb. "[...] when we mention them [the jinn], she gets irritated: one should not pronounce their name, one should not talk about them; she spits to ward off the harmful effect of our words. On the other hand, *she described with pleasure her relationship with the 'moulouks'. She is both man and woman, because the angel who possesses her is a man,* and he is sometimes in love with a woman, but she can only marry a man. It is, besides, her dearest wish."[12] This last paragraph of Taïeb's case study hinted at the existence of bisexual feelings, strengthened by the patient claiming that a female angel, "young and pretty", had "given her her breast and required the patient

---

9   The patient claimed, for example, to be able to "reduce days by an hour [...]." Ibid., 120.
10 On the figure of the ṭālib, the "sorcerer", see p. 31 and p. 174, FN 171.
11 Ibid., 119. Emphasis in the original.
12 Ibid., 120. Emphasis in the original.

to do the same".[13] However, the sexual conflict implied in both these comments went either unnoticed by Taïeb, or was deemed too unimportant to remark upon. Instead, Taïeb focused on the implausibilities in the patient's account of her life and on the traditional Islamic aspects of the patient's hallucinations.

Nevertheless, in the context of both the overall dearth of colonial diagnoses discussed in Chapter 3 and the idea of "missing diagnoses" which will be analysed in this chapter, Suzanne Taïeb's case studies serve as a counterpoint, showing the existence of a diagnostic variety in colonial psychiatric practice. This case study also shows that some patients displayed a wide variety of symptoms, indicating that they suffered from several different disorders, both mental and physical.[14]

5.2 Unfashionable Diagnoses

After looking at the diseases diagnosed in Muslim women in Chapter 3, this chapter looks at those diseases that were, supposedly, not diagnosed. Comparing the situation in North Africa with historical research on the medical situation in Europe, and especially France, highlighted the absences within the diagnostic categories and provided the analytical focus of this chapter on absence and scientific neglect.[15] Many of the reasons given for the absence of Muslim women from general psychiatric care, raised in previous chapters, also apply to this chapter's analysis of three specific non-diagnoses (as one might call them) – general paralysis, puerperal insanity[16] and hysteria, chosen either because of the level of interest shown in their absence by French colonial psychiatry or because they were traditionally "female disorders".[17] The explanations given in the theoretical texts for the absence of these diagnoses mirror the range of conflicting perspectives and interests in French psychiatry, with French colonial psychiatry reflecting

---

13 Ibid., 119.

14 On this topic, see also the introductory case study to Chapter 3, p. 105.

15 The literature used as a means of comparing the situation in North Africa to that in France comprised many of the classics of the history of medicine, but of especial importance were Jan Goldstein's, Ian Dowbiggin's and Patricia Prestwich's research on French psychiatry; Hilary Marland's and Irvine Loudon's articles on puerperal insanity; and Andrew Scull's monograph on hysteria. Goldstein, Console and Classify; ibid., Hysteria Diagnosis; Dowbiggin, Back to the Future; ibid., Degeneration; ibid., Inheriting Madness; Prestwich, Family Strategies; ibid., Female Alcoholism; Marland, Disappointment and Desolation; Loudon, Puerperal Insanity; Scull, Hysteria.

16 The term chosen here, along with "puerperal mania", was used in the 19th century. In the later colonial period, the same problems were mainly described as "puerperal psychoses".

17 About the consequences of the gendering of disorders, see for example: Jordanova, Mental Illness, 111.

the scientific arguments in France. Contextualising Muslim women within the changing environments of specific diagnoses – disputed by different strands of psychiatry and undergoing enormous developments – informs the broader questions of this work. The causes of general paralysis, the "disease of civilisation", were heavily debated during French colonialism in North Africa.[18] First, it was defined as never occurring in Muslims, then as being introduced by the French as an unfortunate side effect of the *mission civilisatrice* and finally as having always been widespread, but hidden in its "typically Muslim form". Puerperal insanity, seen as common in Europe, was almost never diagnosed in Muslim women, who were often viewed as better, more natural mothers than European women. Hysteria was diagnosed in Muslims, male and female, though only rarely in the early colonial period, and was eventually defined as an aspect of the common character of the "North African race", whereas in Europe it was long seen as a female disorder. The theoretical explanations for the absence of each of these disorders in the French colonial sources will be examined in this chapter and compared to the female Muslim case studies specifically dedicated to them.

5.3 General Paralysis: Alcohol, Syphilis and Civilisation

Although general paralysis of the insane,[19] the tertiary and final, i. e. fatal,[20] stage of syphilis, was discovered and defined by Antoine Laurent Bayle in 1822, the origins of the disorder remained controversial for almost another century. In 1872 the dermatologist Alfred Fournier voiced the theory that general paralysis was connected to syphilis, but as allegedly highly syphilitic regions like North Africa had very low rates of general paralysis, this theory was disputed[21] until Hideyo Noguchi proved

---

18 Many psychiatrists mentioned these disagreements and detailed the arguments of both sides. Pascalis, Paralysie générale, 43; Aboab, Contribution, 9; Maréschal/Chaurand, Paralysie générale, 247; Marill/Si Hassen, Paralysie générale, 435 f.; Hadida et al., Augmentation, 466.

19 In English also known as general paresis of the insane. General paralysis was a neurosyphilitic disorder encapsulating "all syphilitic afflictions of the central and peripheral nervous system [...]." Aboab, Contribution, 10. See also: Showalter, Female Malady, 110 f.; Prestwich, Family Strategies, 803.

20 Pascalis, Paralysie générale, 33. In 1916 the British psychiatrist John Warnock wrote about the situation at Egypt's ʿAbbāsiyya Hospital: "Pellagra is the chief reason for our high death-rate, but syphilis (general paralysis) helps." Warnock, Twenty-First Annual Report, 442. In French asylums, general paralytics often died within a year of their admission. Prestwich, Family Strategies, 803.

21 In 1902 Pierre Battarel wrote in his dissertation on "General Paralysis among the Native Muslim Algerians" that the connection between syphilis and general paralysis was "one of the most controversial [questions] of our times [...]." Battarel, Quelques remarques, 35.

the connection in 1913.[22] The symptoms of general paralysis, according to the psychiatrist Élie Pascalis in his 1893 dissertation on "General Paralysis in Arabs",[23] included "either mania with agitation, or the various forms of hypochondriac delirium, or the delirium of persecution",[24] and severe motor problems (i. e. paralysis, speech impediments, trembling)[25] which were "as considerable as the mental troubles".[26]

From the beginning of French medicine's interest in North Africa, there had been a focus on syphilis, which was strongly linked with immorality and responsible for many medical problems not directly related to syphilis.[27] It was believed that most – if not all – North Africans were syphilitic, with both hereditary and "acquired" syphilis being widespread,[28] and it was claimed that as, unlike in Europe, it was not a shameful disorder in North Africa, syphilitics did not suffer from stigmatisation.[29] In the sources, many moralistic explanations for the wide distribution of syphilis can be found, focusing on "deviant" forms of sexuality in Muslims. In 1854, for instance,

---

22 Berthelier, Homme maghrébin, 58.
23 Pascalis wrote the first of a series of dissertations dedicated to general paralysis in particular – and neurosyphilitic disorders in general – in Muslims. Others dealing specifically with general paralysis were Battarel's 1902 dissertation on "General Paralysis in Native Algerian Muslims" and Olry's 1940 dissertation on "General Paralysis in Muslim Natives of Tunisia". Dissertations on neurosyphilitic disorders included Laurens' 1919 dissertation on "Nervous Syphilis in the Native Mohammedans of Algeria", Aboab's 1921 dissertation on "Neurosyphilis of Native Muslims of North Africa", Goëau-Brissonnière's 1926 dissertation on "Nervous Syphilis in the Native Algerian Muslim" and Benkhelil's 1927 dissertation on "Neuropsychiatric Afflictions and Neurosyphilis in the Native Algerian Muslim".
24 Pascalis, Paralysie générale, 7.
25 These physical symptoms were often described in the case studies of female Muslim general paralytics. Meilhon, Contribution, 391; 393; Pascalis, Paralysie générale, 30; Taïeb, Idées d'influence, 122 f.; Olry, Paralysie générale, 54.
26 Pascalis, Paralysie générale, 8.
27 Perrin, Essai, 22; Gournay, Arabes et la médecine, 31; Tremsal, Siècle, 33; Poitrot, Statistiques et remarques, 1070; Charbonneau, Climat pathologique, 655; Thierry, Œuvre, 65. One of these other problems was apparently frequent miscarriages among Muslim women. See for example: Montaldo, Mortalité infantile, 103; Malmassari, Avortement, 97; Lataillade, Coutumes, 58. See also: Summers, Intimate Colonialism, 793.
28 Chellier, Voyage, 38; B., Médecine au Maroc, 382; Susini, Quelques considérations, 17; Le quartier réservé de Casablanca, 1245; Marie/Godin, Malades musulmans à Paris, 42; Woytt-Gisclard, Assistance, 114; Charbonneau, Climat pathologique, 655. See also: Léonard, Médecine et colonisation, 486. In the early colonial period, no statistical evidence for the distribution of syphilis was compiled to support the claim of its omnipresence. In 1961, however, Assicot et al. claimed that 8.1% of all Muslim patients in Blida Psychiatric Hospital suffered from syphilis, compared to 1.4% of all Europeans. They added that, among Muslims, syphilis was more frequent in male than female patients. Assicot et al., Causes principales, 273.
29 Lafitte, Contribution, 79; Monnery, Pratique, 68; Goëau-Brissonnière, Syphilis nerveuse, 63.

Adolphe Armand wrote in his book "Medical Algeria" that the frequency of syphilis was due to the rate of "relationships against nature", by which he meant "pederasty, [...] the general vice of the Arabs".[30] Armand Richardot added in his 1896 dissertation on "Medical Practices of Native Algerians" that the frequency of syphilis was caused by "Arab mores", among which he chiefly enumerated "[male] circumcision, pederasty, [and] prostitution".[31] In the colonial imagination, Muslim prostitution – which was believed to be widespread – was seen as the main reason for syphilis infections, due to prostitution being "cheap", unregulated and therefore dangerous.[32]

North Africa, with its omnipresence of immoral syphilitics and, simultaneously, its absence of general paralysis, was used in French psychiatric circles as the "Arab argument"[33] by those opposing Fournier's theory of syphilis causing general paralysis. Many psychiatrists working with North Africans presented their personal experiences as proof against Fournier's theory.[34] In 1902 Battarel, for example, deduced from his own experiences that "[...] syphilis has always existed among the Arabs, it is very frequent among them and it does not seem to us to be the cause of general paralysis itself."[35]

5.3.1   Immunity

Many French colonial doctors reported on the rarity of general paralysis in North Africa,[36] among them Voisin and Richardot in 1896, Levet and Bouquet in 1909, Porot in 1912, Lemanski in 1913, H. Thierry in 1917, Lacapère in 1918, Monnery in 1924, and M.-J. Thierry as late as 1953.[37] Muslim immunity from general paralysis became a trope,

---

30   Armand wrote that "pederasty" had its "main cause in the sequestration of women, who are the property of a small number [of men]. [...] There is, indeed, a certain amount of Arab prostitutes in the cities of Algeria, but they are only within the reach of a minimal portion of the male and single population, whose venereal appetites are strongly excited by the influence of a hot climate, after having ended precocious puberties." Armand, Algérie médicale, 416. See also: Bulliod, Étude, 11 f.; 51. Victoria Thompson analysed the notion of homosexuality as the "Arab vice" in a recent article. Thompson, 'I Went Pale', 26.

31   Richardot, Pratiques médicales, 19.

32   Astruc, Pratiques révulsives, 43. See also: Malmassari, Avortement, 103.

33   "Argument des Arabes" in French. Vernet, Chronique, 13 f.

34   See for example: Pascalis, Paralysie générale, 43.

35   Battarel, Quelques remarques, 38.

36   It was believed that some "races" were quasi-immune to general paralysis. E. M. Green, in a 1914 article on "Psychoses among Negroes", discussed the misconception of the rarity of general paralysis among "the negro race". Green, Psychoses among Negroes, 705.

37   Voisin, Souvenirs, 90; Richardot, Pratiques médicales, 20; Levet, Assistance, 239 f.; 243; Bouquet, Aliénés en Tunisie, 25 f.; 129; Porot, Tunisie, 71; Lemanski, Mœurs arabes, 109; Thierry,

not only for colonial psychiatrists, but also for specialists of neurosyphilitic disorders in France. Jean Olry summarised this situation in 1940: "Since then [a publication by Emmanuel Régis' which touched on the issues of general paralysis, probably "Practical Manual of Mental Health" in 1885] every book on general paralysis included a paragraph recalling the rarity of the disease among Arabs."[38]

As discussed in Chapter 3, published statistical evidence on colonial North Africa, containing both gender and ethnic categories, was rare. Arguably the best available source of statistics was the effort by Reboul and Régis for the 1912 Tunis Congress. Livet, who contributed his findings from the Civil Hospital of Mustapha in Algiers between 1900 and 1910 to their report, observed that 2.66% and 6.98% of all diagnoses given to Muslim men and women respectively were for general paralysis.[39] Because of the small overall number of female Muslim patients in French psychiatric care, this high percentage represented only three Muslim women. The remaining evidence from French asylums collected by Reboul and Régis all reported no female Muslim cases of general paralysis,[40] and a summary of their reports resulted in the following distribution among the different ethnical and gender groups: of all diagnoses of general paralysis given, 62.5% concerned European men (who comprised 32.68% of the overall colonial patient population in the asylums analysed by Reboul and Régis), 22.79% European women (32.44%), 6.62% Jewish men (5.52%), 2.21% Jewish women (3.74%), 3.68% Muslim men (19.53%), and 2.21% Muslim women (6.09%).[41] Therefore, all groups, apart from European and Jewish men, were underrepresented in the diagnoses of general paralysis, with Muslim men receiving the fewest diagnoses in proportion to their total patient population.[42]

Étude, 41; Lacapère, Vue d'ensemble, 147; Monnery, Pratique, 72; Thierry, Œuvre, 65. Others commented on the absence of all neurosyphilitic disorders in North Africa. Coudray, Considérations, 48; Montpellier, Problème, 451.

38 Olry, Paralysie générale, 21. See also: Susini, Quelques considérations, 22; Sutter et al., Aspects algériens, 895. In other colonial contexts, the rarity of general paralysis was also upheld. The British psychiatrist John Carothers, for instance, mentioned in 1951 that general paralysis was rare in Kenya. Carothers, Frontal Lobe Function, 16.

39 Livet did not give percentages but the actual numbers of patients. Livet, Aliénés algériens, 70; Reboul/Régis, Assistance, 51. Compare Appendix B, Fig. 8c, p. 273.

40 Reboul/Régis, Assistance, 52 ff. Compare Appendix B, Fig. 8d, p. 274 to 8g, p. 277 . In the same hospitals, the numbers for European patients, especially males, were extremely high. In Aix-en-Provence, in 1910, it amounted to 22.96% of all diagnoses given to European men. Ibid., 52.

41 Ibid., 51–4. Compare Appendix B, Fig. 9a/9b, p. 278.

42 Further research produced very different results. In a 1949 article on nervous syphilis in Morocco, it was stated that between 1935 and 1939, 2.77% of all Jewish and 7.25% of all Muslim admissions had been general paralytics. Blancardi et al., Syphilis nerveuse, 227.

The explanations for this relative absence of general paralysis among Muslims reflected the variety of theories explored by psychiatry in the 19th century. Abel-Joseph Meilhon stated in 1891 that until 1877 not a single Muslim patient had been admitted to the Montperrin asylum in Aix-en-Provence for general paralysis, which made him consider whether "the Arab race" was immune to it.[43] It was a question of a special Muslim "immunity", not simple misdiagnoses, because Meilhon's colleague in Aix-en-Provence, Élie Pascalis, showed in 1893 that while general paralysis had not been diagnosed for Muslim patients before 1877, French colonial patients were admitted to Aix-en-Provence as suffering from the condition.[44] The doctors responsible for the patient selection in Algeria were therefore clearly able to diagnose the disorder correctly.

It was even proposed that general paralysis was more frequent among colonial settlers than those living in Europe.[45] Meilhon explained this special Muslim "immunity" through the "idiosyncrasy of the race", by which he meant the Muslim lifestyle and temperament, and religious regulations prohibiting the consumption of alcohol.[46]

However, the main reason for the North African immunity to general paralysis was seen to be the "lack of intellectual overwork" among Muslims.[47] In 1868 Jobert, for example, listed no general paralytics among 665 mad Muslim Algerians, which he explained through the hot Algerian climate and also "the nakedness of thought in populations delayed in civilisation. The good is by the side of the evil here."[48] In the words of Armand Richardot in 1896, general paralysis was "the sad privilege of races of a superior intellectual level",[49] and, according to Pascalis in 1893, it seemed "to be

---

43 Meilhon, Contribution, 385.

44 Pascalis, Paralysie générale, 15. Pascalis concluded in 1893 that general paralysis was still "relatively infrequent among them [the Arabs], since we found barely 5 general paralytics among 100 ordinary patients, a proportion significantly inferior to that generally established in the asylums." Ibid., 17. Jobert mentioned in 1868 that he had seen several cases of general paralysis among Europeans, and in 1912 Reboul and Régis mentioned general paralysis as one of the common disorders for European settlers. Jobert, Projet, 14; Reboul/Régis, Assistance, 13.

45 For instance, one psychiatrist, Ch. Marcel, wrote in 1906: "Finally, note the extreme gravity of nervous diseases, especially of insanity and general paralysis which, among the Europeans in the colonies, are five times more frequent than in France." Marcel, Fréquence comparée, 278.

46 Meilhon, Contribution, 385. Repeated verbatim by Meilhon in his 1896 article. Ibid., Aliénation mentale, part 6, 345.

47 Discussed under the heading of "Lack of Intellectual Overwork" as a characteristic of North African normality. See pp. 50 – 54.

48 Jobert, Projet, 14. The idea that the climate influenced the development of general paralysis seems to have been mentioned by Collardot in his untraceable article from 1864. See: Delasiauve, Review of Collardot, 118.

49 Richardot, Pratiques médicales, 36.

truly frequent only in societies where civilisation has reached its maximum and its utmost intellectual development".[50] Adopting these psychiatric theories, the idea that Muslims were protected from general paralysis by their lack of intellect was accepted by most colonial experts in the early colonial period.[51]

5.3.2 Moral Corruption

At the turn of the century, it was proposed that although general paralysis had been rare or even inexistent at the beginning of the colonisation of North Africa, this was no longer the case after years of French influence. Was the process of civilisation therefore to blame for the rise in numbers among Muslims? In 1897 the Austrian psychiatrist Richard Freiherr von Krafft-Ebing coined the famous phrase of "civilisation and syphilisation" causing general paralysis,[52] repeated by many French colonial psychiatrists.[53] The "lack of intellectual overwork", due to lower levels of civilisation, was now used to explain the relative absence of general paralysis in "syphilised" North Africans.[54] In 1918, for example, Antoine Porot took up this idea because he had not encountered a single case of "native *general paralysis*" in the war, even though he acknowledged that syphilis was widespread. The "immunity" of North Africans against general paralysis could, therefore, not be due to a Muslim resistance to syphilis. He contemplated whether psychiatry should explain this immunity through "[...] the almost constant absence of anxiety in the native and turn the anxious overwork into the pathogenic factor of general paralysis on the syphilised brain?"[55] Syphilis alone

---

50 Pascalis, Paralysie générale, 5. Meilhon's analysis of the professions of his patients suffering from general paralysis seemed to agree with this assumption. He found in 1891 that among the eleven male general paralytics in Aix-en-Provence – the female patients had no profession –, seven had professions that demanded a certain education, which allowed the Arabs to "mingle with the cerebral life of the Europeans, adopting their mores, their customs, their excesses [...]." Meilhon, Contribution, 388. Other psychiatrists objected to this idea. In 1902 Pierre Battarel pointed out the existence of healthy, intelligent Muslims who became, for example, doctors and constantly used their brains without becoming general paralytics. Marill and Si Hassen stated in 1951 that their research into Muslim general paralytics had shown that their professions were rather modest. Battarel, Quelques remarques, 25; Marill/Si Hassen, Paralysie générale, 449. See also: Laurens, Contribution, 44 f.

51 For example: B., Médecine au Maroc, 382.

52 Bloch, Erstes Auftreten, 30.

53 Sicard, Étude, 81; Benkhelil, Contribution, 58; Poitrot, Statistiques et remarques, 1070. See also: Bégué, French Psychiatry in Algeria, 537.

54 Lacapère, Vue d'ensemble, 147; Maréschal/Chaurand, Paralysie générale, 249

55 Porot, Notes, 384.

was not responsible for general paralysis, in Porot's opinion – "anxious overwork" had to coexist with syphilis in order for the disease to develop.

Apart from "overwork", the progress of civilisation was measured, in the context of general paralysis, by the spread of "European vices" among North Africans. Adolphe Kocher gravely stated in 1883 that Arabs had only adopted the vices of civilisation,[56] and the emergence of general paralysis, "which seemed reserved for civilised nations", was proof of this moral decay under French influence.[57] Pascalis repeated this sentiment in 1893: "Letting themselves be overcome by our civilisation today, the Arabs willingly retain only the vices from it, and this explains how general paralysis, appearing only in 1877, seems to be gradually spreading since then."[58] Given time, Arabs would embrace civilisation's vices, abandon the protective mechanisms of their own traditions and become general paralytics, according to the psychiatrist and Charcot student Gilbert Ballet, who joined a discussion on general paralytics in 1898, as reported in the *Annales Médico-Psychologiques*.[59] This opinion was also summarised by Maxime Laignel-Lavastine in a review written on Georges Sicard's 1907 dissertation on the "Frequency of Nervous Disorders among Native Algerian Muslims": "Placed in conditions of existence which bring him closer to the European, the Arab is struck in equal proportions [by general paralysis and *tabes dorsalis*]. It is therefore soon likely that civilisation, from which the Arabs mainly adopt the vices, will constitute in them an altogether favourable ground for the development of nervous afflictions."[60]

Civilisation, it was realised, could, at least in this context, not be construed as a completely positive term. Jean Sutter, for instance, carefully listed in his 1937 dissertation the medical advantages and disadvantages of the French *mission civilisatrice*, with general paralysis among the latter. While the Algerian Muslims had generally benefitted from the civilising process, civilisation – with its accompanying gifts of new vices – had introduced formerly unknown disorders to the North African clinical tableau. Among these vices, alcoholism – adopted by Muslims and erroneously assumed by French colonial psychiatrists to cause general paralysis – played an important role.[61] The theory of alcohol as a pathogenic factor in general paralysis explained the rising patient numbers of already "syphilised" North Africans who, in contact

---

56   Kocher, Criminalité, 1 f.; 72. This sentiment was repeated by others. Meilhon, Aliénation mentale, part 4, 34; Gervais, Contribution, 47; Thierry, Étude, 57.

57   Kocher, Criminalité, 72.

58   Pascalis, Paralysie générale, 42.

59   Semalaigne, Anatomie pathologique, 465.

60   Laignel-Lavastine, Review of Sicard, 624. *Tabes dorsalis* is another neurosyphilitic disorder.

61   Sutter, Épilepsie mentale, 76. See also: Desruelles/Bersot, Assistance aux aliénés en Algérie, 594; Olry, Paralysie générale, 35; 73. For France, see for example: Prestwich, Female Alcoholism, 327. Among the case studies on female Muslim general paralytics, very few patients were described as alcoholics. Olry, Paralysie générale, 53; 55.

with French civilisation, acquired formerly inexistent forms of morbidity. However, Meilhon pointed out as early as 1891 that the theory of alcoholism causing general paralysis did not fit the clinical reality encountered among Muslims. He stated that, while prohibited,[62] the consumption of alcohol was widespread among Muslim men in Algerian cities, but added that "[...] yet, among those intoxicated natives, only a small number, our statistics show, fall into general paralysis."[63]

Nonetheless, many colonial psychiatrists remained advocates of the theory of general paralysis being caused by the increasing alcoholisation (as one might label it) of the Maghreb. In 1893, for example, Élie Pascalis proposed that "among our Arabs, we must assign a significant role to alcoholism. It then becomes easy to explain the time delay in its appearance and the relative rarity of general paralysis among the Arabs."[64] In a paper for the 1937 Congress in Nancy on "General Paralysis in Tunisia" – 25 years after Noguchi proved that syphilis bacteria caused general paralysis –, Maréchal and Chaurand stated that, in their opinion, the absence of alcoholism was "a crucial factor" in the former rarity[65] and the "undeniable increase in the number of general paralyses" in recent years.[66]

5.3.3 Muslim General Paralysis

Some authors, however, insisted that theories on the rarity of general paralysis among Muslims were based on misconceptions.[67] This faulty information was only "dispelled" by new numerical data gained in the psychiatric hospitals constructed in the 1930s.

---

62 Meilhon, Contribution, 385. See also: Ibid., Aliénation mentale, part 6, 345. In 1902, Pierre Battarel attacked Meilhon for accentuating the prohibition of alcohol: "Mr Meilhon, who may have only known the Arabs from the other side of the Mediterranean, could hardly realise their taste for alcohol, particularly for anisette and absinthe." Battarel, Quelques remarques, 29. Battarel himself believed that alcoholism played a significant role in the development of general paralysis. Ibid., 33. On the topic of Muslim North Africans drinking absinthe, see also: Studer, Green Fairy in the Maghreb.
63 Meilhon, Contribution, 387.
64 Pascalis, Paralysie générale, 41.
65 Maréchal/Chaurand, Paralysie générale, 248.
66 Ibid., 250.
67 The personal experience of the French psychiatrist Auguste Marie, for example, had proven that general paralysis was quite common among Arabs. Goëau-Brissonnière referred to a paper given by Marie at the 1922 meeting of the Société de Médecine in Paris, in which Marie described a visit to Egypt in 1904 and how he had been given British statistics covering more than 1,000 cases of Muslim general paralytics over 30 years. Goëau-Brissonnière, Syphilis nerveuse, 47. See also: Marie, Sur quelques aspects, 761; Duclaux, Report, 1056; Ceillier, Report, 1353.

In 1955, for instance, Élie Hadida, François-Georges Marill and Maurice Porot presented a paper on neurosyphilis in North Africans at the Nice Congress, stating that
between 1901 and 1925 there had been only twelve cases of North African general
paralytics, while 529 cases had been reported between 1926 and 1955. They concluded
that "it is therefore not possible anymore, at present, to evoke the 'excessive' rarity of
nervous determinations in syphilis among North African Muslims."[68]

This strand of colonial psychiatry saw itself as fighting against "legends", "prejudices", and "popular opinions"[69] disseminated by ill-informed authors, such as the
general doctors responsible for the collection of patients to be shipped to France,
who, according to the psychiatric experts, were not trained to recognise symptoms
of general paralysis.[70] Moreover, general paralysis was hidden, according to Goëau-
Brissonnière, by the "mores, customs and religious beliefs of the indigenous populations".[71] This mixture of non-specialists misdiagnosing patients and of Muslims somehow "hiding" general paralytics became, over time, the general theory to explain the
changing numbers.[72] Antoine Porot asserted in 1943 that the superior knowledge
psychiatrists had gained from working in the new psychiatric institutions invalidated
earlier assumptions and that new numerical evidence relativised the theory of general
paralysis being rare in North Africa.[73]

In 1959 Jean Sutter, Maurice Porot and Yves Pélicier published the aforementioned article on "Algerian Aspects of Mental Pathology", in which they concluded
that, apart from the "lack of means of investigation" in pre-hospital times, North
African general paralysis was different from that observed in Europe due to its

---

68 Hadida et al., Augmentation, 467. In a paper presented at the 1937 Nancy Congress, Maréschal
    and Chaurand reported on the situation at the Manouba Psychiatric Hospital between Decem-
    ber 1931 and December 1936. In those five years, there had been 45 general paralytics (8.57%)
    out of a general hospital population of 525, and among the 287 Muslims, 23 patients (8%) suf-
    fered from general paralysis. Maréschal/Chaurand, Paralysie générale, 248. See also: Marill/
    Si Hassen, Paralysie générale, 454.

69 Goëau-Brissonnière, for instance, talked about the "persistent prejudice" of the rarity of general
    paralysis in "certain scientific circles" in 1926. Goëau-Brissonnière, Syphilis nerveuse, 47.

70 Laurens, Contribution, 9; Peyre, Maladies mentales, 195.

71 Goëau-Brissonnière, Syphilis nerveuse, 190. This concealment could be literal. Jean Olry stated
    in 1940 that female Muslim general paralytics were hidden by their families, which led to the
    misconception of general paralysis being more frequent among Muslim men. Olry, Paralysie
    générale, 68.

72 In this paper, Maréschal and Chaurand stated in 1937 that "general paralysis *is a specialist diag-
    nosis*", which could be, and had been, misinterpreted by non-experts. With the introduction of
    psychiatric hospitals, home to the real experts, the number of diagnoses would undoubtedly
    rise. Maréschal/Chaurand, Paralysie générale, 249 f. Emphasis in the original. The same was
    stated by Henri Aubin in 1939. Aubin, Introduction, 199.

73 Porot, Œuvre psychiatrique, 372.

"poverty of delusional ideas".[74] They claimed that it had been especially difficult for untrained observers to identify general paralysis among Muslims because they did not display the same characteristics as European general paralytics.[75] Antoine Porot and Jean Sutter described the differences between European and North African general paralysis in 1939: "With regard to native *general paralysis*, we must rise first of all against the dogma of its nonexistence. Native G. P. exists; it is even very far from being exceptional; but it is, from a mental point of view, quite different from classic schemas and this explains partly [why] it remained unrecognised for so long [...]."[76] These differences included the absence of euphoria, megalomania and self-criticism among Muslim patients, and the rapidity of their mental deterioration.[77] An analysis of the case studies, on the other hand, could not confirm these characteristic absences, as some female Muslim general paralytics were described as suffering from "ideas of grandeur" and persecution mania.[78] In the case study introducing Chapter 3, for example, Battarel's 1902 report on a female general paralytic was discussed. Battarel's patient, brought up in a Catholic orphanage, claimed she had married the King of Annam and that one of her sons was Jesus Christ.[79] Another of his patients claimed she was pregnant, "without any symptom of pregnancy", and that she had the rank of an Arab general.[80]

---

74 Sutter et al., Aspects algériens, 895.
75 Meilhon, for example, stated as early as 1891 that "whereas in France the general paralytic is very easy-going", Arab general paralytics were violent. Meilhon, Contribution, 388. This theory was repeated by Pascalis in 1893 and Battarel in 1902. Pascalis, Paralysie générale, 43; Battarel, Quelques remarques, 22 ff. In the case studies of female Muslim general paralytics, however, few were described as dangerous. Meilhon, Contribution, 391; Taïeb, Idées d'influence, 122.
76 Porot/Sutter, 'Primitivisme', 238. Emphasis in the original.
77 Ibid., 238. This special character of Muslim general paralysis, connected to the normal "mentality" of Muslims, had already been mentioned by Maréschal and Chaurand in 1937. Maréschal/Chaurand, Paralysie générale, 250. By contrast, Marill and Si Hassen stated in 1951 that megalomania and euphoria were frequent manifestations among Muslim general paralytics. Marill/Si Hassen, Paralysie générale, 438; 441. In the case studies of female Muslim general paralytics, only one case was described as having none of these symptoms. Goëau-Brissonnière, Syphilis nerveuse, 134. The same case was reported by Benkhelil. Benkhelil, Contribution, 82 f.
78 Battarel, Quelques remarques, 64; Taïeb, Idées d'influence, 123.
79 Battarel, Quelques remarques, 63 f.
80 Ibid., 65. On the topic of French colonial psychiatrists treating pregnancies without symptoms, among them Battarel's case study, see: Studer, Pathologisierung des Maghrebs.

5.3.4   Female General Paralytics

In France, general paralysis was seen as a clearly male disorder. The Canadian historian Patricia Prestwich, who analysed admissions to the asylums of the department of
the Seine between 1876 and 1914, stated that at the Saint-Anne asylum 20% of male
patients suffered from general paralysis, against 6% among women.[81] In the North
African context, few records mentioned female Muslim cases.[82] Kocher's statistical
evidence for general paralysis at the Civil Hospital of Mustapha for the years 1867
to 1882, for instance, showed that among the European male patients 7.36% were
general paralytics, among European women 3.3%, and among Muslim men 5.19%.
Kocher reported no cases of general paralysis in Muslim women for these 16 years.[83]

As mentioned above, among the data collected by Reboul and Régis for the 1912
Tunis Congress, there were only three female Muslim general paralytics.[84] Nonetheless,
Reboul and Régis concluded that while general paralysis was rarer among Muslims
than among Europeans, the statistics showed the "curious peculiarity among Muslims,
as indeed among the Jews in the statistics, that general paralysis is almost as frequent
in women as in men."[85] Similarly, Pierre Battarel wrote in 1902 that his statistical evidence for the Civil Hospital of Mustapha – eight women among 26 Muslim general
paralytics – was noteworthy.[86] Comparing his findings with French statistics composed
by earlier psychiatrists, who had found ratios of one to eight (Bayle and Krafft-Ebing)
and one to 14 (Louis-Florentin Calmeil and Meilhon),[87] Battarel concluded that the
percentage of female Muslim general paralytics was exceedingly high.[88]

---

81 Prestwich, Family Strategies, 803.
82 Meilhon revealed that between 1860 and 1889 13 general paralytics (2.61%) had been among
    the 498 Muslim patients admitted to the asylum in Aix-en-Provence, and only two of these
    had been Muslim women. Both Pascalis' study of 16 patients in Aix-en-Provence in 1893 and
    Benkhelil's 1927 research of 27 Muslim general paralytics at the Civil Hospital of Mustapha
    covered three female Muslim patients. In 1951, the psychiatrists Marill and Si Hassen published
    results of research into general paralysis among Muslim patients at Blida Psychiatric Hospi-
    tal, concluding that only 8.75% of all Muslim general paralytics had been women. Meilhon,
    Contribution, 384 f.; Pascalis, Paralysie générale, 32; Benkhelil, Contribution, 67–90; Marill/
    Si Hassen, Paralysie générale, 448.
83 Kocher, Criminalité, 70. Compare Appendix B, Fig. 8a, p. 271.
84 Livet, Aliénés algériens, 70; Reboul/Régis, Assistance, 51–4. Compare Appendix B, Fig. 9a/9b,
    p. 278.
85 Reboul/Régis, Assistance, 51.
86 Battarel, Quelques remarques, 20.
87 Ibid.
88 Ibid., 21. This was also observed in Egypt. In 1917 there were eleven female patients among 58
    diagnoses of general paralysis, "this proportion of female general paralytics being greatly in
    excess of what occurs most commonly in England [...]." Report for the Year 1917, 133. See also:

Nonetheless, the evidence of Reboul and Régis, and Battarel, was in the minority – most personal accounts mentioned no female Muslim general paralytics, either before the construction of psychiatric institutions in North Africa or after. In 1951, for example, François-Georges Marill and Abdennour Si Hassen conducted a study of general paralysis in the psychiatric service of the general hospital in Constantine and in Blida Psychiatric Hospital. The study of admissions in Constantine between 1935 and 1942 showed that, in comparison with their respective total patient population, European, Jewish and Muslim men (5.43%, 7.25% and 2.95%) had higher proportions of general paralysis than women (1.48%, 2.99% and 2.38%).[89] While the proportion for female paralytics was much lower in Blida between 1937 and 1949, the same general gender difference could be observed for men (6.29%, 5.1% and 3.38%) and women (0.33%, 0.87% and 0.74%).[90] In 1939 André Donnadieu summarised research conducted at Berrechid Neuropsychiatric Hospital on Moroccan general paralytics. Over a four-year period (1935 to 1938), there had been 24 cases of general paralysis out of a total Muslim hospital population of 424 (5.66%), and all of these cases concerned men.[91] Donnadieu pointed out that this "extreme rarity among native women" was surprising as they were "frequently affected by syphilis".[92] As late as 1950, R. P. Poitrot, who conducted research on cases of neurosyphilis at the same hospital, concluded that there had been only seven female cases of general paralysis between 1940 and 1949, and all had been European.[93] Similarly, a study of mental disorders among patients in Blida Psychiatric Hospital covering the years 1958 and 1959 admitted that there were no female Muslim general paralytics among their patient group.[94]

Being equally "syphilised" – though significantly less civilised – than Muslim men, this glaring absence of female Muslim general paralytics was consistently explained by their "primitiveness". In 1893, for example, Pascalis suspected the lack of civilisation among Muslim women to be the reason for their "immunity": "Very common in men, it [general paralysis] is relatively rare in the [Muslim] woman, whose existence is more concentrated, and who, living more in her interior, is not subjected, like man, to the incessant agitation of business and to the on-going activity of the mind."[95] This idea that Muslim women used their brains even less than Muslim men, and were

---

Savage, Lunacy in Egypt, 174. By contrast, only one female patient was among 30 Muslim general paralytics at the ᶜAbbāsiyya Hospital in Cairo in 1909. The Egyptian Government Hospital for the Insane, 167.
89 Marill/Si Hassen, Paralysie générale, 453.
90 Ibid., 453 f.
91 Donnadieu, Situation, 316.
92 Ibid., 318.
93 Poitrot, Statistiques et remarques, 1069.
94 Assicot et al., Causes principales, 268.
95 Pascalis, Paralysie générale, 32.

therefore better protected,[96] was taken up by Witold Lemanski in 1913, who stated that he had not come across a single case of general paralysis in Muslim women in his twenty years' experience as a doctor in Tunisia, adding: "yet the chances of specific contamination are not lacking, as is already known. But only very civilised and very overworked people develop cerebral complications."[97] Lemanski, baffled by the simultaneous distribution of syphilis – shown through his vague allusion to "specific contamination" – and absence of general paralysis among Muslim women, explained the complete absence of female Muslim general paralytics through lack of civilisation and overwork.

Although, among the case studies, most Muslim women were explicitly described as having "no profession",[98] it was assumed that only professionally employed people became general paralytics.[99] Pierre Battarel claimed in 1902 that most female Muslim general paralytics were either prostitutes[100] or servants,[101] the latter because of the civilising influence of contact with Europeans. According to Battarel, this corresponded with experiences in France: "[...] it should also be noted that almost all general paralytics who enter the asylums in France are 'irregular' and not 'legitimate' women who have been more exposed than other women of the same status of fortune to the main factors invoked today for general paralysis: overwork, alcohol, etc. It appears to be the same for our native Algerian women."[102]

The reasons given for the absence of general paralysis among female Muslim patients correspond therefore with the tropes of North African normality discussed in Chapter 1. Muslim women's lives reduced their intellectual faculties and it was obvious, to French observers, that only contact with France or complete moral degradation – as allegedly shown through alcoholism and prostitution – could cause these women to develop the "disorder of civilisation". However, in the colonial imagination, Muslim women not only escaped the pathogenic influence of French civilisation, but, due to complete gender segregation, potential female patients also eluded French awareness. Jean Olry, for instance, stated in 1940 that even if Muslim women, secluded in

---

96 Already discussed, with respect to the general absence of insanity among Muslim women, under the heading of "Lack of Intellectual Overwork", p. 50.

97 Lemanski, Mœurs arabes, 119 f.

98 Pascalis, Paralysie générale, 29; Meilhon, Contribution, 391; 393; Battarel, Quelques remarques, 64.

99 Compare p. 189, FN 50, where Meilhon stated that most of his male Muslim patients belonged to "educated" professions.

100 Battarel, Quelques remarques, 27 f.

101 Ibid., 27; 63. One of the cases described by Suzanne Taïeb concerned a woman who had worked for European employers. Taïeb, Idées d'influence, 124.

102 Battarel, Quelques remarques, 28.

both the countryside and the cities, developed general paralysis, the French had no means of noticing.[103]

Summarising, it can be said that while the colonial psychiatrists were divided over practically every aspect of general paralysis, from its rarity to its reasons and symptoms, they agreed on it being a topic worthy of debate. The other two missing diagnoses discussed in this chapter were of less importance in the colonial worldview.

5.4 Puerperal Insanity: The Perfect Mothers

In the 19th century, puerperal insanity was directly connected to the physicality of procreation and included all mental disorders developed by women because of different aspects of pregnancy, parturition and the postpartum period, as it was believed that, during pregnancy and just after childbirth, women were in an especially delicate state.[104] Those suffering from puerperal insanity were depressed, had attacks of mania, and often attempted to commit suicide or even to kill their child.[105]

In 1857 the French psychiatrist Louis-Victor Marcé published an article in the *Annales Médico-Psychologiques* on puerperal insanity in which he summarised its causes, including, among others, heredity,[106] the number of previous pregnancies, exhaustion through breastfeeding and weaning, previous bouts of insanity, the advanced age of the mother, the woman's "moral state" during pregnancy, the "return of menstruation" after giving birth, and the pains, terrors and attendant medical complications of childbirth.[107] In the 19th century most women had multiple pregnancies and many experienced physical complications during and after birth, but, according to the psychiatrist Victor Parant in 1888, puerperal insanity only occurred in women with a "nervous predisposition", who were "under conditions favourable to the explosion of madness" and in whom "an accident provokes this explosion".[108] He further specified

---

103 Olry, Paralysie générale, 91.

104 The psychiatrist Idanof, for example, wrote in 1893: "there is no doubt, in fact, that during pregnancy and the puerperium the nervous system of women finds itself in exceptional conditions." Idanof, Contribution, 168. The interest in puerperal insanity has to be seen, as Jacqueline Leckie argued, in the broader context of the "medicalization of sexuality [...]." Leckie, Unsettled Minds, 111.

105 Marland, Disappointment and Desolation, 306. For England, see also: Showalter, Female Malady, 57 f. In cases of infanticide, puerperal insanity was seen as a mitigating circumstance, but only if testified by a psychiatrist. Ibid., 313.

106 "First among the predisposing causes we place, as with all mental diseases, heredity." Marcé, Études, 570.

107 Ibid., 583.

108 Parant, Folie puerpérale, 67.

that this "nervous predisposition" was often caused by degeneration. Summarising the theories of the British psychiatrist Archibald Campbell Clark,[109] Parant wrote: "Puerperal insanity, understood in this way, is a true disease of degeneration. The patient who presents it is a degenerate, either in her nervous system, or in her functional organism [...]."[110] This role of degeneration sheds light on a fact related by Hilary Marland in a recent article on puerperal insanity in the 19th century. According to Marland, puerperal insanity was simultaneously associated with rich women "enfeebled by their idle existence and heightened sensitivity, unable to withstand the strains of pregnancy and childbearing", and the poor classes, who endured harrowing circumstances.[111] In Europe, both the overly sensitive lady and the exhausted working-class multipara, each degenerates in their own way, suffered from puerperal insanity.

5.4.1   Puerperal Problems in North Africa

In the published colonial sources, the disorder of puerperal insanity among Muslim women was almost never remarked upon. While the diagnosis itself seems to have been rare, one can only find a couple of statements explaining its absence among Muslims or references to the situation among European women.[112] Puerperal insanity was almost completely absent from the published colonial sources, even though North Africans themselves thought that people were especially susceptible to attacks of jinn during what the Moroccan psychiatrist Rita El-Khayat described in 1978 as "rites of passage": birth, puberty, marriage and pregnancies.[113] These socially accepted demonic possessions following childbirth could probably have been interpreted by French colonial psychiatrists as puerperal insanity, but it seems that they seldom were.

The accounts of colonial doctors working on childbirth in North Africa focused on the severe medical conditions, which the colonial worldview ascribed to the ignorance of traditional Muslim midwives,[114] and the doctors were surprised that physical accidents during childbirth did not occur more often.[115] Overall, most experts agreed

---

109 He referred specifically to the article "Aetiology, Pathology and Treatment of Puerperal Insanity", published in the *Journal of Medical Science*, later the *British Journal of Medicine*, in 1887.
110 Parant, Folie puerpérale, 80.
111 Marland, Disappointment and Desolation, 309.
112 Meilhon, Aliénation mentale, part 2, 206; Lemanski, Mœurs arabes, 120. These exceptional comments are analysed in detail below.
113 El-Khayat, Tradition et modernité, 70. See also: Cherki, Frantz Fanon, 120.
114 The incompetence of these midwives was stressed by, among others: Richardot, Pratiques médicales, 40 f.; Bouhadjeb, Accouchement, 11; Thierry, Étude, 61; Lacascade, Puériculture et colonisation, 11; Comby, Médecine française, 980; Lataillade, Coutumes, 9.
115 Amat, M'zab, 281.

that, contrary to popular opinion, North African women were not immune to physical problems connected with childbirth.[116] Joseph-Marie-Fernand Lafitte even claimed in 1892 that Tunisian women probably suffered to a greater degree from physical accidents during labour than European women "because of the miserable conditions of their existence".[117] Although few experts doubted that Muslim women regularly suffered from mechanical accidents and unhygienic conditions during childbirth, the experiences of colonial psychiatrists showed that very few of these women developed puerperal insanity.[118] Kocher's statistical evidence for the Civil Hospital of Mustapha from 1867 to 1882 recorded that puerperal insanity amounted to 4.67% of all diagnoses among European women, but only 1.23% of all Muslim women – i. e. out of 18 observed cases, only one concerned an Arab woman.[119] Meilhon encountered just one case of puerperal insanity among the Muslim patients at the Montperrin asylum in Aix-en-Provence, which he published as one of his case studies in his 1896 article, and in it commented on the astonishing rarity of the disorder among Arab women.[120]

The reason for this rarity was localised in the character of Muslim women. As discussed in Chapter 1 under the heading of "Muslim Women as Wombs", they were often seen as perfect mothers – both their nature and social customs forced them to adhere to their role as procreators.[121] In 1913 Witold Lemanski explained the absence of puerperal problems through the suitability of Muslim women for motherhood: "Puerperal insanity is also very rarely seen. [Muslim] Women have such a high conception of motherhood that their spirit becomes, if possible, yet more phlegmatic and calm: their uncomplicated ideas do not become confused in the maze of delusions."[122] According to Lemanski, this idealised natural motherhood – lost in Europe through emancipation –, in addition to the simplicity of their minds, explained the low numbers of puerperal insanity among Muslim women.

The numbers of cases seem to have risen with the construction of institutions in North Africa, although this growing acceptance of North African patients developing

---

116 Louis Lataillade, for example, stated in 1936 that accidents of childbirth did occur among Muslim women: "Whatever one pleases to repeat, the Moorish women are not immune to the evils which afflict European women." Lataillade, Coutumes, 160.

117 Lafitte, Contribution, 116.

118 The same was observed in Egypt. The British psychiatrist John Warnock stated in 1924 that "puerperal insanity occurs among Egyptian women, but is more common among Europeans." Warnock, Twenty-Eight Years, 597.

119 Kocher, Criminalité, 70. Compare Appendix B, Fig. 8a, p. 271.

120 Meilhon, Aliénation mentale, part 2, 206.

121 This was repeated by postcolonial doctors and psychiatrists. The Algerian psychiatrist Mahfoud Boucebci, for instance, wrote in 1982 that Algerian women were still defined by their role as mothers. Boucebci, Psychopathologie sociale, 204.

122 Lemanski, Mœurs arabes, 120.

puerperal problems can only be glimpsed through remarks in reports on, nominally, unrelated topics. In 1926, for example, one of Antoine Porot's students, Don Côme Arrii, presented in his dissertation on "Criminal Impulsivity among Native Algerians" the case study of an unmarried young Algerian woman accused of murdering her newborn child, and her responsibility for that crime was examined. He stressed the medical importance of a crisis she had suffered after imprisonment: "It was a fit of manic agitation typical of hysterical manifestations. These fits [...] may very well arise after childbirth, [but] they can also be seen on the occasion of incarceration (prison psychosis)."[123] Arrii did not mean to suggest that this young woman had murdered her child in a fit of "puerperal insanity" – her crisis had, on the contrary, only been triggered by her experience of imprisonment. Rather, this casual connection between North African patients and the diagnosis of puerperal psychosis showed that notions of a North African immunity against puerperal psychoses were no longer upheld.[124]

By 1954 the diagnosis of puerperal insanity seems to have been quite common and was unquestionably accepted by the colonial psychiatrists as a widespread disorder among Muslim women. G.-A. Manceaux, Jean Sutter and Yves Pélicier stated in a paper on "Melancholic States in the North African Native" at the Paris Congress: "Among indigenous women, the importance of the puerperium appeared considerable [as a pathogenic factor of melancholia], contrasting with the modest role of menopause, which is the opposite of what can be observed in European women."[125] This "importance of the puerperium", i. e. the state of a woman during and directly after childbirth, as a pathogenic factor was not further explained, nor were figures given to sustain this claim – the never mentioned, never explained absence of the diagnosis of puerperal insanity in the Maghreb was, without discussion, replaced by the claim that mental problems caused by the puerperium were rather frequent among North African women.

---

123 Arrii, Impulsivité criminelle, 86.
124 Another author casually mentioning puerperal psychoses was Eliane Demassieux, who wrote in her 1941 dissertation on "Social Service in Psychiatry" that Algeria had a maternity hospital for puerperal psychoses, pregnancies of "young female psychopaths" and "those tainted with syphilis [...]." Demassieux, Service social, 47.
125 Manceaux et al., États mélancoliques, 271. Zulmiro de Almeida mentioned this Muslim peculiarity in an article written in 1975 and explained the absence of menopausal problems through the fact that the "rural Muslim woman awaits rather impatiently the time when she will begin to fully enjoy her existence and a higher social status. Until then, she remains a kind of 'spoiled or badly-behaved child' to whom the right to speak is rarely given. Emancipation, freedom and maturity only come to her completely at the age of 45 years." Almeida, Perturbations, 254. De Almeida alluded to the collection of articles on psychiatry in Algeria from the 1969 special issue of Information Psychiatrique and directly quoted one of them by describing Muslim women as being treated as "spoilt or badly-behaved" children. Réflexions sur la pathologie mentale féminine en Algérie, 885 f.

During the struggle for independence, the numbers of puerperal psychoses apparently rose even further in Algeria. In the appendices of the "Wretched of the Earth", Frantz Fanon published a selection of case studies in 1961, one of them describing a French female patient suffering from puerperal psychosis. Fanon used this as an opportunity to discuss "puerperal psychoses among refugees", by which he meant the 300,000 Algerians on the Tunisian and Moroccan borders, displaced by the Algerian War of Independence:[126] "It was predictable, given the malnutrition which reigns in the camps, that pregnant women show a particular predisposition to the emergence of puerperal psychoses. [...] Frankly, there are few Algerian refugees who, having given birth, do not develop mental disorders."[127] Apart from the malnutrition and deplorable hygiene in these camps, Fanon cited the experiences of Muslim women during the War of Independence as a major cause of puerperal psychosis. Among the different symptoms displayed by these Algerian refugees were fury, depression accompanied by suicide attempts, and anxiety attacks. These women suffered delusions of persecution, "aggression against the French, who want to kill the unborn or newly born child, or a sense of imminent death, the patients then imploring invisible executioners to spare their child..."[128]

However, it was only in the last two years of the French colonisation of North Africa that scientific interest in puerperal problems suddenly increased. In 1961 Assicot et al. named malnutrition, puerperal problems and reactions to external factors, i. e. to the Algerian War of Independence, as the main reasons for mental troubles in Algerian Muslims.[129] Statistical evidence they had compiled at Blida Psychiatric Hospital covering 1958 and 1959 showed that 12.5% of all female Muslim patients suffered from puerperal problems, whereas no European cases were reported for the same period. They were the only colonial experts who addressed the sudden increase in puerperal problems in the decade preceding their article – but failed to explain it: "In addition to the relative frequency, we should note the current resurgence, since in 1950 there were only 3.8% of puerperal psychoses [among Muslim women]."[130]

In 1962 Michèle Chappert wrote her dissertation on the topic, and in the same year J. Mares and R. Barre composed an article on the puerperium, published in the *Annales Médico-Psychologiques*. Chappert as well as Mares and Barre took the numerical importance of puerperal problems among Muslims to be self-evident,[131] and Mares

126 Fanon, Damnés, 266.
127 Ibid., 267.
128 Ibid., 267 f.
129 Assicot et al., Causes principales, 262. Assicot et al. also dedicated one of their case studies to puerperal problems. Ibid., 278 f.
130 Ibid., 276.
131 Chappert, Contribution, 10; Mares/Barre, Quelques aspects, 31.

and Barre showed their surprise at the absence of scientific research conducted on the topic.[132] The research of Mares and Barre covered one of the services at Blida Psychiatric Hospital for both Muslim and European female patients between 1960 and 1961. However, they only analysed the Muslim cases of puerperal insanity among those, as they were interested in Muslim particularities in disorders[133] and as the symptoms displayed by European women "match those normally encountered in metropolitan France".[134] Their study revealed that among all female Muslim admissions in that period, 13.93% involved puerperal psychoses, which was significantly higher than in France.[135] According to them, the high prevalence of puerperal psychoses among Muslim women was explained through their "emotional immaturity", which apparently was, *inter alia*, due to Algeria's patriarchal society, the absence of female education, hostility between spouses,[136] marriage between partners who had not known each other prior to their wedding, and the fact that Muslim women were taken from their familiar surroundings after their wedding and placed into the milieu of their in-law families.[137]

While colonial psychiatrists prior to 1961 only rarely mentioned the disorder in their theories, statistics or case studies, postcolonial Maghrebi psychiatrists writing in the 1970s maintained that puerperal psychoses were either extremely frequent in North Africa[138] or at least as common as in Europe.[139] The statistics composed by

---

132 They stated: "A number of studies have already highlighted the many peculiarities of Muslim psychopathology, but very few, to our knowledge, have concerned themselves with the accidents related to the puerperium." Ibid.

133 Ibid., 31. In contrast, Chappert stressed that she was mainly interested in the differences between Muslims and Europeans regarding the reasons, manifestations and symptoms of puerperal psychoses. Chappert, Contribution, 12.

134 Mares/Barre, Quelques aspects, 31.

135 Ibid., 32. Astonishingly, Mares and Barre referred to data provided by the 19th century psychiatrists Jean-Étienne Dominique Esquirol and Louis-Victor Marcé, among others, in their comparison of Muslim numbers to the situation in France.

136 Ibid., 45 f.

137 Ibid., 47. Similar reasons were given by Michèle Chappert. Chappert, Contribution, 15.

138 In 1972, for example, the Tunisian psychiatrist Sleïm Ammar even wrote that "a few years ago" puerperal psychoses had "dominated, together with hysteria, all female mental pathology" in Tunisia. Ammar, Aperçu, 704.

139 In their 1975 article "Puerperal Psychoses in the Moroccan Milieu", Taïeb Chkili and A. El Khamlichi detailed their experiences at the Razi Psychiatric Hospital in Salé, from April 1969 to June 1972, where they treated 100 women suffering from puerperal disorders among 2,025 women hospitalised, or 4.94% of all diagnoses, with the average number in the international context amounting to about 4%. They concluded that their findings on Morocco coincided with this average proportion. Chkili/El Khamlichi, Psychoses puerpérales, 376. Interestingly, the French psychiatrist J.-J. Maupomé, who was chief-physician at the Psychiatric Hospital in Salé, estimated the percentage of puerperal psychoses for Morocco in 1970, one of the years

Maghrebi psychiatrists clearly proved the frequency of the disorder, but allusions to the sudden increase in numbers, occurring just before independence, or to the fact that until the final years of French colonisation the diagnosis had been comparatively rare were missing. It is therefore debatable whether the absence of information on puerperal troubles in the colonial sources before 1961 mirrored the actual situation or, as seen in previous chapters, merely the interests of colonial psychiatry.

The explanations for the high numbers of puerperal psychoses suggested by postcolonial Maghrebi psychiatrists corresponded to those proposed by Mares and Barre discussed above. In October 1969 the journal *Information Psychiatrique* published an issue exclusively on Algeria, in which the unnamed psychiatrists focused, among other topics, on puerperal insanity.[140] One article, "Reflections on the Female Mental Pathology in Algeria", listed precocious marriage, frequent pregnancies, inadequate food, lack of hygiene in deliveries and the "ease of unilateral divorce" as reasons for the frequency of puerperal psychoses.[141] Other postcolonial psychiatrists blamed a mixture of social and economic factors for the frequency of puerperal psychoses in the independent Maghreb states, such as early marriage, the social state of women, the high birth rate, financial difficulties.[142] All these explanations fitted the picture that colonial psychiatrists had drawn of Muslim female normality discussed in Chapter 1, yet the connection between these social circumstances and puerperal insanity was only made once the numbers of afflicted patients were deemed significant. J.-J. Maupomé, in his 1970 article, attributed the frequency of puerperal psychoses mainly to boredom, due to the restrictions placed upon Muslim women by traditions: "We cannot talk about the hysterical base structure [of Moroccan Muslims] without noting the large number of puerperal psychoses (10% of female hospitalisations) [...]. Pregnancies, birth, breastfeeding in themselves valorise women only little [...]. Let us remember that they do not manage the budget and are only little concerned with the household. The tasks called 'feminine', including sewing, are generally performed by men. For them [Muslim women] illness remains [the] only means of being."[143]

As discussed above, Witold Lemanski, one of the few colonial authors who discussed the rarity of puerperal insanity among Muslim women, had pointed to these

covered by Chkili and El Khamlichi's study, as 10% of the total hospital population. Maupomé, Quelques aspects, 50.

140 In an article on the "Particularity of Algerian Pathology", for instance, they wrote that puerperal psychoses were frequently encountered in Algeria. Particularités de la pathologie algérienne, 880.

141 Réflexions sur la pathologie mentale féminine en Algérie, 886.

142 Chkili/El Khamlichi, Psychoses puerpérales, 387. See also: Ibid., 376; 386; Berthelier, Incidence psychopathologique, 19; Boucebci/Yaker, Aspects généraux, 358;19; Boucebci, Aspects de la psychiatrie, 189. See also: Rahim/Al-Sabiae, Puerperal Psychosis, 510.

143 Maupomé, Quelques aspects, 50.

same "facts" in 1913, i. e. fulfilment in being a mother and lack of external stimuli, to explain the diagnostic absence of the disorder.[144] The interpretation of the static life of normal Muslim women changed, therefore, from being a protective force against the development of insanity to being morbid in itself, thus suiting the psychiatric zeitgeist.

5.4.2 Selectively Representative

In the source material examined for this chapter, only four case studies of Muslim women suffering from puerperal problems were found in the period of almost complete silence on the topic before 1961, one of which concerned a patient who was "wrongly" assumed to suffer from puerperal mania before being diagnosed as a melancholic hypochondriac.[145] Moreover, it is debatable whether any of these case studies could be construed as representative of a greater, unnamed majority of cases, as all three involved minority groups or were exceptional because of extreme circumstances. Indeed, one might ask whether puerperal problems were only ever diagnosed in patients either falling outside the category of "normal" Muslim women or being brought to light due to extreme circumstances. However, twenty case studies on women suffering from puerperal problems can be found between 1961 and 1962, almost a fifth of all case studies concerning female Muslim patients between 1891 and 1962. These case studies were representative both of the frequency of the disorder in their numbers and of the female Muslim patients in their symptoms and social backgrounds.[146] The earlier cases, however, from the period when puerperal insanity was rare as a diagnosis and consequently undiscussed in the accompanying theories, represented exceptions and should therefore be analysed in depth.

Chronologically, the first of these early case studies on female Muslim patients suffering from puerperal problems could be found in Meilhon's 1896 article, as mentioned above. He explicitly stated that it was the only case of puerperal insanity he encountered in the patient records in Aix-en-Provence or personally treated while working in the asylum. He described her as suffering from puerperal insanity, with delusions, hallucinations and depressed states, having tried to kill her newborn child. This case was unique because the patient had been baptised, though Meilhon did not state whether she was born a Christian or later converted,[147] which placed her in a minority in Algeria and set her apart from Muslim North Africans. It is appropriate

---

144 Lemanski, Mœurs arabes, 120.
145 Meilhon, Aliénation mentale, part 3, 367.
146 Assicot et al., Causes principales, 278 f.; Chappert, Contribution, 32–55; Mares/Barre, Quelques aspects, 35–40.
147 Meilhon, Aliénation mentale, part 2, 205 f.

to ask whether her family would, had she been Muslim, have brought her into the stigmatising reach of colonial psychiatry for problems that could, within Islamic circles, be comfortably interpreted as demonic possession following childbirth. Further, it should be stressed that it was the extreme nature of her actions – attempted infanticide – that brought her into colonial psychiatric care, not the mental disorder per se.[148]

In 1939 Suzanne Taïeb documented a case of puerperal insanity among her collection of 30 case studies on Muslim women. It concerned a 22-year-old woman suffering from confusion and melancholia, triggered by the puerperium. Taïeb described her thus: "[...] little docile, she is more reticent with regard to hallucinations. She sees people who wish her ill, 'that's all.'"[149] After two years in the psychiatric service, the patient admitted that she had formerly been ill and traced her illness to a specific moment, when an evil jinn had possessed her. Although she was treated by a traditional healer, her situation deteriorated and she was finally admitted into psychiatric care after "the patient tried to destroy herself at home by scalding herself, here by strangling herself [...]."[150] While this patient's experiences of childbirth and demonic possession could be seen as mirroring those of many Muslim women suffering from puerperal problems, her attempts to kill herself in such especially horrific and unignorable ways make it difficult to view her medical history as representative of other, unmentioned cases.[151]

In 1959 J. Henry and Michel Assicot, whose article on modern treatments was discussed in Chapter 4,[152] presented the case of a schizophrenic suffering from puerperal psychoses. They pointedly called the 29-year-old patient "Miss",[153] even though she was admitted "for a schizophrenic post-puerperal development" after giving

---

148 On the other hand, some psychiatrists stressed the frequency of infanticide among Muslim women. For example: Bertherand, Médecine et hygiène, 296; Brierre de Boismont, Review of d'Escayrac de Lauture, 150. See also: Al-Issa, Psychiatry in Algeria, 244.

149 Taïeb, Idées d'influence, 89.

150 Ibid., 90.

151 As mentioned, suicide attempts were deemed relatively common among women suffering from puerperal insanity. Both colonial and postcolonial psychiatric literature described suicide attempts as being very frequent among Muslim women suffering from all kinds of psychiatric problems. Suicide was seen to be another of the "vices of civilisation", increasing by contact with France. Bertherand, Suicide, 153; Tablettes, 95; Payn, Pénitenciers indigènes, 301. For the propensity of Muslim women towards suicide attempts, see: Kocher, Criminalité, 148 f.; Fanon, Damnés, 267. Postcolonial situation: Maupomé, Quelques aspects, 54; El-Khayat, Tradition et modernité, 74; Okasha/Lotaif, Attempted Suicide, 74; Ifrah, Maghreb déchiré, 133; Al-Issa, Psychiatry in Algeria, 243; Douki et al., Women's Mental Health, 187.

152 Compare Chapter 4.4.1 "Physical Treatments".

153 The four other patients were described as "Madame" by Henry and Assicot. Henry/Assicot, Le 7044 RP, 692 ff.

birth.[154] This designation suggests that the patient was an unmarried Muslim mother. Unmarried mothers were, because of the stigma attached to extramarital relations and illegitimate children in Islamic societies, usually cut off from the care of their families.[155] Therefore, the patient described by Henry and Assicot patient could only ever be representative of a minority of cases.[156]

In conclusion, it can be said that psychiatric interest in puerperal psychoses only started in the last years of the colonisation of Algeria. Previously, Muslim women were almost never diagnosed with the condition, yet colonial psychiatrists had not particularly noticed this glaring absence and, therefore, neglected it in their written reports – a microcosm of the general treatment of female Muslim patients by French colonial psychiatry. The diagnosis of hysteria, which had initially been equally neglected, was brought to the attention of the colonial psychiatrists through the experiences of the World Wars.

5.5 Hysteria: Disease of the "Race"

Hysteria, as defined in the early 19th century, could include seizures, fainting, paralyses and the so-called *globus hystericus* (*boule hystérique* in French) – the feeling of a ball rising in the throat, causing a sensation of suffocation or strangulation.[157] The eminent psychiatrist Jean-Martin Charcot, Professor of Diseases of the Nervous System in Paris, described the degenerative disorder of hysteria as having four distinct phases, which he defined in 1872 and observed in detail in the female hysterics of the Salpêtrière.[158] After a phase of seizures, a period of contortions started. The third phase displayed deep emotions, while the fourth was defined by hallucinations or delusions.[159] According to Charcot, these phases were universal and his description

---

154 Ibid., 694.

155 See for example: Douki et al., Women's Mental Health, 183.

156 Among Henry and Assicot's case studies, this patient was exceptional in being the only one who proved to be "incurable" despite electroshock, insulin shock and drug therapy. Henry/Assicot, Le 7044 RP, 694.

157 Showalter, Female Malady, 130; Goldstein, Hysteria Diagnosis, 210 f. The *globus hystericus* was still described as a symptom of hysteria in Egypt by Okasha et al. in 1968. Okasha et al., Preliminary Psychiatric Observations, 952.

158 In the first volume of his "Lessons on Disorders of the Nervous System", published in 1872, he had already discussed hysteria. Charcot, Leçons, 243–337.

159 Scull, Hysteria, 115. Charcot held public lectures with demonstrations of these phases by hysterical patients. Andrew Scull stated in his 2009 "biography" on hysteria that Charcot turned hysteria into "a spectacle and a circus [...]." Ibid., 104. See also: Goldstein, Hysteria Diagnosis, 221; Gelfand, Charcot in Morocco, 2.

was "valid for all countries, for all epochs, for all races".[160] Under Charcot, hysteria became a popular diagnosis in France. Jan Goldstein's research shows this sharp increase in diagnosis – while between 1841 and 1842 only 1% of all women admitted to the Salpêtrière and Bicêtre were diagnosed with hysteria, this number rose to 17.8% for the years 1882 and 1883.[161] Hysteria, as understood by Charcot, reached its peak around 1900 in the West, with numbers declining afterwards.[162]

Historically, hysteria had long been described as a female disorder.[163] In Hippocratic and Galenic medicine, it was associated with women's reproductive organs, especially the uterus.[164] In the 19th century, it was re-interpreted as a nervous disorder, though still often connected with the particularities of women's bodies. In this understanding of hysteria, men could, organically, develop the disorder, but usually did not. As early as 1843, an article in the *Annales Médico-Psychologiques* stated that "hysteria is, in short, for us, an essentially nervous disease, independent of the uterine influence, and which would as well develop in men as in women if the nervous impressionability was the same in both sexes."[165] The implied conclusion was that the "nervous impressionability" in men and women was not the same and that, therefore, women were more likely to suffer from hysteria.[166] Only the experiences of World War I, with vast numbers of "shell-shocked" soldiers displaying symptoms of hysteria, changed this notion.[167]

---

160 Charcot, Leçon d'ouverture, 336. As quoted in: Scull, Hysteria, 115 f.

161 Goldstein, Console and Classify, 322.

162 Parle, Witchcraft or Madness, 127; Scull, Hysteria, 130. Freudian hysteria started with Freud's 1893 book on the "Physical Mechanism of Hysterical Phenomena", and he published on hysteria until 1909 ("General Information on the Hysterical Attack"). As seen in Chapter 4.4.2 "Psychotherapy", Freud's psychoanalytic principles were not implemented in North Africa, and while his theories had a general influence on French colonial psychiatry, his re-interpretation of hysteria was not adopted.

163 In 1910, for instance, in a dissertation on "Female Criminality in France", the author Henri Lacaze described hysteria as an "almost exclusively female" psychosis. Lacaze, Criminalité féminine, 113. See also: Smith-Rosenberg, Hysterical Woman, 668; Showalter, Female Malady, 129; Jordanova, Mental Illness, 111. This was repeated, as late as 1987, in the "Psychiatric Handbook for Maghrebi Practitioners". Douki, Hystérie, 109.

164 Scull, Hysteria, 25.

165 Clinique de M. Chomel, 108.

166 Nonetheless, cases of male hysteria were observed. For example in 1875: Fabre, Hystérie chez l'homme, 354. Goldstein described two cases of male hysteria against 89 female cases at the Salpêtrière and Bicêtre for the years 1882 and 1883. Goldstein, Hysteria Diagnosis, 209. Charcot opened a service for male hysterics at the Salpêtrière in 1882. Scull, Hysteria, 125.

167 Showalter, Female Malady, 164; Scull, Hysteria, 9. It is interesting that in the North African context of the 1940s, hysteria, still associated with femininity in the popular opinion, was described as being frequent among Muslim men, including Muslim soldiers. Susini, Aspects

From a clinical perspective, hysteria was, during its heyday in France in the last quarter of the 19th century, rare among North Africans and other colonised populations. The few statistics available showed it to be infrequent or even absent,[168] and a number of colonial doctors remarked upon its apparently surprising rarity.[169] Jean-Marie Collomb, for example, wrote in his 1883 dissertation on "Hygiene and Pathology in Assam and the Tong-Kin": "[...] when we study the lifestyle, the habits of the inhabitants [i.e., of the colonised], it is surprising not to meet them [epilepsy and hysteria] more frequently; I am inclined to believe that they [the inhabitants] carefully hide these diseases and, most of the time, when they are affected by them, they remain locked up."[170] As seen in Chapter 2, the fact that patients were locked up in their own homes, and therefore hidden from psychiatric eyes, was generally used to explain the low numbers of people suffering from mental illness in North Africa.[171] Other explanations for the more specific absence of hysteria were based on assumptions of what Muslim normality constituted – it was, for instance, suggested that the Muslim nervous system was "unflawed" due to under-use.[172]

---

cliniques, 17; Manceaux et al., Hystérie, 2; Louçaief, Manifestations hystériques, 35. This should be seen in the broader context of what Edward Said described as the de-masculinisation of Muslim men in Orientalist writing. Said, Orientalism, 6. For a discussion of this, see also: Vaughan, Curing their Ills, 19; McClintock, Imperial Leather, 14; Lazreg, Eloquence of Silence, 53; Massad, Desiring Arabs, 9.

168 Adolphe Kocher, who included the category of hysteria in his statistics covering the years 1867 to 1882 at the Civil Hospital of Mustapha, reported that among European men only 0.65% (3 patients) were diagnosed as suffering from hysteria and among Muslim men only 0.97% (2 patients). Among European women, the diagnosis of hysteria was given to 6.87% (25 patients) and among Muslim women to 2.47% (2 patients). Kocher, Criminalité, 70. Compare Appendix B, Fig. 8a, p. 271. In the statistical evidence collected by Meilhon in 1896 and by Reboul and Régis for the 1912 Tunis Congress, the category of hysteria was absent. Meilhon, Aliénation mentale, part 2, 191; Reboul/Régis, Assistance, 51–4. Nonetheless, among Meilhon's case studies were three Muslim women with hysterical manifestations, although two of them suffered mainly from other disorders. Meilhon, Aliénation mentale, part 2, 201; part 4, 40; part 6, 353.

169 Richardot, Pratiques médicales, 36; Astruc, Pratiques révulsives, 48.

170 Collomb, Essai, 45. Epilepsy and hysteria were often named together. In 1872 Charcot himself stated that observers were struck by the similarities between epileptic and hysterical attacks. He therefore decided to call the "convulsive phase" "hystero-epilepsy". Charcot, Leçons, 321. See also: Meilhon, Aliénation mentale, part 6, 353.

171 See p. 83.

172 See for example: Laurens, Contribution, 44. Laurens, in 1919, disagreed with this notion and thought that Muslim disadvantages – consanguinity, precocious marriages, marriages of old men to young girls, hashish, tobacco, opium, "genital overwork", the climate, masturbation and the rigours of Islam – made up for any "lack of overwork". Ibid.

With the rise of the *École d'Alger*, the idea of North African hysteria as a rarity was replaced with a new theory in the published sources. Proponents of the School claimed that hysteria was, contrary to earlier beliefs, very frequent.[173] Even prior to the *École d'Alger*, however, there had been voices asserting that hysteria was common in North Africans. In 1907, for example, Georges Sicard quoted an unnamed article by Henri Gros[174] in his dissertation: "The frequency of neuroses is noted and very categorically affirmed by Mr Gros. He has met in his consultations only two cases of hysteria, but he had the opportunity to see them [cases of hysteria] more often and 'his impression is that hysteria is a common disorder in native women.'"[175] This discrepancy between professional experience – only two observed cases – and "knowledge",[176] which somewhat discredited Gros's statement, was only resolved with the rising numbers of Muslim patients after World War I, when experience started to approach "knowledge". In 1918 the *"frequency* of, and *predisposition to, pithiatic accidents and reactions* [...] in these primitive men" had been stressed by Antoine Porot as one of the "psychological surprises" of World War I.[177] This newly observed – not, as in Gros's case, merely suspected – frequency of hysteria became part of Porot's construction of the North African primitive, and was translated into the scientific vocabulary of the *École d'Alger*.[178]

In 1947 two publications were released on hysteria in North Africa: Robert Susini's psychiatric dissertation, and an article which he published together with his doctoral supervisor G.-A. Manceaux and the psychiatrist Charles Bardenat in the *Annales Médico-Psychologiques*. Both publications focused on the frequency of hysteria among Muslims in general and Muslim soldiers in particular. In the years for which records

---

173 Hysteria was often believed to be frequent not only among North Africans but among all "Oriental races". In 1938, for instance, Louis Lauriol stated that the frequency of hysteria was connected with "race" and that "some more emotional, more impressionable people are particularly subjected to it (Malagasy, Malays, Muslims, North Africans...)." Lauriol, Quelques remarques, 29. See also: Mazel, Visite, 16; Rouquès, Report, 305; Humann, Troubles mentaux, 1085. Postcolonial North African psychiatrists, including those from Egypt, shared this opinion. Boucebci/Yaker, Aspects généraux, 358; Ammar, Ethnopsychiatrie (1975), 320; 325; Al-Issa, Psychiatry in Algeria, 244; Okasha, Focus on Psychiatry, 266.

174 According to Sicard, this article was published in the journal *Bulletin Médical de l'Algérie* in 1906. Sicard, Étude, 70 f.

175 Ibid. The same passage by Gros was also quoted by Benkhelil in 1927. Benkhelil, Contribution, 18 f.

176 These discrepancies between "knowledge" and "experience" in the scientific treatment of Muslim women will be discussed in the conclusions of this book.

177 Porot, Notes, 380. "Pithiatism" is another word for hysteria, formed by Joseph Babinski in 1901. Scull, Hysteria, 130.

178 See, for example: Porot/Sutter, 'Primitivisme', 241.

exist – 1939 to 1940 and 1943 to 1945 –, there had been 500 Muslim men with hysterical problems (29.41%, among a total hospital population of 1,700 Muslim patients) while among the Europeans there were only 70 cases (2.59%, among a total hospital population of 2,700) in the Neuropsychiatric Ward of the Maillot Military Hospital in Algiers. Through this direct comparison with Europeans, according to Susini, "we realise even more readily the frequency of pithiatism in the native".[179] Because of the assumption that all North Africans shared certain "primitive" characteristics, these experiences with individual Muslim North African soldiers could be used to describe the normality of all Muslims. The dogma of hysteria's omnipresence in North Africans became so widespread that, in 1959, Sutter et al. stated that all observers before them had emphasised the frequency of hysterical manifestations,[180] quietly dismissing all those who had, on the contrary, stressed its rarity or even its absence.

5.5.1 Primitive Hysteria

North African hysteria, part of the "North African character", was more loosely defined than clinical European hysteria. Antoine Porot defined Muslim North African normality as early as 1918 and characterised it by credulity, suggestibility, fatalism, superstitions and an intellectual resistance expressed through stubbornness. While not clinically hysterical, this normality predestined Muslim North Africans towards violent hysterical reactions that led "[…] to the production of crude formulas, the veritable hysteria of the savage, violent and brutal crises, rhythmic movements of head and neck, indefinite persistence of caricature-like attitudes [i. e. postures], reminiscent of simulation, all intermingled with ideas of possession (by spirits, by the jinn), with no real delusional concept. The pithiatism of the natives completes his resemblance to our ancient medieval hysterias by the frequent collective factor and the easy tendency towards spreading by contagion."[181]

This last remark about the medievalism of North African hysteria is familiar from the previous chapters. Both colonial and postcolonial psychiatric texts maintained the trope that manifestations of hysteria in North Africa were "old-fashioned" and many psychiatrists commented on the fact that hysterical North Africans displayed

---

179 Susini, Aspects cliniques, 17. See also: Manceaux et al., Hystérie, 2.
180 Sutter et al., Aspects algériens, 893.
181 Porot, Notes, 381. This paragraph was echoed in articles which Porot wrote in 1932 with Arrii and in 1937 with Sutter. Porot/Arrii, Impulsivité criminelle, 591; Porot/Sutter, 'Primitivisme', 229; 237.

the characteristics of the "grand hysteria" defined by Charcot in the 1870s.[182] In 1947, for instance, Manceaux et al. stated that "the *big theatrical crisis* which has practically disappeared from European hospitals, makes us relive [...] the heyday of hysteria of Charcot's time."[183] In 1956 Pierre Maréschal wrote: "Another feature of Tunisian psychiatry seemed to me to be the relative frequency of hysteria in its most classic forms, described by Charcot (passionate attitudes, anaesthesia [loss of sensation in the skin], paralysis, secondary states [crepuscular states], coprolalia [the compulsive utterance of obscenities], neuropathic crises, vaticination [prophesying], etc...) [...]."[184]

In 1947 these coarse, Charcotesque crises were also described by Susini as the "most frequently observed manifestation" of hysteria in North Africans, representing "the simplest, most primitive and crudest form of emotional expressions, stripped of any cultural contribution. [...] It is a spectacular accident, which the native knows well and [which] he attributes, in almost all cases, to the action of evil spirits [that] can take various forms and which he calls 'jinn.'"[185] Susini stated that, as the hysterical patients he encountered had shown all the characteristics of the "primitive mentality" defined by Porot, Muslim peculiarities should be taken into account in the treatment of North African hysterics.[186] Susini concluded by claiming, "this implies therefore the existence of a mental constitution specific to the North African native, which would favour the outbreak of hysterical disorders. And so we understand well the frequency of this affliction and the difficulties of treatment."[187] Not only did the "racial" characteristics of the "primitives" define the hysterical patients treated by French colonial psychiatry, but Susini even stated that "we are sometimes surprised to only find in

---

182 Postcolonial psychiatrists: Ammar/M'Barek, Hystérie, 485; Berthelier, Incidence psychopathologique, 33; Particularités de la pathologie algérienne, 880 f.; Bensmail et al., Considérations, 400. The same was also observed in other Muslim countries, like Sudan, Iraq and Libya. Elsarrag, Psychiatry in the Northern Sudan, 946; Al-Issa/Al-Issa, Psychiatric Problems, 19; Pu et al., One Hundred Cases, 606.

183 Manceaux et al., Hystérie, 4. Emphasis in the original. See also: Bardenat, Criminalité, 323.

184 Maréschal wondered whether the existence of sexual taboos in North Africa, which he compared with the situation in Charcot's France, explained these delayed manifestations. Maréschal, Réflexions, 79.

185 Susini, Aspects cliniques, 29. Manceaux et al. also stressed the "coarseness" of Muslim hysterical symptoms. Manceaux et al., Hystérie, 3.

186 Susini regretted that, because of the "generally massive, coarse and brutal" ways through which hysteria was expressed by North Africans, doubts about the "sincerity of the patient" were common and warned other psychiatrists that the sincerity of the North Africans "could not be estimated [...] with the scale of our judgement, our knowledge and our beliefs". Susini, Aspects cliniques, 18. The same weariness of simulation in hysteria was voiced by Manceaux et al. Manceaux et al., Hystérie, 26–9.

187 Susini, Aspects cliniques, 89.

the patients the characteristics of the native mentality in general, without any other superimposed mental stigmata."[188] Therefore, in the view of certain psychiatrists, some hysterical patients only suffered from being North Africans.

As already seen in quotes from Porot's 1918 article and Susini's 1947 dissertation, it was assumed that North Africans suffering from hysteria interpreted their disorder as a form of possession and attended traditional exorcism ceremonies to be cured.[189] In these psychiatrically untreated forms of demonic possession, hysteria was deemed to be extremely common among North Africans, and in the eyes of French colonial psychiatrists both these ceremonies and the disorders they sought to heal were hysterical symptoms.[190] In 1911, for example, an article, "Medicine in Morocco", was published in the journal *Presse Médicale*, in which the author, named only as R. B., wrote that the North African belief in the supernatural "encouraged" certain forms of hysteria, namely the "exaggerated religious practices, cherished by the different Moroccan populations: such as these strange reunions, which certain religious orders celebrate several times a year in public squares and in the streets."[191] The article therefore proposed that this shared belief in the supernatural generated hysterical manifestations not just in individuals but whole populations. H. Thierry explained in 1917 that these "religious orders" – i.e. the exorcism practising Sufi-brotherhoods, for North Africans one of the choices offering cures to the insane – were veritable reservoirs of hysteria: "In Morocco there is a sect, which is called Aïssaouas; they hallucinate and run through markets and indulge in every imaginable eccentricity; they eat glass, roll on hot coals, swallow scorpions, beat their skulls with bronze axes, burn themselves with hot irons, plunge knives into the skin and feel nothing. One can see them twist, while yelling, with haggard eyes, foaming at the mouth, then dance to the tambourines until they fall exhausted. For the Moroccans, the Aïssaouas are possessed by jinn: for us, they are clearly hysterical."[192]

---

188 Ibid.

189 Brault, Pathologie et hygiène, 58; Legey, Essai, 146 f.; 153; Desruelles/Bersot, Assistance aux aliénés chez les Arabes, 701. Many of the medical experts observed that this was not only the case in Islam. Armand Richardot, for example, wrote in 1896 that Muslim healing ceremonies could be compared to Catholic miracles at Lourdes, but, he argued, religious healing ceremonies were a thing of the past in Europe: "Formerly, the sudden healing of hysterical contractures and paralyses was a therapeutic miracle. Science today has shown that these phenomena were not organic, but purely dynamic, the miracle no longer exists [...]." Richardot, Pratiques médicales, 17.

190 See: Thierry, Étude, 18.

191 B., Médecine au Maroc, 382.

192 Thierry, Étude, 20.

5.5.2   Hysterical Muslim Women

As discussed, hysteria was seen to be a female disorder in Europe, and some psychiatric sources believed the same could be said for North Africa, usually without providing statistics or even personal experiences to support their claim.[193] As already mentioned, Georges Sicard recounted in 1907 how Gros was under the impression that hysteria was frequent in Muslim women, despite only ever having treated two actual cases.[194] Some French doctors and psychiatrists suspected that the character, lifestyle and beliefs[195] of Muslim women predisposed them more towards hysteria than Muslim men. In 1854, for example, the French doctor Adolphe Armand suspected that the circumstances of the lives of Muslim women – imprisoned in harems, in an immoderate climate, and genetically lustful – induced hysteria and epilepsy.[196]

Other psychiatrists were struck by differences between the numbers of female hysterics in North Africa and France and tried to explain why North African women were less susceptible than European women, often resorting to common knowledge about Muslim women's normality being different to European women's normality. In 1892 the French doctor Lafitte, for example, wrote about the situation in Tunisia: "I have never observed [cases of] hysteria, except two or three times in a harem. The precarious condition of women, their role as slaves, as beasts of burden, as things, finally, to which they are condemned, stands in opposition to their development

---

193 Kocher's statistics were an exception, showing, as mentioned, that while only 0.87% of all male Muslim cases at the Civil Hospital of Mustapha between 1867 and 1882 were diagnosed as hysterics, 2.47% of all Muslim women received the same diagnosis. In fact, there had been two male and two female Muslim cases of hysteria, but the difference in overall patient numbers accounts for the difference in the percentages. Kocher, Criminalité, 70. See Appendix B, Fig. 8a, p. 271. It was also thought that hysteria was frequent in women in other Muslim countries, such as the Ottoman Empire in 1866. Les aliénés dans les hôpitaux de Constantinople, 501.

194 Sicard, Étude, 70 f. See p. 209.

195 It was reported, for instance, that Muslims believed women to be especially susceptible to demonic possessions, which were often interpreted as hysteria by French observers. Menouillard, Mejnoun, 477; Thierry, Étude, 17. See also: Limbert, Spirit Possession, 425.

196 Armand, Algérie médicale, 443. See also: Taïeb, Idées d'influence, 78. This was also maintained in postcolonial psychiatric literature on Muslim women. The psychiatrist M. E. Elsarrag, for example, wrote about Northern Sudan in 1968: "Hysteria is predominantly a female disease. It would not be unfair to say that the average Sudanese woman has a hysterical personality by Western standards, in the sense that she is highly emotional and loves to display emotions of various kinds on a superficial level – she loves theatricalities. [...] It is small wonder that hysterical manifestations occur readily in the Sudanese woman." Elsarrag, Psychiatry in the Northern Sudan, 946.

of mental abilities."[197] Witold Lemanski, who often denigrated European females through comparisons with Muslim females, also thought the simple lives that Muslim women led protected them from hysteria. Echoing Lafitte, he stated in 1900 that the isolation of Muslim women, together with their natural timidity, hindered the "full development" of their "mental faculties" and prevented the emergence of such nervous diseases as hysteria.[198]

Lemanski claimed that Islam shielded Muslim women from "religious madness, so frequent among hysterical Christian women",[199] and from "hysteriform or epileptiform attacks of alcoholic origin".[200] Above all, the traditional lifestyle, devoid of the consequences of a hasty emancipation, fortified Muslim women against hysteria: "Arab women do not undergo any of the fatigues of the European woman, who frequents balls, theatres, churches, casinos, games, who, after staying up late, sleeps badly, eats and drinks too much, who does not even want to stop when she carries a new being within her. Neurasthenia, hysteria, epilepsy are the frequent results of this existence without measure, without reason, without hygiene. Madness, for the descendants, is the result of these aberrations. [...] The rapid emancipation of Arab women would be a mistake for Muslims, as well as for Christians: one of the biggest arguments against it would precisely be the scarcity of female madness in the Orient."[201]

These voices explaining the rarity of hysteria among Muslim women all predate the World Wars. As mentioned, the experiences of both conflicts cemented the idea of a primitive form of hysteria as part of the North African character, common to men and women, and a typically female hysteria was no longer discussed. Postcolonial North African psychiatrists, however, reverted to describing hysteria as a mainly

---

197 Lafitte, Contribution, 86. Among the two case studies on Muslim female hysterics found while researching this chapter, one was from a poor background associated with Lafitte's description of female Muslim normality. Meilhon, Aliénation mentale, part 4, 40. The second was described by George Sicard as "*a civilised native woman*", suffering from hysteria and syphilis. Sicard, Étude, 45. Emphasis in the original.

198 Lemanski, Psychologie, 93. In 1913 he repeated that hysteria was rare among the "still elementary" Muslim "nervous pathology", showing that he thought hysteria to be a disease of civilisation: "It is feared that this relative immunity will disappear the day important changes alter the Qur'anic rules. One can reason by analogy. In some Tunisian Jewish families, where ease allows making sacrifices for the children, I have often seen young girls of 15 or 20 years suffering from hysterical or neurasthenic symptoms as a result of emotions, of overwork." Lemanski, Mœurs arabes, 112 f.

199 Ibid., 115.

200 Ibid., 111. While Muslim women respected the prohibition of alcohol, Lemanski regretted that "all Muslims are not as sober as their wives [...]." Ibid., 111 f.

201 Ibid., 109 f.

female disorder.[202] Sleïm Ammar and Ezzeddine M'Barek, for instance, claimed in a 1961 article about "Hysteria in Tunisian Girls and Women" that the harsh treatment of young Tunisian girls of bygone days, "subjected to an education [which is] tyrannical and rigorous to the extreme", had caused hysteria in them, and attacked "the veil, the obscurantism and the total lack of education", polygamy and arranged marriages.[203] They observed that, since independence, Tunisian women had been given more rights, which influenced the psychiatric tableau that Tunisia presented, with "rough hysterical conversions" gradually being replaced by "the neuroses of character and situation so frequent in Europe".[204] Nonetheless, the idea that hysteria was somehow hidden in North Africans remained. In 1972, for example, Sleïm Ammar explained that the passivity of Tunisian women effectively masked nervous disorders, like hysteria.[205]

This idea of Muslim women "normally" behaving in an almost hysterical way, though not medically diagnosed with hysteria, further blurred the already vague borders between insanity and normality. It was feared that "misunderstandings" occurred in diagnosis – women suffering from mental problems might be labelled as "normal" and therefore as not requiring treatment, while "normal" women might be diagnosed as hysterical and find themselves institutionalised.[206] The legal consequences of these misdiagnoses were of an even greater importance. As mentioned in the discussion of puerperal insanity, Porot's student Don Côme Arrii, in his 1926 dissertation, reported at length on the case of a young unmarried woman who allegedly murdered her newborn child. Porot, who was the psychiatrist called as an expert witness, deemed her to be mostly responsible for her crime, i. e. "normal" and not "mad", despite her *"manic, hysteriform crisis after incarceration"*,[207] her "tendency to hysterical imbalance"[208] and her "tendency towards confabulation and lies that we find in all hysterics".[209] The fact that Porot, in court, did not deem the accused to be "insane", despite these symptoms of hysteria, serves as further proof that hysteria was almost officially established as a

---

202 Al-Issa/Al-Issa, Psychiatric Problems, 19; Bensmail et al., Considérations, 400; Okasha/Lotaif, Attempted Suicide, 73.

203 Ammar/M'Barek, Hystérie, 481.

204 Ibid. Later in their article, they further specified: "The more liberal attitude of families, a more buoyant education of young girls, makes them less and less subject to coercive and 'infantilising' structures. Hysteria declines in young Tunisian girls." Ibid., 486.

205 Ammar, Aperçu, 688.

206 Meilhon, for example, stated in one of his case studies in 1896 that a female alcoholic had been described as suffering from hysteria. He himself could not verify this diagnosis as the woman was demented when he started to observe her, and "all hysterical manifestation had disappeared". Meilhon, Aliénation mentale, part 4, 40.

207 Arrii, Impulsivité criminelle, 84.

208 Ibid., 86.

209 Ibid.

character trait of the "race", as her wild hysterical reactions seem to have been accepted as part of the personality of any sane Muslim woman.

5.6 The Absence of Diagnoses

This analysis of these three disorders shows that all were described as absent in Muslim women for different reasons, to different degrees and in different ways, illustrating the different layers of the psychiatric construct of Muslim women and the interest colonial psychiatry had in them. It is noteworthy that in the published sources analysed for this book, save for the very last years of the French colonial presence in the Maghreb, twelve case studies were dedicated to the allegedly non-existent diagnosis of general paralysis[210] – more than for the two "female disorders" of puerperal insanity[211] and hysteria[212] combined.

The "gender-neutral" disorder of general paralysis proved to be of greater interest to the French colonial psychiatrists than the other two for several reasons. Questions about its causes were at the forefront of contemporary psychiatric developments and its distribution illustrated the forces of a "racialised" notion of civilisation.[213] In addition, its connection to syphilis prompted discussions of the deviant sexualities of North Africans, who contracted syphilis through their "Arab vices" without suffering from general paralysis, while the disorder was instrumentalised to demonstrate that North Africans could not be assimilated into French society, as each of the different phases in the theoretical treatment of Muslim general paralysis exemplified the

---

210 Pascalis, Paralysie générale, 29 f.; Meilhon, Contribution, 391; 393; Battarel, Quelques remarques, 63 f.; 64; 65; Goëau-Brissonnière, Syphilis nerveuse, 134 f.; Taïeb, Idées d'influence, 122 f.; 124; Olry, Paralysie générale, 53 f.; 54; 55. Pascalis repeated in 1893 two of Meihon's 1891 case studies, and Benkhelil repeated in 1927 the same case as Goëau-Brissonière in 1926. Pascalis, Paralysie générale, 19 f.; 22 f.; Benkhelil, Contribution, 82 f.

211 There were only the three case studies already discussed on p. 204. Meilhon, Aliénation mentale, part 2, 205 f.; Taïeb, Idées d'influence, 89 f.; Henry/Assicot, Le 7044 RP, 694.

212 There were five case studies on hysterical female Muslim patients. Among these, three were not classified as hysterics, but as suffering from other disorders. Classified as hysterics: Meilhon, Aliénation mentale, part 4, 40; Sicard, Étude, 45 f. Other disorders: Meilhon, Aliénation mentale, part 2, 201; part 6, 353; Arrii, Impulsivité criminelle, 84–7.

213 For many authors, "race" was an obvious variable in the equation. In 1949, for instance, Blancardi et al. wrote on Morocco: "The racial factor is the first that comes to mind [when trying to explain the rarity of general paralysis]." Blancardi et al., Syphilis nerveuse, 226. Others disagreed with "race" having an influence on the formation of general paralysis. Benkhelil wrote in 1927 that, given the ethnical diversity in North Africa, "race" seemed to him to be a negligible factor in the absence of general paralysis in North Africa. Benkhelil, Contribution, 58.

civilisational "gap" between North Africans and Europeans.[214] First, general paralysis was assumed to be a purely civilisational malady, sparing uncivilised, yet "syphilised", "races", while the civilised French had to remain morally upright – refraining from both alcohol and syphilis – in order to escape its infection. After proof was found that the disorder was caused by the allegedly "omnipresent" syphilis bacteria, the relative absence of general paralysis in North Africa was explained by the "absolute" absence of civilisation and the rising numbers by the increasing presence of civilised French "vices". Finally, the building of psychiatric institutions in North Africa led to a newly discovered frequency of "Muslim general paralysis", but the disorder itself was still described as "uncivilised", i. e. primitive, and inherently different from European forms of the disorder.

In the context of puerperal insanity and hysteria, on the other hand, it can be argued that the absence of information was due to the lack of written testimonies on Muslim women, not the absence of the disorders themselves. This lack of written evidence seemed to be almost independent of the numerical situation, remaining rather static over a time period stretching from the assumed absence of the diagnoses to the accepted ubiquity of both disorders. The sudden importance of the disorders in the postcolonial statistics suggests an actual absence during colonial times was improbable.[215]

Explanations for the absence of puerperal insanity can be found in the general lack of interest French colonial psychiatrists showed in their female Muslim patients and in the difficulty presented to male French experts by Muslim segregation. It is possible that cases of puerperal insanity in Muslim women were, in the eyes of colonial psychiatrists, too close to European cases already described by metropolitan psychiatrists to deserve special mention,[216] but, in that case, colonial statistics should at the very least have furnished evidence of puerperal problems among Muslim women in asylums and psychiatric hospitals.

---

214 The use of psychiatric findings in the debate over the assimilability of North Africans will be discussed in the conclusions of this book.

215 This "sudden" importance cannot be explained purely through an increase in patient numbers. While it is clear that more Tunisian women took advantage of psychiatric institutions after independence, the same cannot be said for Algeria and Morocco, where the absence of female patients remained an issue for postcolonial authors. Particularités de la pathologie algérienne, 880; Bouricha, Service, 740; Ammar, Hôpital, 664; Bensmail et al., Considérations, 394; Möbius, Entwicklung der Psychiatrie, 16; Douki et al., Women's Mental Health, 187.

216 Mares and Barre mentioned in 1962 that they could exclude European cases from their study of puerperal psychoses in Algeria as they were too similar to those encountered in France – therefore their focus on Muslim patients points to their symptoms being essentially different from Europeans. Mares/Barre, Quelques aspects, 31.

The absence of puerperal psychoses was more likely due to French hospitals rarely treating pregnant Muslim women. French doctors were almost never contacted when it came to childbirth, as Muslim (and French) midwives were the first port of call. The few births where male doctors were present were usually catastrophic affairs, with severe physical complications often leaving mother or child, or both, dead. It is therefore possible that the psychiatrists did not write on puerperal madness because they never came into contact with normal pregnancies, let alone pregnancies with non-physical complications. In this explanation, the "invisibility" of puerperal problems Muslim women faced would be due to a) the different levels of segregation in colonial societies, which hid pregnant women, and also those seeking exorcisms, from the gaze of colonial experts and psychiatric care, and b) the colonial assumption that Muslim women were "good" mothers, content with their limited status as mothers and wives, which further inhibited psychiatrists from diagnosing puerperal problems. The aforementioned case study in Arrii's 1926 dissertation about a young unmarried woman,[217] who was "normal" but suffered from hysterical attacks nonetheless, accused of murdering her newborn child, is interesting in this context, because it seems that it was never considered whether this patient could have suffered from puerperal insanity.

In the case of the diagnosis of hysteria, two general points should be highlighted. First, while some early authors focused on questions of hysteria in Muslim women, later authors, exemplified by the publications of Susini and Manceaux et al. in 1947, chose to focus on the prevalence of hysteria and hysterical symptoms in Muslim soldiers. Hysteria was, by that time, no longer purely connected with women in European theories; nevertheless, a strong association with females remained. Both publications, in establishing a connection between Muslim soldiers and a feminine disorder, so soon after North Africans had fought alongside the French in World War II, unfavourably linked Muslim masculinity with notions of not only femininity but of a disordered femininity. Secondly, the initial absence of clinical hysteria, and later omnipresence of hysteria as part of Muslim normality, seems to be due to a clash between a traditional interpretation of certain symptoms as possession and a French biomedical model. The North African interpretation itself was defined as indicating an all-embracing, unhealthy, but normal, Muslim pathology in the colonial sources.

Alleged similarities between hysterical symptoms and "normal Muslim characteristics" were often highlighted and should be taken as an example of the broader pathologisation of North African normality. The naval doctor F. Brissot, for example, wrote in his 1959 article on the "Mentality of North African Muslims" that "[...]

---

217 This same case was mentioned in Porot and Arrii's 1932 article on "Criminal Impulsivity among Native Algerians" in their discussion of responsibility among criminals. Porot/Arrii, Impulsivité criminelle, 607.

he [the North African Muslim] will be considered as typically pithiatic: the Muslim has from it [hysteria] the whole lability, the facial and expressional attitudes, the elements of mythomania."[218] This pejorative pathologisation of North African normality endured after the end of French colonial psychiatry, as evinced by the French psychiatrist J.-J. Maupomé writing in 1970 about Morocco, "[...] the underlying hysterical personality, classical, banal, less intellectualised, or less cultural than that of Europeans, is constant. We exaggerate little if we speak of it as the 'common denominator' of all our patients."[219]

---

218 Brissot, Propos, 497. A very similar sentiment can be found in Humann's 1934 article on "Mental Problems among the Natives of the Algerian Sahara", in which he stated, before detailing their characteristics (mythomania, impressionability and a "singular malleability of the mind"), that "this predisposition towards accidents of this kind [hysteria] seems to highlight in the Negroes a particular mental fund [...]." Humann, Troubles mentaux, 1085.
219 Maupomé, Quelques aspects, 49.

Conclusion: Visible Psychiatrists

The previous chapters have demonstrated that, especially during the early French colonial period, it was widely assumed that, in the Maghreb, Muslims in general, and Muslim women in particular, rarely went "insane", and, as a direct consequence, only a negligible percentage of the colonial psychiatric patient population was made up of Muslim women. Accordingly, colonial psychiatric sources dedicated comparatively little space to describing the few female Muslim patients in French care. However, the previous chapters also showed that while there is justifiable doubt about whether female Muslim patients were actually absent from the colonial institutions, it is certain that they were almost completely missing from the accounts thereof. This historical analysis set out to map this absence.

The examination of the published colonial sources has shown that, as anticipated, no female Muslim voices could be found, other than, to a certain degree, in Suzanne Taïeb's 1939 publication, where the fluent Arabic-speaking psychiatrist shared jokes and stories with her patients and reported them carefully in the case studies collected for her dissertation.[1] The other sources usually did not even attempt to report conversations with those being treated; the voices of female Muslim patients, unintelligible in both language and gesture, were not deemed important enough to be recorded. It is precisely because of this general absence of female Muslim voices in the source material that gender-focused, critical historical analyses of colonial psychiatry are necessary – to highlight the unexpected areas where Muslim women were present in the colonial psychiatric sources and institutions, and to challenge both the lack of awareness concerning female Muslim patients and numerous colonial misrepresentations.

The sources mostly remain silent on topics ranging from specific North African interpretations of mental disorders to the hallucinations and delusions professed by individual female Muslim patients. However, this silence is eloquent and suggests a variety of conclusions that may be drawn about French colonial psychiatrists. The chapters of this book offer a systematic critique of the academic discourse on Muslim women in the colonial Maghreb and of the ways in which psychiatric "knowledge" about female sanity and mental health was created. The

---

1 It is refreshing to see the humour and life in Taïeb's case stories. One female patient, for instance, repeatedly talked to Taïeb about the spirits, junūn in Arabic, which possessed her, but one particular day "refused stubbornly" to talk about them, and "pretended to believe that we spoke to her of 'knees' [genoux, in French]...; we used the singular 'jinn', she pretended to understand 'young' [jeune, in French]." Taïeb, Idées d'influence, 120. On these female Muslim interpretations, see also the introductions to Chapters 1 and 5.

sources, silent on so many topics concerning Muslim women, offer an abundance of information on both the production of knowledge and the tangible consequences of this process.

In the colonial psychiatric context, female Muslim patients were seldom chosen as subjects for written treatises. If they were selected as a theme, or to illustrate a broader topic, the focus remained on the "abnormal normality" common to all female Muslims rather than on specific diagnoses or their behaviour as identifiable patients. However, statements by colonial psychiatrists describing Muslim femininity were gravely undermined by the fact that these psychiatrists had little contact with normal Muslim women and were incapable of talking to those they met. Despite this focus on normality, the colonial psychiatric sources cannot inform our understanding of the reality of the lives normal Muslim women led, because the information gained from the colonial psychiatric texts often involves little more than settler prejudices and stereotypes,[2] expressed in a medical – and therefore more authoritative – language. This mirroring of academic discourse and settler stereotypes is underpinned by the fact that many psychiatrists repeated the same tropes without acknowledging their sources, which points to the existence of a canon of colonial prejudices from which colonial psychiatry simply lifted ideas.[3]

These source-related problems – the silence on topics concerning female Muslim patients; texts focusing on an imagined normality of Muslim women, instead of describing patients; the (alleged) physical absence of female Muslim patients from colonial care, without figures to confirm this omnipresent claim – reveal more about those describing than those described; more about those non-describing than those undescribed.

It has already been claimed by historians of medicine that psychiatric sources, especially in colonial contexts, reveal more about the conceptions of the male psychiatrists regarding what constitutes femininity than about the female patients themselves or the lived reality of colonised women.[4] In the context of French colonial psychiatry

---

2 This is, as Kay Adamson remarked in 1978, a problem of most genres of colonial sources on North African women. Adamson, Approaches, 22.

3 For example, in 1979 Emanuel Sivan analysed settler stereotypes in Algeria, and while he did not compare them to academic discourses, the similarities between his description, academic Orientalism and the tropes used by colonial psychiatry are considerable. According to him, the *pied noir* picture of the North African was made up of "five major stereotypes: he is savage, poor, dirty, dishonest, and lascivious". See: Sivan, Colonialism and Popular Culture, 32. See also: ibid. 24 f.; 36 ff. This directly corresponded with the notions of colonial psychiatry, especially under the *École d'Alger,* as discussed in the previous chapters.

4 Megan Vaughan expressed this elegantly in 1983: "In an admittedly rather curious way, a study of European ideas on African psychology and insanity demonstrates the insecurity and

in the Maghreb, I suggest that, while an analysis of the source material allows such a conclusion, this conclusion can also be reached by examining the lacunae within that source material. Colonial psychiatrists – in their worldview dispassionate and impartial experts – were the ones truly analysed in the preceding chapters: their connections to each other, their ideas about themselves, their understanding (and gendering) of hierarchies, politics and religion. These aspects can be observed in what they neglected to write as much as in what they wrote.

What, then, can be said about these psychiatrists as a distinct professional group of colonial "experts" from the information gathered in the preceding chapters? The writings of more than 100 colonial psychiatrists, all focusing on the Maghreb, have been studied for this book, and there can be no question of "unity" among them – they came from different backgrounds, both military and civilian, and had dissimilar outlooks and experiences.[5] Nonetheless, they shared laudable human-itarian concerns[6] and a medical education. Until the establishment of a chair for General and Medical Pathology at the Medical Faculty of the University of Algiers in 1925, almost all psychiatrists working on topics concerning North Africans were born in France,[7] while a few had never lived in North Africa and only knew it from holidays.[8] Antoine Porot, who was the first to hold that chair, and his successors,

---

psychological vulnerability of the Europeans themselves, in a situation where the segregation of cultures seemed necessary for the maintenance of their own sanity and the precarious myth of their superiority." Vaughan, Healing and Curing, 289. For a discussion of this hypothesis, see: Mills, Mad and the Past, 146.

5   In 1989 Ann Laura Stoler rightly criticised the way historical analyses of colonial societies see the colonisers as unified entities. However, while the psychiatrists themselves were very diverse, the colonial psychiatric discourse on Muslim women often seems surprisingly uni-fied. It is therefore important to focus on the debates and controversies within this seemingly homogeneous discourse. Stoler, Rethinking Colonial Categories, 136.

6   It cannot be denied that many colonial psychiatrists had heartfelt humanitarian scruples and thought they could improve the situation of North African patients. Nonetheless, there is a clear discrepancy between their intentions and the often disastrous implementation of reme-dies, for instance the outcry about the situation of patients in Islamic *māristāns* produced the "solution" of shipping patients to France.

7   There were exceptions. Pierre Battarel's father had been a doctor at the Civil Hospital of Mustapha. Battarel, Quelques remarques, 7. Others born in North Africa were Georges Sicard and Victor Trenga. Sicard, Étude, title page; Trenga, Âme arabo-berbère, 4. The few Algerian and Tunisian Muslims studying medicine or psychiatry before the construction of a psychiatric institute at the University of Algiers were also born in North Africa. For example: Benkhelil, Contribution, title page. See also the mini-biographies in Appendix A.

8   As mentioned in previous chapters, these "metropolitan colonial psychiatrists" were reproached for their lack of direct "knowledge" of North African societies by doctors and psychiatrists living and working in the Maghreb. Battarel, Quelques remarques, 29; Levet, Assistance, 239.

had among their students a variety of second-generation French settlers and even some North African Jews and Muslims.[9] Before 1925 practically all these psychiatrists had been trained at a handful of French universities, of which Lyon, Paris and Bordeaux – where Emmanuel Régis taught as Clinical Professor of Mental Diseases at the Medical Faculty from 1884 onward[10] – were numerically the most important.[11]

There was a complex network of relations between these colonial psychiatrists. Many knew one another personally, studying in the same universities, attending the same conferences, working in the same hospitals and writing for the same journals. Between supervisors and doctoral students, between chief physicians and interns, and between the students and the interns, tight relationships developed, and in many cases, friendships were maintained over long periods of time, even after the end of their psychiatric careers. The network of former students around Antoine Porot, who strongly felt they were part of a group even after they were given chairs in different universities in France, is the best example of this camaraderie.[12]

---

9   Among those born in North Africa were, for example, Paul Sauzay, Robert Susini and Jean Sutter. Sauzay, Assistance, title page; Susini, Aspects cliniques, title page; Sutter, Épilepsie mentale, title page.

10 Reboul/Régis, Assistance, title page; Discussion du rapport d'assistance psychiatrique, 177.

11 Other important universities for the education of colonial psychiatrists were Marseille, Montpellier and Toulouse. Of those psychiatrists who wrote dissertations on North Africans, literally none had studied at other universities. Paris, Marseille and Bordeaux were those universities where the civilian colonial doctors were educated. Aubin, Assistance, 168.

12 For example: Sutter, Leçon inaugurale, 443; Michaux, Professeur Antoine Porot (1876–1865), 72.

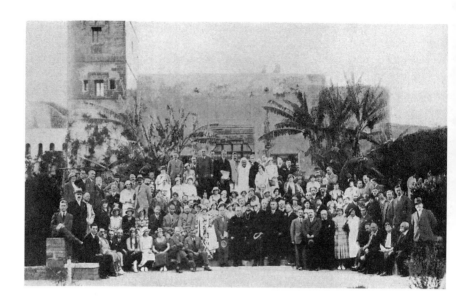

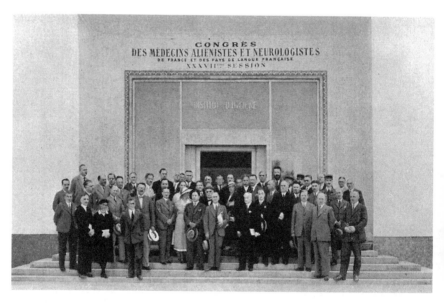

The participating neurologists and psychiatrists of the 1933 Congress in Rabat, photographed at the reception of the Congress at the Kasbah of the Udayas in Rabat and after the last session of the conference. Taken from: Charpentier, Comptes Rendus, between pages 484 and 485, pictures A and C.

The preceding pictures show the participating neurologists and psychiatrists of the 1933 Congress in Rabat, photographed at the reception and after the last session of the conference, posing as a unified group of educated experts. However, not all professional relationships were defined by this sense of kinship and loyalty. There were also discordances and competition between psychiatrists, and not all of them viewed each other as competent, as shown in the forceful scientific debates in the academic journals, and even through downright bickering and personal attacks.[13]

In addition to these academic arguments, colonial psychiatrists were often convinced that their predecessors, for various reasons, had not acquired full command over the scientific tools of research open to the new generation of psychiatrists, and that they therefore had, involuntarily, falsified their published accounts by relying on unsound data. Very few psychiatrists contradicted the opinions presented by earlier psychiatrists, and if they did, it was usually in narrow fields of expertise, such as the frequency of general paralysis, as discussed in Chapter 5.3. Even in criticism, this authority of earlier generations was not generally questioned. William Goëau-Brissonnière, for instance, wrote in 1926 that "not long ago" it had been believed that the psychopathology of North Africans was completely different from that of Europeans – something he disagreed with.[14] He stated, respectful towards his misinformed predecessors: "We do not want to say that our predecessors were poor observers, but simply that the conditions in which they found themselves were particularly unfavourable, not allowing them a sufficient penetration of the Muslim world: besides, it is due to their efforts that we today have this easier access, and it is just, here, to pay tribute to them."[15]

An analysis of this network of connections should not be limited to professional relationships, whether dominated by opposition or loyalty and respect, but should also include the complex way in which "knowledge" was produced within the web formed by the publications of these colonial psychiatrists. Examining the sources in detail, one realises that they quoted and double-quoted each other,[16] taking details

---

13 Antoine Porot and Dumolard, who were contemporaries in Algiers, where Porot worked as a professor and Dumolard as a lecturer at the same university, accused each other of all kinds of misdeeds in a series of articles published in the journal *Hygiène Mentale* in 1925 and 1926. The Tunisian doctor Ahmad Chérif reacted in 1909 to Maurice Boigey's racist "Psychological Study of Islam", published by the *Annales Médico-Psychologiques* in 1908, by refuting each of his hypotheses in an article of the same name and in the same journal.

14 Goëau-Brissonnière, Syphilis nerveuse, 19.

15 Ibid., 20.

16 By double-quoting I mean the situation of psychiatrist A quoting an original source B, and psychiatrist C later quoting psychiatrist A and source B as if they were separate and unrelated. Psychiatrist C thus pretends to have two sources whereas, in fact, there is only one. One example would be the repetition of Constans' 1873 percentages on death rates among Muslim patients,

from other psychiatric texts out of context[17] and borrowing bizarre formulations from other psychiatrists as well as from other academic disciplines.[18] They neglected the compilation and use of statistical evidence[19] and even plagiarised whole paragraphs and pages from predecessors.[20] As regards Muslim women, all of these problematic forms of empirical behaviour, which should be seen as professional forms of bias, helped to make the paucity of existing knowledge more scientifically authoritative through the sheer number of quotations reiterating the same "truth".[21] Below, the perspective of the colonial psychiatrists will be contextualised in two ways. First, the bias in the colonial sources will be examined. Second, the explanations given by colonial psychiatrists for the absence of female Muslim patients will be presented and their context and limitations analysed.

Scientific Bias

One way of analysing these psychiatric reports is to look at different forms of "scientific bias" in the production of "knowledge" and the ways in which this bias hid Muslim women in the published sources. In addition to general problems of unscrupulous

---

discussed in Chapter 3, repeated by Meilhon in 1896, by Gervais in 1907, and by Reboul and Régis in 1912. Linas, Aliénés en Algérie, 492; Meilhon, Aliénation mentale, part 2, 185; Gervais, Contribution, 5 f.; Reboul/Régis, Assistance, 43.

17 See, for example: Livet's complicated calculation of the potential number of Muslim patients in Algeria, discussed in Chapter 3. Livet, Aliénés algériens, 37; Reboul/Régis, Assistance, 49 f.; Abadie, Report, 379; Dupouy, Chronique, 529.

18 Such as the crude and discriminatory formulations on normal Muslim femininity, discussed in Chapter 1, or the formulation of Kocher in 1883 that Muslims only "adopted the vices of French civilisation", discussed in the subchapter on general paralysis (Chapter 5.3). Kocher, Criminalité, 1 f.; 72; Lafitte, Contribution, 22; Pascalis, Paralysie générale, 42; Meilhon, Aliénation mentale, part 4, 34; Matignon, Art médical, 85; Laignel-Lavastine, Review of Sicard, 624; Gervais, Contribution, 47; Thierry, Étude, 57; Porot, Notes, 380.

19 For example: Maréschal, Réflexions, 79.

20 Sometimes it is difficult to tell who copied whom. Louis Margain and Auguste Marie wrote articles on psychiatry in the colonies in 1908 and 1905 respectively, in which Margain seemed to have copied large amounts from Marie's text. However, they were friends and seem to have collaborated on a report for the 1905 Colonial Congress, so an initial text, which they both used for their respective articles, might well have been composed by both of them. For instance: Marie, Sur quelques aspects, 766 f.; Margain, Aliénation mentale, 88 f. At other times, plagiarisms are easy to detect. In his 1932 dissertation, Henri Soumeire copied page after page of Henri Bouquet's 1909 dissertation, and Sextius Arène plagiarised large parts of his 1913 dissertation from Lucien Bertholon's 1889 article on the "Criminal Anthropology of Tunisian Muslims".

21 See Studer, 'Pregnant with Madness'.

quoting and the dismissal of statistics, actual scientific misconduct can be found in a significant number of the sources examined in this book. Three mechanisms of misconduct have been identified and used to group thematic "clusters" of conclusions – the focus on normality, the gaps between "knowledge" and "experience", and the gaps within the body of colonial "knowledge" itself.

Focus on Muslim Normality

One of the biggest issues of colonial psychiatry was that French colonial psychiatrists expected normal North African Muslims to be "abnormal". This expectation explains their fascination with Muslim normality and, deriving from this, the importance given to normality in the theoretical treatises on the psychopathology of North Africans. Megan Vaughan argued in her 1991 book "Curing their Ills" that in Europe the "mad" had to be presented as different from the "normal", for the combined sake of identity and security, whereas the colonised were already othered per se, so further differentiating between "normal" and "abnormal" was unnecessary.[22] Instead of a distinct boundary between the sane and the mad, as in Europe, the defining borders in the colonial context were "race" and, where Muslims were concerned, religion (which was used almost synonymously with "race"). Both borders levelled out any differences within the colonised populations. From the point of view of French colonial psychiatry, this affiliation to an imaginary single unit (the Maghreb), this uniformity of the colonised meant that "normal" North Africans shared more irrational character traits with "abnormal" North Africans than with "normal" Europeans.

In Chapter 5, this marked differentiation between North Africans and Europeans through the pathologisation of Muslim normality could be observed in what was written about Muslim manifestations of hysteria. Psychiatrists claimed that while Muslim patients seldom suffered from the psychiatric disorder of hysteria, hysteria could often be described as an accompanying symptom in a variety of mental disorders, or even as a widespread character trait of "normal" North Africans, prone to hysterical reactions. In addition, the claim that hysteria manifested itself in 20th century North Africans in forms that had disappeared from French patients at the turn of the century emphasised the perceived, deep distinction between Muslims and Europeans, patients and non-patients alike, by associating North Africans with remnants of long discarded and outgrown theories.

These descriptions, of colonised normalities as abnormal, functioned through the attribution of morbid character traits and the use of a deeply pathological vocabulary,

---

22   Vaughan, Curing their Ills, 10. For othering in the context of French colonial psychiatry, see
       also: Collignon, Construction, 176 f.; Keller, Colonial Madness, 124.

such as that shown in the psychiatric discussion of normal Muslim women, discussed in Chapter 1, who were described as having profoundly abnormal brains or souls, as lacking understanding, reason and intelligence, and as being, pathologically, on the same level as children, animals or even inanimate objects. Female Muslim normality was described in terms that made it clear to European observers that, judged by Europeans standards, North African women were highly pathological. French colonial psychiatrists were not the first to describe North African women in this way – there was already a tradition of travel literature, romantic fiction and general medical jargon which used the same Orientalist images in their depictions of Muslim femininity. The scientific writings of French colonial psychiatrists only reinforced what was "already known" about Muslim women and made the "common knowledge" shared by European settler communities acceptable to a wider academic and social field.

These characteristics of female Muslim normality were explained through the primitivity of both Muslim women and their husbands, which was expressed through them treating their wives "barbarically". The commentaries on normal Muslim femininity in Chapter 1 can be roughly categorised as those that were judged as positive (for instance, Muslim women being good mothers) and those seen as negative (for instance, being treated as animals). While the latter were due to Muslim society – dominated by Muslim men –, the former were "natural qualities" of all uncorrupted women. The sources provide abundant information about the psychiatric conceptions of a "universal" femininity, evinced by their repeated comparisons between Muslim and French women. To some degree, the picture drawn of Muslim women in the colonial psychiatric sources consisted of criticisms of too developed, too demanding, deeply unfeminine French women, who had preferred, so to speak, the cultivation of mental problems over the fulfilment of their "natural roles".[23] Overall, this construct of female Muslim normality had no independent features,

---

23   In his 1913 book "Arab Mores", Witold Lemanski described in detail what enlightenment and emancipation would entail for the mental state of simple Muslim women by evoking the origins of psychiatric problems in European women: "There are few unbalanced women in Islam: there are no such original women, such eccentrics, furiously engaged in sports, journalism, 'globe-trotting', in the crusade for the emancipation of women, and also, resulting from this, in the customary habits of alcohol, ether, gambling and other more or less complicated vices. Life at home is the biblical simplification of the natural and philosophical purpose of women. This simplification is incompatible with insanity." Lemanski, Mœurs arabes, 120 f. This comparison should not only be seen as a direct criticism of European women but also as a justification for opposing their further emancipation. Rosemary George suggested in 1993 that comparisons with "'native' women" gave European men the "comfortable belief that the white woman's emancipation was a completed project [...]." George, Homes in the Empire, 116.

as all characteristics reflected grievances concerning threats posed by other groups within the population.[24]

Chapters 2, 3 and 4 focus on patients, i. e. those Muslim women deemed pathological, in a purely psychiatric sense, within the already pathologised field of female Muslim normality. All three chapters portray different aspects of the pathologisation of normality. Chapter 2 analyses which "types" of Muslim women were admitted into colonial psychiatric care. This was the only instance in which colonial psychiatry, instead of claiming that Muslim normality and abnormality overlapped, stressed the crucial differences between "harmless" normal women and potentially dangerous disturbers of the public order.[25] Any Muslim woman caught in the psychiatric net of institutionalised care, by being picked up by the police or through a complaint of a neighbour, whether "insane" or not, would suffer instant pathologisation as a social outcast, as no "normal" woman – always within the narrow field of what constituted normal Muslim femininity in both the colonial and male Muslim imagination – would have behaved in a manner necessitating the intervention of the police and legal system.

Chapter 3 analyses additional layers of pathologisation of the female Muslim patients after admission to the institutions. Certain symptoms, otherwise difficult to contextualise, were summarised under umbrella terms – such as mania, expressed through North African gestures, agitation and lamentations – which were diagnosed by experts who, in most cases, had no understanding of North African languages. "Normal" expressions of distress – understandable in any person, mentally ill or not, picked up by the police and interned in a highly stigmatised institution, where communication between carers and patients was impossible due to a language barrier – were, under these circumstances, interpreted as pathological symptoms of a vaguely defined disorder. Another allegedly typical North African symptom, present in a variety of diagnoses, was "somatisation", which, in the psychiatric theories, was one of the markers differentiating between Muslim and European patients. While "somatisation" explained the absence of Muslim patients,[26] it also pathologised "normal" North African expressions of psychological unease and implied that many apparently "normal" Muslims consulting doctors with vague bodily symptoms were in fact suffering from mental disorders.

Chapter 4 deals with the therapies implemented in the psychiatric institutions, which further pathologised North Africans. After wave after wave of new treatments

---

24 The corrupting power of civilisation has been mentioned in very different historical contexts and corresponds to fears about the decay of the authors' own societies, which are then projected onto a more "primitive", but quintessentially better, society, which is corrupted by contact with the more civilised society. It is less a commentary on the corrupted society than the corrupting one and was usually used to criticise events in the authors' homelands.

25 This change in both vocabulary and concepts was, however, not discussed in the source material.

26 See also p. 243.

introduced in the 20th century, patients were grouped within precise psychiatric categories and, at least in theory, given treatments corresponding to these scientific diagnoses, but even this clearly medical environment employed unsound deductions about the deeply "abnormal normality" of North Africans. It was proposed by some, for example, that North Africans did not feel pain in the same way as Europeans and could therefore bear harsher therapies better, such as electroshocks.[27]

Both the introduction and (lack of) success of therapies were rationalised through the "abnormal normality" of North Africans. In the 19th century, using patients as a work force was seen as therapeutic, but psychiatrists thought North African labour almost unusable due to Muslims being lazy, untrainable and potentially aggressive. This did not mean that their labour was not actually used for the budgetary wellbeing of the French institutions; it only meant that their labour was seen as pathologically different from European labour. These North African character traits, supposedly demonstrated by the normal and the abnormal alike, also suggested that any lack of success in treatments was not caused by flaws in the therapies but rather by the obstinacy of Muslim patients. Equally, Muslim architecture, through its supposed lack of air and light – even though typical French descriptions of Muslim houses usually included a courtyard complete, in many cases, with fountain and garden[28] – was thought to hinder patient improvement. Contrasting North African buildings with French theories on healthy architecture resulted in conventional Muslim houses being described as infectious, potentially morbid and even dangerous for the inhabitants.[29] While this concern about the therapeutics of space would be understandable regarding the development of certain physical disorders – tuberculosis for example[30] –, the

---

27 Brault, for instance, suggested in 1905 that North Africans, like French farmers, apparently "feel pain less keenly", which gave him the possibility to perform surgical procedures on them without anaesthetics. Brault, Pathologie et hygiène, 156. Racy discussed in 1970 the "anecdotal reports and the personal impressions" of some psychiatrists working in what he called the Arab East on the "remarkable tolerance of Arab patients to potent psychiatric therapy", such as electroshock therapy. Racy, Psychiatry in the Arab East, 41.

28 As discussed in Chapter 4.3 on "Morals and Degeneration".

29 The criticism of North African architecture is also interesting in the context of what Richard Keller described as the symbolism of colonial architecture, in which new psychiatric buildings, like Blida Psychiatric Hospital, "add to the prestige of French Algeria". Keller, Colonial Madness, 77 f.

30 Other psychiatrists claimed that it was particularly in the French institutions that Muslims developed – and died of – tuberculosis. Reboul and Régis reported at the Tunis Congress in 1912 that of 35 Senegalese female patients transported to the asylum in Marseille between 1897 and the Congress, 29 had died, "almost all" of tuberculosis. Reboul/Régis, Assistance, 93. Regarding tuberculosis infections among Muslim psychiatric patients, see also: Pascalis, Paralysie générale, 33; Brault, Pathologie et hygiène, 29 f.; Levet, Assistance, 242 f.; Gervais, Contribution, 20 f.;

psychiatric unease with traditional Muslim architecture seems exaggerated and should be seen as part of the broader vilification of the "normal" North African lifestyle.

Difference between Knowledge and Experience

These pathologised definitions of female Muslim normality were part of what was "known" about North Africans, but this "knowledge" did not always correspond with the practical findings of the colonial psychiatrists.[31] The second set of problems in the colonial handling of North African female psychopathology examined in the previous chapters involved exactly this difference between the academic discourse and medical practice, the gaps between "knowledge" and "experience".[32]

In the passages concerning North African women, prefabricated knowledge, dangerously close to – and sometimes overlapping with – what could be described as colonial myths, was often favoured over experience.[33] This knowledge was so specific as to be directly understandable by anyone living in North Africa, "knowing" the region and its people, yet so general as to be applicable to almost any historical or geographical context.[34] Consequently, colonial depictions of "normal", i.e. non-patient Muslim women, simplistic in the extreme, incorporated vast contradictions. While the normal Muslim woman was treated as barely more than a "beast of burden" by her husband, she was also spoilt and pampered, languishing in the golden cages of the harems. While her limited, almost animalistic, mental faculties protected her from

---

Dupouy, Chronique, 528 f.; Sutter, Épilepsie mentale, 75 f.; Porot, M. et al., Tuberculose des aliénés, 398.

31 These contradictions were already mentioned by other historians. Alice Bullard stated in 2001: "However, the distinctly gendered norms of civilization and the deeply powerful patriarchies of the Maghreb and France provoked apparent contradictions in colonial psychiatry." Bullard, Truth in Madness, 123. See also: Vaughan, Introduction, 2.

32 Many of these contradictions were not found within the texts of any single psychiatrist but within the larger frameworks adhered to by psychiatrists. Therefore, some of the contradictions may well be explained through the different – often opposing – strands of colonial psychiatry, or, as in the case of Antoine Porot for example, the evolution of theoretical thinking during one person's career.

33 As discussed in Chapter 3, colonial psychiatry, which saw itself as a thoroughly innovative science, did not really make use of the experience-based tool of modernity, statistics. It was "known", for instance, that fewer Muslim women than men became insane. The collection of statistical evidence, which could only prove what was already "known", but which also had the potential to disprove existing "knowledge", was therefore of only secondary importance.

34 The Orientalist idea that North African and Middle Eastern women were completely timeless and ahistorical – and therefore uninteresting for research based on questions of changes and developments – was discussed by Marnia Lazreg in 1988: Lazreg, Feminism and Difference, 86.

the strains of intellectual overwork, she was scheming and treacherous, betraying her husband out of habit and boredom more than lust. While she was used as an "instrument of pleasure" by her husband, a "genital field", and suffered his unwanted sexual attacks, her nubility was unnaturally precocious and her lust insatiable. Although descriptions of these extremes could be partly based on the professional experiences of the psychiatrists themselves, and the doctors and ethnologists on whose practical knowledge they often relied, such extreme types could not simultaneously represent a unified female Muslim normality. The concept of a unified female Muslim normality – incorporating these contradictory characteristics – was, in this case, the "knowledge", while the "experiences" provided much more multifaceted descriptions of Muslim life, which could reflect the very dissimilar lives of Muslim women from different social classes, as seen, for example, in the case studies.[35]

These glaring contradictions between "knowledge" and experience in those sections of the colonial sources concerning Muslim women are suggestive, as the same accumulation of gaps does not appear in the academic treatment of psychiatric topics concerning Muslim men. This does not imply that the image of Muslim men in the colonial psychiatric sources was by any means less biased or more "truthful" than that of Muslim women. As discussed in Chapter 1, the descriptions of "normal" Muslim men were strongly influenced by practical experiences with patients, which led to an inverse process of pathologisation – practical experience informed theories about Muslim men instead of theories being based on a lack of personal experience. A direct comparison of the theories about normal Muslim men and women allows for the conclusion that there were fewer contradictions in the theoretical net of "knowledge" about Muslim men, but not necessarily more "truths".

In his 1998 article "The Algerian with the Knife", the British historian David Macey examined both the origins and the consequences of this particular "knowledge", this set of preconceived ideas about the behaviour and characteristics of – male – North Africans. Macey argued that this image was consolidated by French colonial psychiatry in its scientific publications. However, the enduring consequences of these theories, still felt today, were not due to the influence of these written efforts, which were only intended to reach an audience composed of experts, but due to the fact that these texts validated common knowledge. Macey wrote: "The doctors of the Algiers School simply knew what everyone knows, and a vicious epistemological circle supplied all the proofs that were needed to demonstrate the validity of the theory."[36]

---

35 Suzanne Taïeb's collection of case studies covered destitute Muslim women, others from simple working-class backgrounds, as well as female patients coming from a certain degree of wealth and education. See, for instance: Taïeb, Idées d'influence, 92; 111–4.

36 Macey, Algerian with the Knife, 166.

Even though Macey mainly wrote about Muslim men, the same applied to Muslim women. This normative "knowledge" about Muslim women, conforming to an instinctively felt reality, also had a function – to demonstrate that North African men were inherently incapable of being civilised. As mentioned in the introduction of this book, the conviction that Muslim women were brutalised by their husbands and victimised by Muslim society was one reason why Muslims were declared unassimilable as a "race".[37] From this perspective, innovations were useless, as North African Muslims were unable to change or adapt, doomed to stay at this primitive level of civilisation, as shown by their continued treatment of Muslim women. Additionally, few colonial authors advocated active improvements in the organisation of Muslim family life with – from their point of view – its deplorable consequences for the helpless North African women, claiming that France had pledged to protect North African traditions and rites.[38]

Some psychiatric experts explained this reluctance to interfere by claiming that changes to the situation of Muslim women, far from bettering their situation, would actually propel them towards mental disorders.[39] Witold Lemanski, for example, described in 1913 the dangers of the path of enlightenment and emancipation: "When the pre-eminence of man, a fundamental Qur'anic precept, ceases to be accepted, the woman will no longer recognise in him the right of high and low justice, she will have accomplished a complete religious revolution, she will have escaped the constraints of the Qur'an; from the darkness of the Middle Ages, she will pass into the lights of

---

37 Arène, Criminalité, 170.

38 Gordon, Women of Algeria, 37. This was untrue. France repeatedly involved itself in many areas that could be interpreted as Muslim traditions – the suspension of the Islamic penal code, the introduction of "French" education, the imposition of a new political organisation etc. The French did, however, take a stand against changes in the private lives of Muslims, fighting against the emancipatory ideas of independence movements. Maher, Women and Social Change, 105; Adamson, Approaches, 23; Dorph, Islamic Law, 171. In reality, basic notions of femininity were shared by French and Muslim men, and the French did not want to provoke Muslim men too far by pushing the importance of women's rights. See for example: Keddie, Problems, 226; Lazreg, Eloquence of Silence, 96.

39 Postcolonial psychiatrists' findings usually showed that the same social problems which had been discussed by the colonial psychiatrists influenced the mental state of female Muslims. Douki et al. claimed in a recent article that the "subordinate position of women in Arab communities" caused various mental problems among them. They went on to describe specific instances of oppression of Muslim women which could lead to mental troubles, many of which should feel familiar after this analysis of colonial psychiatric sources: "Following are a series of culture-related risk factors including education, work, marriage, sexuality, infertility, domestic violence, sexual harassment, birth control etc. which greatly contribute to triggering mental disorders in females or to worsen their course and outcome." Douki et al., Women's Mental Health, 179 f.

modern civilisation, dazed, confused, unbalanced, maybe disillusioned and *unbelieving*. Will it be a good thing?"[40] Torn between ending the subjugation of Muslim women and preventing the emergence of mentally unbalanced, unbelieving masses, Lemanski, and many of his professional colleagues with him, chose the conservation of religion and the resulting subjugation of women. Here, it was feared the "emancipation" of Muslim women would entail the same morbid consequences that the introduction of alcohol had had on Muslim men. Both alcohol and emancipation were imagined as unfortunate side effects of the French *mission civilisatrice*, causing mental illness and degeneration in the "natives", and both needed to be tightly controlled.

These gaps between "knowledge" and "experience" are analysed in each of the preceding chapters, but the most obvious contradiction is shown through the fact that colonial psychiatrists were more interested in defining a pathology of female normality than in writing about their own patients – even though they admitted that they had, as male interlopers, only a small insight into the mysterious world of "normal" women.[41] They insisted they had the authority of experts over those hidden from them, instead of portraying those groups of the female Muslim population which were at their "disposal", so to speak, in the form of patients, in the psychiatric institutions. This led to a variety of contradictory statements. In Chapter 2, for instance, their experiences with mainly criminalised psychiatric patients clashed with the knowledge that Muslim women, unlike Muslim men, never committed criminal acts. Theory dictated that both "normal" and "abnormal" male Muslims shared a penchant for alcoholism and crime, while Muslim women tended towards abstention and meekness, which in turn led towards compliance with the law. However, the personal experiences of the psychiatrists treating patients within the psychiatric institutions contradicted these basic notions of Muslim femininity, as they vividly reported the physical danger posed by female Muslim patients and their various addictions.[42]

---

40 Lemanski, Mœurs arabes, 181 f. Emphasis in the original.

41 This was stated by both male doctors and psychiatrists. Henri Duchêne-Marullaz, for example, wrote in 1905: "She [the Muslim woman] does not like European doctors. These women, who sell themselves for pennies without hesitation, acquire a fierce virtue, from the moment when, from the simple medical point of view, we try to examine them." Duchêne-Marullaz, Hygiène, 51. See also: Perrin, Essai, 51 f.; Richardot, Pratiques médicales, 57; Wolters, Rôle de l'instituteur, 52; Vitoux, Report on the 5th Congrès de Gynécologie, 268. Others claimed that examinations of Muslim women, even very intrusive ones (such as genital examinations), caused no problem. Gomma, Assistance médicale, 109; Wiehn, Service médical, 58; Lévy-Bram, Assistance médicale, 62.

42 Charles Bardenat, for instance, wrote in 1948, referring to his experiences at Blida Psychiatric Hospital, that, while still far below that of any male category, more Muslim women than European or Jewish women were criminally insane: "Without wishing to draw definite conclusions from this fact, we must admit that the native woman – noisier and more destructive

The balance between "knowledge" and experience in the examples above favoured the former over the latter, with "knowledge" not being defined scientifically but existing as part of a pool of general knowledge, a shared settler canon of obviousness, of "felt" truths. In the context of treatments administered to Muslim patients, however, the balance was reversed. Chapter 4 examines how early psychiatric treatments, like work therapy, were eventually dismissed from the theoretical frameworks because they were ineffectual in the face of ever-rising patient numbers, yet persisted in practice. It also discusses later theories which envisaged distinct surgical or drug-treatments for each diagnosis, or at least for each set of general symptoms, while, in practice, new treatments were often tried out on "incurable" North Africans. Paradoxically, both the persistence of outdated therapies and the testing of new therapies independent of the actual diagnoses showed the pragmatism of French psychiatry, with experience-based decisions triumphing over theories. The knowledge, here discredited in favour of experience, was, however, not the same kind of "common knowledge" discussed earlier; these psychiatric theories, which superseded useful treatments like work therapy and demanded distinct therapies for each diagnosis, came from the *Métropole* or even from abroad, and not from within the circle of French colonial psychiatrists. This form of knowledge had nothing to do with the understanding of Muslim societies shared by settlers in North Africa; unsuitable to the colonial reality, it could therefore be dismissed in favour of the experiences of French colonial psychiatrists.

Interest and Disinterest

The third of these forms of "scientific bias" comprises the arbitrary ways in which French colonial psychiatrists composed their theoretical texts. Analysis of the colonial sources in the preceding chapters shows that large sections of the colonial societies, including both normal and abnormal Muslims, were disproportionally present or disproportionally neglected in those sources. As discussed in Chapter 3, in the early years of colonial psychiatry, the lack of interest in Muslim women could be justified with the relative numerical unimportance of female Muslim patients, especially compared with the significant numbers of European patients. However, the numbers of female Muslim patients rose, and by the late 1950s and early 1960s, their numbers in Algerian psychiatric institutions finally overtook those of European women (at least in

in the hospital than her kind in the other ethnic groups – does not reach the harmfulness of the native man, due to the condition as a minor, in which she is kept in her society, living under a strict and quasi-servile dependence." Bardenat, Criminalité, 320.

the public, i. e. non-private and non-paying, institutions).[43] Overall, there were fewer female Muslim patients than there should have been if insanity was in proportion with the general population, but not so few as the colonial neglect would have suggested – an average of 24.49% of Muslim patients in the statistics (published in the academic source material accessible to colonial psychiatrists) were women. Although the numerical situation encountered in the late colonial period was diametrically opposite to that of earlier decades, the lack of interest remained – colonial sources neither offered explanations for the rising numbers nor even acknowledged the new situation. The new presence of female Muslim patients remained as undiscussed as their former relative absence.

The historian Alice Bullard wrote in her 2001 article "Truth in Madness" that "only by tracing the boundaries of the French erasure of North African women can we begin to conceive what was erased; only by examining his [Abel-Joseph Meilhon's] male-centred theory of madness can we begin to ask questions about the female mad."[44] Following Bullard's hypothesis, I propose that studying the topics that colonial psychiatry focused on allows conclusions to be drawn about those it neglected; examining the interest of colonial psychiatry reveals its lack of interest.[45] This book looks at the areas in which this neglect of female Muslim patients was encountered and contrasts them with those topics concerning Muslim women which were not neglected in the source material. Chapter 1 examines those women who were, by definition, absent from colonial psychiatric care because psychiatry primarily existed to authoritatively segregate potentially dangerous abnormality from normality. Considering this strong focus of colonial psychiatry on protecting society from the threats posed by the criminally insane, those portions of society deemed normal should have been uninteresting to colonial psychiatry. However, French colonial psychiatrists did focus on these normal – i. e. non-criminal, non-patient – Muslim women, and their descriptions drew heavily from the pool of common "knowledge" discussed above.

Juxtaposing the focus on this highly pathologised normality with the lack of interest in female Muslim abnormality suggests that the neglect of female Muslim patients was due to there being, in the colonial imagination, no – or, at best,

---

43 Assicot et al., Causes principales, 262 f.; Chappert, Contribution, 20; Mares/Barre, Quelques aspects, 31 f.

44 Bullard, Truth in Madness, 123.

45 The absence of certain topics and the presence of others cannot be defined as scientifically biased per se. It is clear that some topics were deemed more important, or even politically relevant, for the bigger picture than others. Nonetheless, it is only when contextualising the question of an accurate depiction of the reality of female Muslim patients that one realises how deliberate the silence on certain topics seems to be.

minimal – differentiation between normal and mad Muslim women. Since they all behaved in a primitive, irrational way, descriptions of female Muslim patients were subsumed into those of normal Muslim women – even if, as stated above, the experiences gained through everyday contact with female Muslim patients contradicted these notions.[46] From this perspective, descriptions of female Muslim abnormality were simply superfluous – everybody knew what normal Muslim femininity consisted of and even abnormal Muslim women "had" to conform to the rules established about their normality.

These instances of the interest and uninterest of colonial psychiatry were also exhibited in other areas. Chapter 5 focuses on the absence of three different diagnoses – one which, it was supposed, Muslims could only rarely develop (general paralysis), and two that were widespread in Europe at the time (hysteria and puerperal insanity). The latter were chosen because they were conceived either as exclusively female (puerperal insanity) or as predominantly female (hysteria), and because they were rarely discussed in the sources throughout all but the final years of the colonial period. One must therefore differentiate between the very different reasons for the absence of general paralysis on the one hand, and the absence of hysteria and puerperal insanity on the other. In the case of general paralysis, an abundance of texts exists, dedicated to carefully describing this absence, while the written sources remained mostly silent on the topics of hysteria and puerperal insanity.[47] An analysis of the case studies on Muslim women shows that general paralysis, whose absence or rarity was part of the established colonial knowledge, was much more present in the published case studies than the other two disorders, whose occurrence remained largely undiscussed and therefore undisputed. From this, two conclusions may be drawn. If the focus on general paralysis had really been caused by its extreme rarity, one would expect to find more sources on the other two, even rarer, disorders. However, lacking the sensationalist and explosive ingredients of syphilis, alcoholism and civilisation, puerperal insanity and hysteria remained neglected. On the other hand, it shows that habit influenced the choice of theme to a certain degree, as colonial psychiatrists wrote mainly about well-established psychiatric topics – part of the scientific logic of writing about prominent topics in order to garner citations from others. Therefore, the suggestion is that interest – here, interest in certain disorders over others – and a longing for academic respectability dictated what was written about, not any clinical reality.

---

46 See also: Bullard, Truth in Madness, 123.

47 This silence is especially interesting if one considers that the Tunisian psychiatrist Sleïm Ammar stated in 1972 that "a few years ago" hysteria and puerperal problems had "dominated" female mental pathology in Tunisia. The alleged absence of these disorders in colonial North African women must therefore be compared with the predomination of these same disorders among Muslim women in the 1960s and 1970s. Ammar, Aperçu, 704.

Chapters 2, 3 and 4 analyse the practical consequences of the lacunae within the colonial interests – consequences for the selection of patients, the diagnoses given, and the treatments administered. Chapters 2 examines colonial psychiatry's focus on the institutionalisation of marginalised Muslim women. While colonial psychiatry could have changed its admission mechanisms to include non-criminalised women, considerations concerning overcrowding and the budgetary difficulties faced by psychiatric institutions prevented this. Only treating the tip of the iceberg – i. e. marginalised women – and not the suspected, hidden mass of female Muslim patients was economically advantageous and did not represent a social hazard, unlike neglecting potentially dangerous male Muslim patients. "Knowledge" about Muslims therefore influenced the focus of colonial psychiatry (i. e. those threatening French society), which in turn had an impact on the selection of patients. The result was that the French colonial psychiatric system was defined by often subconscious calculations of the ratio of danger posed by individual patients versus available funds rather than by simply wishing to cure people of their mental problems.

Chapter 3 analyses diagnostic fashions, i. e. the overrepresentation of female Muslim patients in certain diseases, such as mania and epilepsy, and the absence of other diagnoses, as demonstrated through a direct comparison of the different numbers of patient groups among the various categories of disorders. Jan Goldstein suggested in 1982 that "a diagnostic preference or preoccupation, if shared by a sufficiently large number of doctors" had, historically, produced diagnostic trends, as "certain equivocal pathological phenomena come to be labelled in a uniform manner".[48] Arguably, these diagnostic trends were, once again, led by the "knowledge" of colonial psychiatry about Muslim normality rather than by actual symptoms, and strengthened by the cumulative authority of a frequently cited diagnosis.

Finally, in Chapter 4, the most serious consequences stemming from colonial interests are examined through the physical reality of the therapies implemented or withheld. In the early colonial period, there was a distinct absence of medical treatments prescribed for North African patients in the asylums of the French South, which was due to the general lack of therapeutic success. In the later period, the introduction of ever more innovative treatments dominated colonial psychiatry, and many of these treatments were tried out on Muslims, even if the sources remained vague about the "races" of those experimented upon. Colonial psychiatry sought successful treatments in order to stop overcrowding, and the resulting financial strains, in psychiatric institutions. To this end, colonial psychiatrists experimented with aggressive therapies in their treatment of Muslim women, while "soft" therapies, such as psychotherapy, were neglected in both the hospitals and the texts.

---

48   Goldstein, Hysteria Diagnosis, 220.

Summarising, it can be said that, thematically, the core interests of French colonial psychiatry changed little over the period studied in this book. Early psychiatric examinations already focused on questions of settler security,[49] budgetary considerations,[50] aspects of civilisation[51] and the humane or inhumane treatments of the colonised insane.[52] This choice of topics – dangers, money, civilisation and humanitarianism – had direct political implications, which went on to influence later colonial psychiatric research.[53] Female Muslim abnormality fell outside these core interests. Meek Muslim women were perceived as posing no threat to French settler societies, and, representing allegedly only a minute percentage of the patients, could not cause overcrowding within the psychiatric institutions. The alleged primitivity and deep lack of civilisation of Muslim women fascinated the French colonial psychiatrists, but, as it was a characteristic of all Muslim women, no special examination of female Muslim patients was warranted. The inhumane treatment of Muslim women – in the traditional *mâristâns* as well as at the hands of their own husbands – was of interest to colonial psychiatrists, but, like primitivity, it was seen to affect more than just female Muslim patients; conditions in the *mâristâns* concerned all Muslim patients, and mistreatment by Muslim husbands all Muslim women. Therefore, since female Muslim patients were viewed in the context of far larger groups, they were eclipsed by those groups and consequently ignored in the texts. Thus the blind spots within the colonial psychiatric net of "knowledge" repeatedly coincided with topics concerning female Muslim abnormality.

---

49   This interest can be seen in the plethora of studies devoted to Muslim criminality, such as Adolphe Kocher's "Criminality among Arabs" from 1883.

50   Early considerations of financial aspects are shown through the repeatedly rejected plans for the construction of institutions in North Africa. See for example: Porot, Assistance psychiatrique, 86; Charpentier, Comptes Rendus, 59 f.; Desruelles/Bersot, Note sur l'histoire, 311 ff.

51   In the earliest psychiatric source, the question of the influence of civilisation was already asked by Moreau de Tours: "Is civilisation, as it has been commonly said, favourable to the development of insanity? If we stick to the vulgar understanding of the word, it is true, from the point of view of pure and simple fact; from the theoretical point of view, the questions could be resolved, *a priori*, in the affirmative." Moreau, Recherches, 124. Emphasis in the original.

52   As shown in reports on the inhumane treatment of Muslim patients in both Muslim and French institutions. For early criticism of the institutions in France, see: Delasiauve, Review of Collardot, 115 f.; Jobert, Projet, 16. For 19th century criticism of Muslim *mâristâns*, see for example: Bertherand, Médecine et hygiène, 22; Moreau, Recherches, 110 f.

53   While these gender-neutral general interests theoretically included Muslim women, the language of the psychiatric studies often explicitly excluded them, as shown in the personification of Muslim danger as a "man with a knife", for example. This image, in the published accounts of colonial psychiatry as well as in other colonial genres, was analysed by David Macey in his 1998 article, "The Algerian with the Knife".

Imagined Absence of Female Muslim Patients

The absence of Muslim women from colonial psychiatric care is the pivotal colonial premise scrutinised in this historical analysis. Colonial psychiatrists claimed
that Muslim women, for a variety of reasons, did not consult psychiatric experts
and therefore did not appear in the colonial institutions. The examination of the
colonial sources, however, suggested that it was primarily an imagined absence. It
is undeniable that Muslim women were underrepresented in comparison to other
patient groups in colonial care, but not to a degree that warranted their extensive
neglect in the sources. We may therefore ask what the reasons were for the absence
of female Muslim patients from colonial psychiatric institutions, why colonial psychiatrists chose to describe the admittedly small group of female Muslim patients in
terms of "absence", and, coming back to the hypothesis proposed earlier that what
is written can say more about those describing than those described, what this says
about French colonial psychiatrists. The reasons given for this "absence" have been
divided into two groups: those reasons which the psychiatrists produced, and which
therefore reveal French colonial psychiatry's self-image; and those reasons of which
they were not aware, because of their particular views and preconceived ideas, and
which therefore reveal French colonial psychiatry's limitations.

Explanations Proposed by Colonial Psychiatrists

Colonial psychiatry's main explanation for the absence of female Muslim patients
was based on the assumption that female Muslim insanity existed but was beyond
the reach of the psychiatric institutions. It was proposed that female Muslim patients
were kept hidden from the colonial psychiatric gaze by a set of restrictions imposed
upon Maghrebi societies by Muslim gender segregation. This conviction, which has
been addressed in each of the preceding chapters, has two components: the first relies
on the assumption that Muslim women were so completely segregated that they
remained outside the field of vision of any Europeans living in the colonies, while the
second presents the issue of Muslim women failing to consult French experts about
their medical problems.

In the colonial imagination, only marginalised Muslim women were allowed to
be "seen", and therefore only their psychopathology could be perceived by the vigi-
lant gaze of colonial psychiatrists.[54] This idea that respectable Muslim women were

---

54 In 1913 the psychiatrists Solomon Lwoff and Paul Sérieux described Moroccan society as fol-
    lows: "Insanity is an often unrecognised disease, especially when it comes to a people like the
    Moroccans, whose intimate life is hidden from us." Lwoff/Sérieux, Note, 696.

deliberately kept away not only from colonial psychiatric institutions but also from all contact with Europeans corresponded with romanticised fantasies of the "caged" Muslim woman. In this explanation, the low numbers of female Muslim patients were due to them not being discoverable by colonial experts because of gender segregation. However, those psychiatrists living in North Africa – as opposed to those working in asylums in France – must have had some contact with Muslim women. Even disregarding social interactions, one imagines that women cleaned their houses and hospitals, and cooked their food, or at the very least would have been observed buying goods in the markets and working the fields,[55] yet many colonial psychiatrists emphasised the complete absence of Muslim women from everyday life. One wonders whether the veil rendered Muslim women "invisible" to colonial European observers, making their shape, as many authors invidiously claimed, almost unrecognisable as human.[56]

The other component of this explanation – Muslim families actively choosing not to consult French medical experts – is more intriguing. It was imagined that a "typically" Muslim prudery (as opposed to their equally "typical" overt sexuality) discouraged Muslim families from handing over potential patients to colonial care, especially during the period when patients were shipped to France, rarely to return. French colonial doctors emphasised the resistance they met in treating Muslim women, and the same problem was encountered by colonial psychiatry.[57] If the medical examination of a woman by a male doctor was difficult for the moral sensibilities of Muslims, how much worse was the institutionalisation of patients on the other side of the Mediterranean and without family supervision?[58] Colonial psychiatrists admitted

---

55 Contemporary travel literature on North Africa, on the other hand, usually stressed the visibility of at least a few – sometimes veiled, sometimes unveiled – Muslim women. See for example: D'Arlach, Le Maroc, 48 f.; Maurin, Saison d'hiver, 126; Celarié, Un mois au Maroc, 62; 100. The urban poor and rural North African families were never able to impose strict gender segregation, as their women had to work, both inside and outside the house. Gordon, Women of Algeria, 39 f.; Hatem, Politics, 255 f.; 264; Lazreg, Feminism and Difference, 90.

56 For example: Matignon, Art médical, 91; Brault, Pathologie et hygiène, 177; Lemanski, Mœurs arabes, 81 f. In 1913 Witold Lemanski also described the veil as follows: "In the modern life of the great cities of the Orient, the Arab woman necessarily comes into contact with modern civilization, but she does not easily let the barrier be crossed which defends her from indiscreet incursions into her intimate life." Ibid., 41 f. These descriptions, showing the disconnectedness many European observers felt when confronted with veiled Muslim women, are found in other genres: Abadie-Feyguine, Assistance médicale, 65; Bugéja, Sœurs musulmanes, 29 f.; 58.

57 Pierre Maréschal claimed in 1956 that such problems had been overcome. He described the earlier state as follows: "Muslims were reluctant to place their wives in the crowded Hospitals, where wearing the veil was impossible and where they [Muslim women] escaped from family supervision." Maréschal, Réflexions, 78. Capitalisation in the original.

58 This North African resistance towards letting women be treated by French colonial experts was described by many authors. Some colonial doctors and psychiatrists even claimed that

that this was an issue they struggled with, but they merely attributed the problem to backward Muslim society, a somewhat limp response when contrasted with the zeal with which they declared their desire for active humanitarianism.

Chapter 1 discusses the two most broadly defined explanations for the absence of female Muslim patients – protection through primitivity and indistinguishability between primitive normality and insanity. Both of these paternalistic explanations relied on the self-image of the French as highly civilised, with some parts of society even being "civilised to excess",[59] while Muslims were described as almost medievally barbaric and primitive. This simplistic, binary worldview was intrinsically linked to both settler notions and belief in the authority of expert knowledge, and it is unsurprising that the theory of the "primitive mentality" of Muslims – explaining what had made the detection of insanity difficult for earlier psychiatrists – was proposed by the first generation of psychiatrists teaching, working and living in North Africa. Their in-depth knowledge about the "mentality" of Muslims simply had to be more complete than that of general doctors pre-diagnosing patients to be shipped to France or psychiatric experts residing on the other side of the Mediterranean.

French colonial psychiatry saw itself, as discussed in Chapter 2, as part of the machinery protecting French societies in North Africa from all sorts of threats and dangers, a worldview, in which colonial psychiatrists were responsible for identifying and controlling the most dangerous – the criminally insane. Colonial psychiatrists set out rules for identifying the "mad" among the masses of the "seemingly mad" and were the only ones able to imprison, effectively, those presenting a danger before they committed a crime. This self-appointed role, catalysed by the increasing settler demands for security, imposed a novel function on colonial psychiatry: it had to neutralise these "threats", pre-emptively institutionalising and controlling those who were both "criminal" and "insane". Since the most visible threats were posed by Muslim men, paying attention to Muslim women – seemingly meek, docile and unable to commit crimes – was unnecessary. In this explanation, Muslim women were absent from psychiatric care, re-defined to suit the needs of the colonies because they were already controlled – indeed, over-controlled – by Muslim society.

---

husbands, faced with paying for their wives' medical treatments, had refused to do so, stating it was "cheaper" to get a new wife than fix the old one. It is difficult to judge how much of this was the colonial imagination and how much was actually "true". Jayle, Faculté de médecine, 101; Lataillade, Coutumes, 162.

59 As discussed in Chapter 1, Witold Lemanski used this expression repeatedly to describe European women in 1913. Lemanski, Mœurs arabes, 104; 109; 124. In the same year, Victor Trenga mirrored this notion, wanting to describe Algeria before "it becomes a myth, buried under the flood of modern banalities of Europeanisations to excess." Trenga, Âme arabo-berbère, 4.

Another explanation, never formulated in the psychiatric sources but still part of the colonial psychiatric worldview, was briefly mentioned in Chapter 3, in relation to the discussion of typically Muslim symptoms in psychiatric disorders.[60] A number of colonial psychiatrists claimed that many Muslims, perhaps the majority, somatised their mental troubles, and that they complained about general physical, but un-organic, pains, instead of expressing these problems through a psychiatrically definable diagnosis.[61] Though this is a coarse generalisation, it provided an additional explanation for the absence of potential patients: colonial psychiatrists were led to believe that a tradition of somatisation caused patients to visit a doctor to heal their physical symptoms instead of visiting a psychiatrist for mental problems which they did not perceive themselves to suffer from. The rivalry between medical doctors and psychiatrists over both potential patients and general authority caused psychiatrists to suspect that "their" patients were withheld from them not only by traditional Islamic healers, but also by French doctors whose lack of psychiatric understanding might prevent them from recognising the somatisation of psychological problems among their consultants.

Explanations "Unnoticed" by Colonial Psychiatrists

Some possible explanations for the absence of female Muslim patients remained outside the psychiatric conceptualisation of both gender relations and the colonial situation. As discussed in Chapter 2, the mechanisms of admission into colonial care, both during and after the period when patients were sent to France, limited the patient population mainly to those who had come into contact with the colonial administration through the police and court systems. While French colonial psychiatrists seemed oblivious to negative repercussions for the patients stemming from their association with psychiatric institutions, the criminalising processes of admission deterred genuine patients, especially Muslim women. While European families, more used to viewing mental disorders as a medical problem, might have contacted psychiatric experts out of concern for the health of potential patients, Muslim families only did so when

---

60 See p. 134, FN 182.

61 The somatisation of psychological problems was part of what Frantz Fanon described in 1952 as the reactions of immigrants to a hostile environment. French psychiatrists perceived somatisation to be part of the "North African syndrome", which Fanon defined as a diagnosis given to Muslims living in France, based on French racist prejudices rather than actual symptoms. Fanon, 'Syndrome nord africain', 14 ff. See also: Keller, Colonial Madness, 164. In the "Psychiatric Handbook for Maghrebi Practitioners", published in 1987, somatisation was still described as an important factor in the psychiatric tableau of disorders in the Maghreb. Bensmail, Généralités, 107.

caring for suffering family members became untenable.[62] With mental disorders interpreted as disturbances of the public order and patients as types of delinquents, both
the patients and their families opposed medical internment for as long as possible.[63]

Muslim women faced stigmatisation once institutionalised, not because they were
officially labelled "mad" – their behaviour was, within traditional interpretations,
socially acceptable as spirit possession – but because only dangerous and deviant
women were interned in colonial institutions: the ostracised antisocial and violent
elements, the drunks, vagrants and prostitutes. Muslim women interned for genuine
mental health issues faced discrimination by association, with tangible and serious
consequences. In the colonial sources, allusions can be found to husbands unilaterally
divorcing interned wives or, especially scandalous in the colonial worldview, taking a
second wife.[64] For these reasons, Muslim families refused to bring potential patients
within the purview of what they experienced as a deeply tainted and tainting system.
Colonial psychiatrists were unaware of this stigmatising impact and never consciously
commented on it. Instead, they interpreted the predominance of marginalised Muslim
women in colonial institutions as a consequence of strict gender segregation – the
prevalence of "criminal women" was the fault of Muslim traditions, which opposed
voluntary admission of the non-criminally insane, and was not attributable to the
French institutions.

A second possible explanation for the absence of female Muslim patients, which
again escaped colonial notice, was that Islamic treatments actually cured mental disorders, which were framed as "possessions". Caught in their dualistic worldview, in

---

62 Despite all protestations to the contrary, colonial psychiatry seemed to quietly acquiesce to
Muslim families looking after insane female family members, as this was financially beneficial
to the chronically strained budgets of the colonial institutions and posed little threat to society.

63 The anthropologist Emmanuelle Tall suggested in 1992 that "African" families only brought
their relations to psychiatrists as a last resort. She stated that "the group accepts its failure [in
healing the patient] and the social death of the hospitalised individual". Tall, Anthropologue,
72. See also: Al-Issa, Psychiatry in Algeria, 242.

64 Dequeker et al., Aspects actuels, 1112; Maréschal, Réflexions, 69. For other Arabic countries,
see for instance: Bazzoui/Al-Issa, Psychiatry in Iraq, 828. From the colonial perspective, this
repudiation was due to the stigma of mental illness, not of psychiatric institutions. For example in: Desruelles/Bersot, Assistance aux aliénés en Algérie, 593, FN 1; Chappert, Contribution, 19. The same has been upheld for the postcolonial situation, both in the Maghreb and
other Muslim states. See for example: Katchadourian, Survey, 24; Al-Issa/Al-Issa, Psychiatric
Problems, 17 f.; 21; Hughes, Psychiatry in Sudan, 46; Al-Krenawi/Graham, Gender and Bio-
medical/Traditional Mental Health Utilization, 226; Douki et al., Psychiatrie en Tunisie, 54;
Salem-Pickartz, Mental Health, 269 f.; Douki et al., Women's Mental Health, 187. Postcolonial
research also found that female relations of psychiatric patients sometimes had difficulties in
finding husbands. Chaleby, Women of Polygamous Marriages, 58; El-Islam, Mental Illness, 133.

which French rational therapies were directly opposed to North African superstitions, colonial psychiatrists did not understand how Islamic traditions could help in treating the insane.[65] For French psychiatrists, Muslim healing techniques only consisted of internment in the traditional *māristāns*, when in fact the North African conceptualisation of mental illness as spirit possession allowed for a range of behaviour that was not normal yet could still be deemed acceptable. Ideologically blinkered, colonial psychiatrists mostly missed the plurality of options open to North Africans suffering from mental problems, ranging from dramatic exorcisms, magic and religion to support and social acceptance of people behaving oddly.[66]

Finally, a third possible explanation missing from colonial interpretations regarding the absence of female Muslim patients involved psychiatrists misinterpreting forms of feminine protest as a peculiar form of "insanity".[67] One example of this can be found in an analysis of insanity caused – or, as the case may be, cured – by marriage. The "custom" of brides being removed from familiar circumstances to live away from family and friends could either have a negative impact on the lives of Muslim women, who developed mental problems because of conflicts with in-laws and particularly husbands,[68] or could, on the contrary, rescue them from repressive social surroundings, which were the origins of their mental malaise. In both cases,

---

65 In 1961, however, L. Couderc mentioned in passing that the healing methods of the *marabouts*, thought to be long discarded, were on the rise in Algeria. Couderc, Conséquences, 257. Postcolonial psychiatrists trained by the French, for example the Tunisian psychiatrist Sleïm Ammar, at first strongly opposed North African healing traditions, and only started to incorporate them into the psychiatric treatment of Muslim patients in the 1970s. In 1955, for example, he described the different practices of exorcism as "witchcraft and magic, and torture [...]." Ammar, Assistance aux aliénés, 24. See also: Boucebci, Psychiatre, 536; Okasha, Mental Health Services in the Arab World, 42. For a discussion of this change in Ammar, see: Keller, Colonial Madness, 203. For traditional healers in other African countries, see: Edgerton, Traditional Treatment, 168.

66 This social acceptance of mental illness is shown through the fact that the traditional healing mechanisms for mental illness usually involved an effort of the community, not just the individual concerned. For the postcolonial situation, see: Aouattah, Maladie mentale, 186; Al-Krenawi, Explanations of Mental Health Symptoms, 58; Al-Issa, Mental Illness, 56 f.

67 The Moroccan sociologist Fatima Mernissi described in 1977 Moroccan women visiting shrines to alleviate mental problems as a form of female empowerment, rejecting psychiatric hegemony over cures. Mernissi, Women, Saints, and Sanctuaries, 103 f.

68 In 1959, for instance, Sutter et al. wrote that marriages between couples who had never met before the wedding were problematic for the mental state of both partners. Sutter et al., Quelques observations, 907 f. This was taken up by postcolonial authors, who claimed that stressful wedding ceremonies and unhappy marriages were common causes of mental troubles among Muslims. See for example: Maupomé, Quelques aspects, 43 f.; Ammar, Aperçu, 687; Chaleby, Traditional Arabian Marriages and Mental Health, 139.

Muslim women might have chosen to protest against the way they were treated (by their own families before their wedding or by their new families afterwards) either through a vocabulary of possession or through somatised physical pains[69] – just as French women might have chosen a psychiatric or neurological vocabulary to express their unease at such a treatment, probably earning them a diagnosis of hysteria or neurosis. However, these manifestations of what psychiatrists would have described in European women as mental troubles meriting internment were socially accepted forms of female protest in North Africa. However, judging from their experiences with misunderstood French forms of female protest, French psychiatrists expected Muslim women to develop psychiatric problems after their marriages and were surprised that Muslim women only rarely developed mental issues based on their ill-treatment at the hands of their husbands or on their separation from their families. Since North African women claiming to be possessed or to feel vague physical pains – the Maghrebi vocabulary of female protest – were not understood as either suffering from a medically curable illness or as being a danger to society, nobody would have contacted the colonial authorities. The social acceptance in North Africa therefore hid these protesters from the French.

In conclusion, colonial psychiatrists explained the absence of female Muslim patients through two sets of theories – that psychiatric problems were rare in Muslims (general absence of insanity), or that those with mental disorders existed, but were hidden from colonial observers (relative absence of patients). The former proposed that Muslim women were too primitive to develop mental illnesses. The latter were represented through such theories as the visibility of only marginalised and non-segregated Muslim women, which claimed that potential female Muslim patients were physically hidden from colonial care or that specifically North African forms of mental problems (such as somatisation), and the "primitive mentality" of North Africans, hid symptoms from the colonial observers by making them in some way unrecognisable. In all of these explanations, colonial psychiatrists saw their own conduct as blameless – "racial" characteristics and Islamic regulations were culpable and responsible for the different forms of absence.

---

69 Möbius, Entwicklung der Psychiatrie, 51. Ethnopsychiatric interpretations of mental problems claim that illness presented an opportunity of empowerment for many women, a way of claiming attention, compassion and understanding from their peers. Maupomé, Quelques aspects, 43 ff.; Bullard, Truth in Madness, 127; 130. In other colonial contexts, hysteria, for example, has been described as an "outlet for gendered social conflicts [...]." This quotation by the historian Julie Parle applies to Zululand between 1894 and 1914. Parle, Witchcraft or Madness, 128. For the postcolonial situation see: El Saadawi, Women and Islam, 205; Constantinides, Women Heal Women, 688. For Europe see: Brown et al., Daughter, 135 f.; 139; Showalter, Female Malady, 14.

Because of the particular worldview of French colonial psychiatrists, some explanations remained unnoticed, thus demonstrating the limitations of the knowledge produced by French colonial psychiatry. They failed to perceive the stigmatising impact their institutions had on female Muslim patients; they were unaware both of the plurality of options open to North Africans suffering from mental illness and of the successes of the traditional therapies; and they interpreted female protest as mental illness in France, and, transplanting this misinterpretation into the colonial context, were amazed at the absence of these "universal" forms of insanity.

It is not unreasonable to suggest that the disparity between how colonial psychiatrists described their female Muslim patients and the reality of the situations throws their accuracy in other areas into doubt. If administrative concerns and, more particularly, pejorative settler "knowledge" had such an influence on something as important as the selection, treatment and depiction of female Muslim patients, it stretches credulity that other areas upon which colonial psychiatry impinged remained utterly free of similar bias. It is striking how few critics or historians of French colonial psychiatry have remarked on the absence of female North African patients from psychiatric sources, accepting, instead, the colonial claim that they were simply absent from psychiatric care. The result has been a lack of awareness about these significant gaps, which in itself then adds another layer of concealment over colonial female Muslim patients.

In 1907 the psychiatrist Camille-Charles Gervais expressed regret about the fate of a female Muslim patient who died in Aix-en-Provence from pulmonary tuberculosis without the hospital staff or the responsible psychiatrist even knowing her name: "She appeared on all the records under the name: 'X..., native Muslim woman'! That is all that is said of this poor creature!"[70] The shortcoming of colonial psychiatry was a failure to perceive the presence of Muslim women; the shortcoming of postcolonial writing is a failure to recognise the absence of Muslim women, for even the fact that this nameless patient was once ignored is ignored today.

---

70 Gervais, Contribution, 45.

Appendix A:
Mini-Biographies of Colonial Authors
on Insanity among North African Muslims[1]

Abadie-Feyguine, Hélène: 1881–?; Russian-born doctor who lived in Algeria. She focused on Algerian women; medical dissertation on the "Medical Assistance of Native Women in Algeria" at the University of Montpellier in 1905.

Aboab, Joseph: 1894–?; born in Oran. French neurologist; medical dissertation on "Neurosyphilis in Native Muslims of North Africa" at the University of Algiers in 1921.

Amat, Charles: Doctor in the French army. Wrote a book on the situation of the M'zab region in Algeria in 1888, where he established part of the medical service.

Ammar, Sleïm: 1927–1999; Tunisian psychiatrist. Assistant physician at the Manouba Psychiatric Hospital in Tunis under **Pierre Maréschal** and **Tahar Ben Soltane**; from 1960 to 1988 Chief Physician and director at the Razi Hospital (formerly Manouba Psychiatric Hospital); he was also professor of Psychiatry and Medical Psychology at the Medical Faculty of the University of Tunis. Richard Keller called him "Tunisia's most prominent psychiatrist in the postcolonial era".[2] He published articles on a variety of subjects, but in the context of this book, only those published before Tunisian independence or with a historical perspective are relevant. In 1955, for example, he wrote an article on the "Assistance of Lunatics in Tunisia" for the Journal *Information Psychiatrique*. He also wrote a series of articles on "Ethnopsychiatry and Transcultural Psychiatry" for the Journal *Tunisie Médicale* in the 1970s; and in 1987, he wrote a chapter on the "History of Maghrebi Psychiatry" for the "Psychiatric Handbook of the Maghrebi Practitioner", edited by the Tunisian psychiatrist Saïda Douki, the Moroccan psychiatrist Driss Moussaoui and the Algerian psychiatrist Farid Kacha.

Arène, Sextius-Pierre: 1888–1977; lived in Tunisia from an early age. French psychiatrist. He went to the Military School of Health in Lyon. Psychiatric dissertation on the "Criminality in Arabs from a Medico-Legal Point of View in Tunisia" at the University in Lyon in 1913. Was a major-general in World War II.

Armand, Adolphe: French military doctor; studied at the Faculty of Medicine at the University of Montpellier. Wrote a book on "Medical Algeria" in 1854.

Arrii, Don Côme: 1900–?; French psychiatrist. Psychiatric dissertation on "Criminal Impulsivity among Native Algerians" at the University of Algiers in 1926; student of **Antoine Porot**. His was one of the first psychiatric dissertations at the newly created institute of General and Medical

---

1 The data in the biographies was mainly taken from the information on authors provided on the title pages of dissertations and articles, from obituaries, and from Pierre Morel's "Biographical Dictionary of Psychiatry". Publication details can be found in the bibliography.

2 Keller, Colonial Madness, 171.

Pathology at the University of Algiers. In 1932 he collaborated with Antoine Porot on an article on the "Criminal Impulsivity in the Native Algerian". He was one of the early key members of the *École d'Alger*.

Assicot, Michel: French psychiatrist; worked at Blida Psychiatric Hospital; wrote a number of articles on his experiences with patients at Blida, for instance a 1959 article on the drug Nozinan in "Chronic Psychoses and Particularly in Schizophrenia" with his colleague **J. Henry**, and in 1961 he was one of nine authors of an article on the "Principal Causes of Psychiatric Morbidity among Algerian Muslims".

Aubin, Henri: French psychiatrist; student of **Emmanuel Régis**. Military doctor in the 'colonial troops'; led neuropsychiatric services in Oran (successor of **Louis Livet**) and Algiers; taught neuropsychiatry at the School of Colonial Health in Marseille. Aubin was a legate from the Ministry of Colonies at the Nancy Congress in 1937. His focus was on comparative psychiatry and he was one of the founders of what is commonly called ethnopsychiatry. His most important articles in the context of this book were on "Native Psychiatric Assistance in the Colonies" in 1938, an "Introduction to the Study of Psychiatry in Blacks" in 1939, "Outlines of an Ethno-Psychopathology" in 1945 and a description of the "Psychopathology of Native North Africans" in **Antoine Porot's** "Alphabetical Handbook of Clinical and Therapeutic Psychiatry" in 1954.

Bardenat, Charles: French psychiatrist; medical dissertation at the University of Algiers in 1934; student of **Antoine Porot**. He worked first as an intern, finally as Chief Physician in Blida Psychiatric Hospital, leading one of its four divisions (with **Jean Sutter**, **Maurice Porot** and **Jean Olry** leading the other three). One of the key members of the *École d'Alger*. In 1948, he wrote the influential article "Criminality and Delinquency in the Mental Alienation of Native Algerians". He remained interested in criminal psychopathology, as shown by his collaborations with Antoine Porot, with whom he published a book entitled "Medico-Legal Psychiatry" in 1959 and a second book on the "Abnormal and Mentally Ill in Criminal Justice" in 1960. He also wrote on other aspects of what he conceived of as a "typically Muslim" psychopathology – for example, in 1947, together with **G.-A. Manceaux** and **Robert Susini**, on "Hysteria in the Native Algerian", or, in 1955, as one of five authors, on "Heroin abuse in the Region of Algiers". He was also interested in new methods of treatment, as shown by his collaborations on an article concerning the effects of electroshock treatment in 1942 ("Reflections on 3,000 Electroshocks Practiced in the Psychiatric Services of Algeria") and on shock therapy in 1955 ("Two Years of Practice of Shock Methods with Premedication").

Barre, R.: French psychiatrist; worked at Blida Psychiatric Hospital. In 1962, he wrote an article with **J. Mares**, his colleague at Blida, on "Psychiatric Accidents of the Puerperium among Algerian Muslim Women".

Battarel, Pierre: French psychiatrist; born in Algiers, son of E. Battarel, who had been a doctor at the Civil Hospital of Mustapha. Psychiatric dissertation on "General Paralysis in Native Algerian Muslims" at the University of Montpellier in 1902.

Benkhelil, Abdesselam: 1899–1964; born in Constantine, Algeria. Algerian psychiatrist. He wrote a psychiatric dissertation on "Neuropsychiatric Afflictions and Neurosyphilis in the Native

Algerian Muslim" at the University of Algiers in 1927. He was a student of **Dumolard**. Politically active, he fought for Algerian independence, and went to prison for his convictions in 1945.

Ben Soltane, Tahar: Tunisian Chief Physician of one of the services at the Manouba Psychiatric Hospital in Tunis; director of the Manouba from 1956 to 1960 after the departure of **Pierre Maréschal**, who called Ben Soltane his friend and colleague in an article from 1956.[3] Interested in new treatments, demonstrated through his participation in a paper given at the Montpellier Congress in 1942 entitled "Results of Electroshock Treatments Applied to 340 Patients at the Psychiatric Hospital of La Manouba (Tunisia)".

Bersot, Henri: Psychiatrist in Le Landeron, Switzerland. He published widely on aspects of child and adolescent psychiatry and neuropsychiatry, both in French and German. He wrote, in collaboration with **Maurice Desruelles**, a number of articles and Congress papers on the history of psychiatry in North Africa in 1938 and 1939.

Bertherand, Émile-Louis: French doctor; opened the Muslim Hospice in Algiers in 1850 and worked for the *Bureaux des Affaires Arabes* in several Algerian cities from 1848–1855. President of the Society of Medicine in Algiers. In 1855 he published his important book on "Medicine and Hygiene among the Arabs", in which he wrote about his personal experiences with insanity among Muslim Algerians. In the secondary literature, he is often confused with his brother, Alphonse Bertherand, also a French doctor in colonial Algeria, who in 1842 also wrote a book on medicine in Algeria, especially in Blida, entitled "Memoires of Medicine and Medical Surgery".[4]

Bertholon, Lucien: 1854–1914; French doctor. He was a student of the eminent forensic psychiatrist Alexandre Lacassagne, based at the University of Lyon. He finished his medical studies in 1877 at the Val-de-Grâce Military Hospital in Paris and worked as a military doctor in Tunisia from 1881. He was also Chief Physician of the Tunisian prisons. Founded the Journal *Revue Tunisienne* in 1894 and wrote an "Outline of Criminal Anthropology of Tunisian Muslims" in 1889.

Boigey, Maurice Auguste Joseph: 1877–1952; French doctor. Medical dissertation at the University of Lyon in 1900. He worked as an intern at the hospitals in Lyon before becoming a military doctor in North Africa. His most important work in the context of this book is an article published in the *Annales Médico-Psychologiques* in 1908, a "Psychological Study of Islam". This article has been described as the most overtly racist and aggressive article of French colonial psychiatry,[5] a fact already acknowledged by some colonial psychiatrists, for instance **William Goëau-Brissonnière** in 1926.[6] Boigey's article prompted an outraged response by **Ahmad Chérif** the following year, also published in the *Annales Médico-Psychologiques*. Boigey also worked on

---

3   Maréschal, Réflexions, 74 f.
4   Compare, for instance, Léonard's and Lorcin's texts: Léonard, Médecine et colonisation, 490; Lorcin, Imperialism, 672.
5   Berthelier, À la recherche, 131; Bennani, Psychanalyse, 67; Gouriou, Psychopathologie et migration, 47.
6   Goëau-Brissonnière, Syphilis nerveuse, 67 f.

topics such as "Hospitals in a Muslim Country" and birthing rituals in the Sahara in 1907 as well as "Marriage among Muslim Tribes of Africa" in 1911.[7]

Bouquet, Henri: 1884–?; French psychiatrist. Worked as both extern and intern in hospitals in Lyon, and as intern at the French Civil Hospital in Tunis. Psychiatric dissertation on the "Alienated in Tunisia" at the University of Lyon in 1909; student of **Antoine Porot**, both in Lyon and in Tunis. Chief Surgeon at the French Civil Hospital in Tunis. He also wrote an article in 1931 on the relationship between "Medicine and Colonialism" for the *Exposition Coloniale Internationale* in Paris.

Brault, Jules-François-Marie-Joseph: 1862–1916; professor of Clinical Medicine of Hot Countries and of Syphilitic and Skin Diseases at the University of Algiers. He wrote extensively on the topic of tropical hygiene and venereal diseases among North Africans. In 1905, for example, he wrote a book, "Pathology and Hygiene of Native Muslims of Algeria", in which he presented his theory that nervous diseases were rare in Algerians in particular and in Muslims in general.

Brunswic-Le Bihan: Chief Surgeon, and from 1903 director, of Sadiki General Hospital in Tunis. Famously opened the doors of Sadiki in 1904 and set the lunatics free, in protest of the conditions they endured in his own hospital. He wrote two articles on these conditions – in 1904 he published "Medical Assistance of Natives in Tunisia and Medical Aids" and in 1905 "Sadiki Hospital and Native Medical Assistance in Tunisia".

Bugéja, Marie: Born in Algeria; French feminist journalist. She wrote a book on Muslim women in 1931 ("Our Muslim Sisters"), in which she attacked French writers for using and perpetuating stereotypes on Muslim women, claiming that they had, as men, no access to Muslim women.[8]

Chappert, Michèle: 1935–?; French psychiatrist. Psychiatric dissertation on "Puerperal Psychoses" at the University of Paris in 1962, based on her personal experiences at Blida Psychiatric Hospital. She and **Suzanne Taïeb** were the only female clinical psychiatrists who could be found working in colonial North Africa during the research for this book.

Chaurand: Worked at Manouba Psychiatric Hospital, Tunis. Wrote a series of articles together with **Pierre Maréschal**, director of the Manouba at that time, on general paralysis in North Africa (for example: "General Paralysis in Tunisia" in 1937).

Chérif, Ahmad: 1878–?; born in Moknine, Tunisia. Tunisian doctor; medical dissertation on the "History of Arab Medicine in Tunisia" at the University of Bordeaux in 1908. Chief Physician of the Quarantine Lazaretto in Beirut. Wrote an answer to, and refutation of, **Maurice Boigey**'s "Psychological Study on Islam" under the same title in the *Annales Médico-Psychologiques* in 1909.

Constans, Augustin: French psychiatrist; Chief Physician of the Montperrin asylum in Aix-en-Provence. Brother-in-law of the one-time Governor-General of Algeria, Aimable Jean-Jacques Pélissier. In 1874, he was one of a committee of three inspectors general of the French national asylum system, together with **Lunier Ludger** and **Dumesnil**.

---

7 Information has been taken from H. L. Rocher's obituary of Boigey. Rocher, Maurice Boigey, 558.

8 Bugéja, Sœurs musulmanes, 81.

Couderc, L.: French psychiatrist; Chief Physician of the Neuropsychiatric Service in Oran. Wrote an article in 1955 on "Psychiatric Assistance in the Department of Oran" and one in 1961 on the "Consequences of the Current Conditions of Psychiatric Assistance in Algeria".

Coudray, Jean: 1886–?; French doctor. Medical dissertation on the "Sadiki Hospital and the Native Surgical Pathology in Tunisia" at the University of Montpellier in 1914. Worked as an extern in Tunis and later as assistant surgeon at Sadiki General Hospital.

Delasiauve, Louis Jean François: 1804–1893; French psychiatrist at Bicêtre and, from 1865, director of the Salpêtrière, where he focused on the treatment of epileptics and mentally retarded children.[9] Wrote a review in 1865 of a report by Collardot (who was, at that time, assistant physician at the Civil Hospital of Mustapha in Algiers) on the psychiatric situation in Algeria.

Demassieux, Eliane, born Paulian: French psychiatrist; psychiatric dissertation on "Social Service in Psychiatry" at the University of Algiers in 1941; student of **Antoine Porot**. Worked as a social worker in the Psychiatric Out-Service of the Civil Hospital of Mustapha but not as a clinical psychiatrist like **Michèle Chappert** and **Suzanne Taïeb**.

Desruelles, Maurice: French psychiatrist at the asylum of Sainte-Ylie (Jura). Together with **Henri Bersot**, he wrote a series of articles on the history of psychiatry in North Africa in 1938 and 1939.

Dilhan, Aug.: French ethnologist. Wrote an anthropological account of Tunisia ("Ethnology of Tunisia") in 1866, which he revised in 1872 and published in 1873 in the *Mémoires de la Société d'Ethnographie*.

Donnadieu, André: French psychiatrist; psychiatric dissertation at the University of Bordeaux in 1932. He was, together with **C. A. Pierson**, head of Berrechid Neuropsychiatric Hospital. He mainly worked on the question of the influence of civilisation and civilisational disorders on the psychopathology of Moroccans, as shown by articles on such topics as alcoholism, neurosyphilis and "Psychosis of Civilisation", published in 1939 and 1940.

Duchêne-Marullaz, Henri: 1882–?; born in Blida, Algeria. French doctor; medical dissertation on the "Hygiene of Algerian Muslims" at the University of Lyon in 1905.

Dumesnil: French psychiatrist; in 1874, he was one of a committee of three inspectors general of the French national asylum system, together with **Augustin Constans** and **Lunier Ludger**. He also wrote for the *Annales Médico-Psychologiques* regularly – for example, in 1882 a review of an article, written by the eminent British psychiatrists A. R. Urquhart and William Samuel Tuke, entitled "Two Visits to the Asylums in Cairo".

Dumolard: French neurologist; Chief Physician at the Neurological Service of the Civil Hospital of Mustapha. Wrote articles on psychiatric issues, such as the "Subject of Psychiatric Assistance in Algeria" in 1926. He was one of those opposing the theories of **Antoine Porot**'s *École d'Alger*, by claiming that the psychopathology of North Africans was similar to that of Europeans. The personal attacks between him and Porot found their way into a series of articles in the journal *L'Hygiène Mentale* between 1925 and 1926.

---

9   Morel, Dictionnaire, 76.

Fanon, Frantz: 1925–1961; born in Martinique. French psychiatrist. Studied medicine and psychiatry at the Medical Faculty of the University of Lyon and worked as one of four chief physicians at the Blida Psychiatric Hospital in Algeria from 1953 to 1956. He had to leave Algeria in 1956 and worked at the Manouba Psychiatric Hospital and at the Charles Nicolle Hospital (before 1946, it had been the French Civil Hospital) in Tunis from 1957 to 1959. Although best known for his political texts, he also wrote profusely on psychiatric topics. In the context of this book, it is important to note that even before moving to North Africa, he had come into contact with North African psychiatric patients in Lyon, which motivated him to write an article on what he called "The 'North African Syndrome'" in 1952. Between 1954 and 1959, he wrote, in collaboration with interns and colleagues from both Blida and the Manouba, a series of articles on the treatment of North African patients in French colonial psychiatric institutions. In 1961 his book "The Wretched of the Earth" drew on his professional psychiatric experiences in North Africa, and he published a collection of case studies in its appendices.

Fribourg-Blanc, André: 1888–1963; French psychiatrist. Psychiatric dissertation at the University of Lyon in 1912; student of the eminent forensic psychiatrist Alexandre Lacassagne. Moved to Morocco as a military doctor in 1914 and worked for the Ministry of Colonies from 1925 onwards. He was a professor at the Military Hospital in Val-de-Grâce, Paris, and was, in this capacity, president of the Marseille Congress in 1948. In 1927 he wrote an article on the "Mental State of Natives in North Africa and their Psychopathic Reactions".

Gentile, J.: French psychiatrist; worked at Blida Psychiatric Hospital. Wrote an article on "Alcoholism and Mental Troubles in the Native Muslim Algerian" in collaboration with **Maurice Porot** in 1941.

Gervais, Camille-Charles: Born in Guadeloupe; French psychiatrist. Psychiatric dissertation on the "Diet and Treatment of the Indigenous Insane in Algeria" at the University of Lyon in 1907. He worked as an extern in hospitals in Marseille and as an intern in Aix-en-Provence. Later he became Director of Public Health in Algeria.

Gillot, Victor: 1872–1952; French doctor. Professor of Infantile Clinical Medicine and Hygiene at the University of Algiers. He also worked on questions of neurosyphilis and general paralysis and supported the theory that insanity, and all nervous disorders, were rare among North Africans.

Goëau-Brissonniere, William: 1900–?; French psychiatrist. Psychiatric dissertation on "Nervous Syphilis in the Native Algerian Muslim" at the University of Algiers in 1926. Student of **Dumolard**.

Gomma, François: French doctor; medical dissertation on the "Medical Assistance in Tunisia" at the University of Bordeaux in 1904. He worked as an extern at hospitals in Toulouse and as an intern at the French Civil Hospital in Tunis.

Gros, Henri-Réné-Louis-Augustin-Eugène: French doctor; medical dissertation at the University of Lille in 1883. He was physician at the Native Infirmary at Rébeval, Algeria. He worked on questions concerning the Muslim medical assistance and frequency of certain diseases, for example neuroses or general paralysis in North Africans.

Hadida, Élie: Worked as a doctor in Algiers; focused on questions of venereal diseases. Became professor of Clinical Medicine of Hot Countries and of Syphilitic and Skin Diseases at the University of Algiers after **Maurice Raynaud**. Presented a paper with **François-Georges Marill**

and **Maurice Porot** on the "Apparent Increase in the Frequency of Parenchymal Neurosyphilis among the Native North Africans" at the 1955 Congress in Nice.

Henry, J.: French psychiatrist; worked at Blida Psychiatric Hospital. Wrote an article on the effects of the drug Nozinan in "Chronic Psychoses and Particularly in Schizophrenia" with his colleague **Michel Assicot** in 1959.

Humann: Chief Physician of Native Assistance in Ain Salah and in Tamanrasset, Algeria. He published an article on "Mental Troubles of Natives in the Algerian Sahara" in 1934.

Igert, Maurice: Military doctor; moved to Morocco in 1924. Chief Physician at both the Military Hospital and the Pavilion of Neuropsychiatry at the Civil Hospital of Casablanca, where he focused on new treatments. He was also a student of **René Laforgue** and became a psychiatrist-psychoanalyst. He proposed notions of a typically Moroccan psychopathology ("Introduction to the Moroccan Psychopathology" or "Moroccan Cultural Milieu and Neuroses", both in 1955).

Jeanselme, Édouard: Doctor and professor in Paris, with interests in colonial (psychiatric) questions. His focus was on the Far East; he worked, among other things, on the rarity of certain diseases (like neurosyphilis) among the colonial populations. He wrote an article on the "Condition of Lunatics in French, English and Dutch Colonies of the Extreme Orient" in 1905.

Jobert, A.: Medical officer in the French navy; doctor of colonisation in Guelma, Algeria. In 1868 he wrote an article on "Creating a Special Establishment for Lunatics in Algeria", calling for an end to the transfers of patients to France.

Kocher, Adolphe: French psychiatrist. Psychiatric dissertation on the "Criminality among Arabs from the Point of View of the Medico-Judicial Practice in Algeria" at the University of Lyon in 1883; student of the eminent forensic psychiatrist Alexandre Lacassagne. Worked in the Civil Hospital of Mustapha in Algiers.

Lacapère, Georges: French doctor; expert on questions of syphilis in North Africa. He published, for example, a series of articles on different aspects of syphilis in the journal *Annales des Maladies Vénériennes* between 1919 and 1922 and wrote a book on "Arab Syphilis (Morocco-Algeria-Tunisia)" in 1923.

Lafitte, Joseph-Marie-Fernand: French doctor. Law degree; medical dissertation, entitled "Contribution to the Medical Study of Tunisia", at the University of Bordeaux in 1892. Worked as an intern at hospitals in Bordeaux; worked as doctor to Crown Prince Taïeb-Bey and at the Saint-Louis Hospital in Tunis.

Laforgue, René: 1894–1962; French psychiatrist-psychoanalyst. Student of Sigmund Freud; assistant of Clinical Psychiatry at the Faculty of Medicine in Paris. First president of the *Psychoanalytical Society of Paris*. Moved to Morocco in 1947 or 1948, where he stayed until 1956. Published a series of articles in the journal *Maroc Médical* (for example on the "Psychosomatic Aspect of Neuroses" in 1953 and on "Psychosomatic Medicine" in 1955). Laforgue established the only psychoanalytic school in the colonial Maghreb.

Lamarche: French psychiatrist; Chief Physician of the Pavilion of Nervous Diseases at the French Civil Hospital in Tunis. Wrote a paper on the "Medical Assistance of Lunatics in Tunisia" with **Pierre Maréschal**, director of the Manouba Psychiatric Hospital, for the Nancy Congress in 1937.

Lasnet, Alexandre: French doctor, who had been stationed in Madagascar, Indo-China, the Antilles, Congo, and Equatorial and West Africa, fighting epidemics. Chief Medical Officer in Algeria; founder and director of the Public Health Office of Algeria in 1932. In this capacity, he was credited, together with **Antoine Porot**, with founding psychiatric assistance in Algeria.[10] Together with Antoine Porot, he gave a paper on the "Organisation of Psychiatric Assistance in Algeria" at the Limoges Congress in 1932.

Laurens, Étienne-Paul: 1893–?; born in Zemmora, Algeria. French psychiatrist. Psychiatric dissertation on "Nervous Syphilis in the Native Mohammedans of Algeria" at the University of Algiers in 1919.

Lemanski, Witold: French doctor; Chief Physician at the French Civil Hospital in Tunis. He worked extensively on questions of hygiene and insanity in Tunisia (he wrote, for example, a book on "Settler Hygiene, or Handbook of Europeans in the Colonies" in 1902) and was later seen to be one of the pioneers of psychiatric interest in North Africans.[11] He was one of the few experts interested in the psychopathology of Muslim women, as shown by an article on the "Psychology of the Arab Woman" published in the *Revue Tunisienne* in 1900 and by a chapter dedicated to the same topic in his 1913 memoir "Arab Mores".

Levet: French psychiatrist; worked at the asylum in Aix-en-Provence; Chief Physician of the asylum of Charenton. Wrote an article for the *Annales Médico-Psychologiques* on the "Assistance of the Algerian Mad in a Metropolitan Asylum" in 1909.

Lévy-Bram, Abel: Algerian doctor; medical dissertation on the "Medical Assistance for Natives of Algeria, particularly the Medical Assistance of Women and Children" at the University of Paris in 1907.

Livet, Louis: French psychiatrist; worked as an extern at the hospitals of Lyon and as an intern in Algiers. Medical dissertation on the "Algerian Mad and their Hospitalisation" at the University of Algiers in 1911. In his dissertation, he attacked the system of transporting patients from Algeria to France. Director of the psychiatric service in Oran from 1933 onward.

Luccioni, Joseph: French jurist; legal dissertation at the University of Algiers in 1942. Chief of the Administration of Habous [religious endowments] in Morocco. In 1953 he wrote an article on the "Maristans of Morocco", published in the *Bulletin Économique et Social du Maroc*.

Lunier, Ludger-Jules-Joseph: 1822–1885; French psychiatrist. Nephew of the prominent French psychiatrist Jules-Gabriel-François Baillarger, who had been one of the founders and directors of the *Annales Médico-Psychologiques*. Worked with **Jacques-Joseph Moreau de Tours** in the French asylum of Ivry.[12] He wrote a number of reviews and reports in the *Annales Médico-Psychologiques* on a variety of subjects which are relevant in the context of this book, for example on the "Gradual Increase in the Numbers of Lunatics and its Causes" in 1870. In 1874 he was one

---

10 Dequeker et al., Aspects actuels, 1107; Aubin, Assistance, 153; Desruelles/Bersot, Assistance aux aliénés en Algérie, 588.

11 Vadon, Assistance, 13.

12 Morel, Dictionnaire, 162.

of a committee of three inspectors general of the French national asylum system, together with **Augustin Constans** and **Dumesnil**.

Lwoff, Solomon: French psychiatrist; he was, together with **Paul Sérieux**, Chief Physician of the asylums of the department of the Seine. Both were sent on a "mission" to Morocco by the Ministry of the Interior and the Ministry of Public Education in 1910. They then published a series of articles on their experiences, for example on "Lunatics in Morocco. Moristans and Prisons" in 1911, and, in 1913, a "Note on the Organisation of the Assistance of Lunatics in Morocco".

Manceaux, G.-A.: French doctor and psychiatrist; early focus on pathological anatomy. Succeeded **Antoine Porot** as Professor for Clinical Neurology and Psychiatry at the University of Algiers in 1946. He was in turn succeeded by **Jean Sutter** in 1959. Published widely on the psychopathology of North Africans. He wrote, for example, articles with **Charles Bardenat** and **Robert Susini** on "Hysteria in the Native Algerian" in 1947, and with Jean Sutter and **Yves Pélicier** on "Melancholic States in the North African Native" in 1954. He was also interested in the development of new treatments, as shown by his publication of articles on shock therapies.

Maréschal, Pierre: French psychiatrist; second director of the Manouba Psychiatric Hospital in Tunis from 1935 to 1956 after **Georges Perrussel**. He wrote profusely on a variety of psychiatric topics related to a specifically North African psychopathology – in 1937 alone, he published articles on "Heroin Abuse in Tunisia", on "General Paralysis in Tunisia" with **Chaurand**, and on the "Medical Assistance for Lunatics in Tunisia" with **Lamarche**. In 1956 he published an article on his professional experiences in Tunisia in the journal *La Raison*, entitled "Reflections on Twenty Years of Psychiatry in Tunisia". He had to resign from his job as head physician of the Manouba because of what René Collignon vaguely described as "several scandals".[13]

Mares, J.: French psychiatrist; worked at Blida Psychiatric Hospital. Wrote an article on "Accidents of the Puerperium in Algerian Muslim Women" together with one of his colleagues at Blida, **R. Barre,** in 1962.

Margain, Louis: French psychiatrist; published an article on "Mental Alienation in the Colonies and Protectorates" in the journal *Revue Indigène* in 1908; specialised on the situation in the Dutch Colonies.

Marie, Auguste: 1865–1934; French psychiatrist; student of **Auguste-Félix Voisin**. Chief Physician at the asylum of Villejuif in 1900;[14] travelled to Algeria in 1893 and to Egypt in 1904 and visited the psychiatric institutions there (the Civil Hospital of Mustapha in Algiers and the ʿAbbāsiyya Hospital in Cairo). Most famous for his three-volume edited collection of articles, "International Treatise on Pathological Psychology", published between 1910 and 1912. He wrote profusely on the psychopathology of the colonised, especially concerning their adequate institutionalisation. This interest finally shifted to include questions of immigration, as shown by his last publications in 1934, with one article focusing on the questions of "Immigration and Mental Hygiene" and one, together with Pierre Godin, on "Muslim Patients in Paris".

---

13   Collignon, Psychiatrie coloniale, 538, FN 37.
14   Morel, Dictionnaire, 168.

Marill, François-Georges: French psychiatrist; worked at Blida Psychiatric Hospital. Wrote an article on "Progressive General Paralysis in the Native Muslims of North Africa" with **Abdennour Si Hassen** in 1951 and one with **Elie Hadida** and **Maurice Porot** on the "Apparent Increase in the Frequency of Parenchymal Neurosyphilis in Native North Africans" in 1955.

Matignon, Raymond-Joseph: 1871–?; French doctor. Medical dissertation on "Medical Art in Tunis" at the University of Bordeaux in 1901. Worked as an intern in Bordeaux and at the French Civil Hospital in Tunis.

Mazel, Jean de Labretoigne du: French doctor and psychiatrist. In 1921, he visited the *māristān* of Sidi Fredj in Fes for the Service of Health and Public Hygiene in Morocco and wrote a report on his experiences, published in 1922. Together with Jules Colombani (first Director of Public Health in Morocco from 1926 to 1934), he was credited with establishing psychiatric assistance in Morocco. First director of the first psychiatric hospital in Morocco, Berrechid. Also creator and first director of the Pavilion of Neuropsychiatry at the Civil Hospital of Casablanca.

Meilhon, Abel-Joseph: French psychiatrist. Psychiatric dissertation at the University of Bordeaux in 1886; student of **Emmanuel Régis**. Assistant physician and later director at the asylum of Montperrin in Aix-en-Provence and finally at the asylum of Montauban in 1896. Charged with the care of Algerian patients transferred to France and institutionalised in the asylum of Aix-en-Provence. Meilhon published two important articles on his experiences with these Muslim North African patients in the *Annales Médico-Psychologiques*: on the "Study of General Paralysis Considered in Arabs" in 1891 and his nosological study entitled "Mental Alienation in Arabs" in 1896.

Monnery, Maurice: 1893–?; French doctor. Intern at the French Civil Hospital in Tunis. Medical dissertation on the "Practice of Social Hygiene and Medical Action in Tunisia" at the University of Lyon in 1924.

Montaldo, Pierre: 1905–?; born in Bône, Algeria. French doctor; medical dissertation on "Infant Mortality in Algeria" at the University of Algiers in 1933.

Moreau de Tours, Jacques-Joseph: 1804–1884; student of the famous French psychiatrist Jean-Étienne Dominique Esquirol. Doctor at the Bicêtre Hospital in Paris; together with Bénédict Augustin Morel, one of the founders of the theory of degeneration in the 1850s. Accompanied one of Esquirol's wealthy patients on a three-year journey through the "Orient" (Egypt, the Levant, Asia Minor and Malta) and published an article in the *Annales Médico-Psychologiques* entitled "Research on the Alienated in the Orient" in 1843, one of the founding texts of French psychiatric interest in Muslims. He also studied hashish addiction in these countries, tried hashish himself and compared its impact with insanity. Consequently, he wrote a book on "Hashish and Mental Alienation" in 1845. In 1887, his son, Paul Moreau de Tours, published an article on "Lunatic Asylums in the Orient" in the *Annales Médico-Psychologiques*, heavily relying on his father's testimony.

Naudin, Lucien-Joseph-Victor: 1890–?; French psychiatrist. Psychiatric dissertation on "Colonial Psychiatry" at the University of Bordeaux in 1913, focusing mainly on the French colonial army.

Olry, Jean: French psychiatrist; psychiatric dissertation on "General Paralysis in Muslim Natives of Tunisia" at the University of Marseille in 1910. Worked at the Manouba Psychiatric Hospital;

Chief Physician of one of the four medical divisions at Blida Psychiatric Hospital alongside **Jean Sutter, Charles Bardenat** and **Maurice Porot.**

Pascalis, Élie: French psychiatrist. Psychiatric dissertation on "General Paralysis in Arabs" at the University of Montpellier in 1893. Worked at hospitals in Marseille and at the asylum in Aix-en-Provence, where he was a colleague of **Abel-Joseph Meilhon**, on whose 1891 research on general paralysis in Arabs Pascalis heavily relied.

Pascalis, Gérard: French psychiatrist; worked at Blida Psychiatric Hospital; named by **Jean Sutter** as one of the promising psychiatrists of the modern generation in 1959.[15] Later became professor of psychiatry in Kabul, then in Reims. He worked on a number of articles together with Jean Sutter: in 1956 they wrote about the effects of an anti-psychotic drug ("Psychological Effects of Chlorpromazine") and in 1959, they wrote, together with **Robert Susini** and **Yves Pélicier**, on "Nuptial Psychoses in Algerian Muslims".

Pélicier, Yves: 1925–1966; French doctor and psychiatrist, focusing first on bacteriology at the Faculty of Medicine at the University of Algiers, then on psychiatry. Worked at the Faculty of Medicine at the University of Algiers under **G.-A. Manceaux.** Later became professor of psychiatry at the University of Rouen, then Paris. Key member of the second generation of the *École d'Alger*. In 1959, for example, he wrote a paper with **Jean Sutter** and **Maurice Porot** on "Algerian Aspects of Mental Pathology". He was also interested in new treatments, like shock therapy, as shown in his collaborations with G.-A. Manceaux.

Périale, Marise: French travel writer and journalist who wrote several general travel accounts on Morocco. In 1934 she described her visit to one of the traditional asylums in Salé, Morocco, in an article entitled "Maristane of Sidi Benachir, Commonly Called 'the Madhouse'" in the *Bulletin de l'Enseignement Public au Maroc.*

Perrin, Gabriel: French doctor; intern at the Civil Hospital of Mustapha. Medical dissertation on the "Medicine of Arabs and the Medical Assistance of the Algerian Natives" at the University of Toulouse in 1895.

Perrussel, Georges: French psychiatrist; from 1914 onward, Chief Physician of the French Civil Hospital in Tunis after **Antoine Porot**; Chief Physician at the Tékia in Tunis from 1924 until 1931. Played an important role in the construction of the Manouba Psychiatric Hospital, whose first Chief Physician he was once it opened in 1932. He was the official delegate of the Tunisian Government at the 1933 Congress in Rabat. Wrote an article on the "Assistance of Psychopaths in Tunisia" in 1931.

Pierson, C. A.: French psychiatrist; lived in Morocco for 25 years. Together with **André Donnadieu,** Chief Physician of the Neuropsychiatric Hospital of Berrechid until 1946; Chief Physician of the Pavilion of Neuropsychiatry at the Civil Hospital of Casablanca. The Moroccan Ministry of Health encouraged him to obtain a second degree in law. He wrote general articles on psychiatry in Morocco, for example on "Psychiatric Assistance in Morocco" in 1955, together with **R. P. Poitrot** and **Rolland,** who both succeeded him as directors of Berrechid.

---

15   Sutter, Leçon inaugurale, 443.

Poitrot, R. P.: French psychiatrist; physician at the Neuropsychiatric Hospital of Berrechid from 1938 onward and Chief Physician after **C. A. Pierson** left in 1946. Worked on a variety of psychiatric subjects, for example on "Nervous Syphilis in Morocco" in 1950 and "Climatological Influences at the Neuropsychiatric Hospital of Berrechid" in 1953. Wrote an article with C. A. Pierson and his successor at Berrechid, **Rolland**, on the "Psychiatric Assistance in Morocco" in 1955.

Porot, Antoine: 1876–1965; French psychiatrist; psychiatric dissertation at the University of Lyon in 1904. Moved to Tunisia in 1907 and worked there until 1914; founded the first psychiatric service in North Africa in 1910 (Pavilion of Observation and Treatment of Nervous and Mental Diseases of the French Civil Hospital in Tunis), which was inaugurated at the 1912 Tunis Congress. He also founded the Journal *Tunisie Médicale* in 1911. In 1916 he was appointed as Chief Physician of the Neurological Centre of the 19th military region in Algiers. He then became professor of General and Medical Pathology (renamed as General Pathology and Clinical Psychiatry in 1934) at the University of Algiers from 1925 to 1946. He was also the technical health advisor for psychiatry for the Algerian government. He wrote extensively on aspects of the primitive psychopathology of North Africans but also on more general psychiatric questions such as the organisation of a psychiatric service in North Africa. His article "Notes on Muslim Psychiatry", published in the *Annales Médico-Psychologiques* in 1918, was the founding text of the *École d'Alger*, and Porot's person and personal interests dominated the *École d'Alger*. Today, he is most famous because of **Frantz Fanon**'s direct criticism of him and of his school of thought. Antoine Porot was, for example, fascinated by questions of North African delinquency and published, together with his student **Don Côme Arrii**, an article on "Criminal Impulsivity among Native Algerians" in 1932, the article being a summary of Arrii's 1927 dissertation. He developed the idea of a special North African "primitivism" further, and published, with his student **Jean Sutter**, an article on the "'Primitivism' of North African Natives" in 1939. But he was also interested in addictions among North Africans and in new methods of psychiatric treatment, as shown by his articles on electroshock therapy (for example "Reflexions on 3,000 Electroshocks Performed in the Psychiatric Services of Algeria", published with a group of students in 1942, among them his son **Maurice Porot**). He stayed active even after he left Algeria in 1946 – he edited, for example, the various editions of the "Alphabetical Handbook of Clinical and Therapeutic Psychiatry", first published in 1952.[16]

Porot, Maurice: 1912–?; son of **Antoine Porot**, close friend of **Jean Sutter**. French psychiatrist; medical dissertation at the University of Algiers in 1938, where he was first a student of Aubry (Professor of Clinical Medicine). Worked as an intern at the hospitals of Algiers and at the Psychiatric Hospital of Blida before he became director of one of its four divisions, with Jean Sutter, **Charles Bardenat** and **Jean Olry** leading the other services. He later became Professor of Neuropsychiatry at the Faculty of Clermont-Ferrand. His personal interest seems to have encompassed new treatments – he published on lobotomies ("Prefrontal Leucotomy in Psychiatry" in 1947);

---

16 Information was taken from the obituary for Antoine Porot, written by Michaux. Michaux, Professeur Antoine Porot (1876–1965), 71 f.

on drug treatments (for example, with G. Duboucher on the "Cure of Alcoholics through Antabus" in 1952); and on electroshock therapies (for example, the article "Reflexions on 3,000 Electroshocks Performed in the Psychiatric Services of Algeria", which he published in 1955 together with his father and four of his father's students). After the War of Independence started in Algeria, he researched the psychological reactions to the war in articles published in 1956 and 1958. Like many of Antoine Porot's other students, he never fully distanced himself from the theories of a typical Muslim psychopathology, as shown, for example, in his 1959 article, written with Jean Sutter and **Yves Pélicier**, on "Algerian Aspects of Mental Pathology".[17]

Reboul, Henry: French psychiatrist and military doctor in the 'colonial troops'; director of Public Health in Indo-China. Edited the report "Assistance of Lunatics in the Colonies" for the 1912 Congress in Tunis, together with **Emmanuel Régis**, where **Antoine Porot** was the general secretary.

Régis, Jean-Baptiste-Joseph-Emmanuel: 1855–1918; French psychiatrist. From 1884 Clinical Professor of Mental Diseases at the Medical Faculty of the University of Bordeaux, where he taught mainly naval and colonial doctors. He composed the immensely influential "Practical Manual of Mental Health" in 1885. Under his overview, hundreds of students worked on questions of mental health.[18] He also worked on general paralysis in the colonies and formed the theory that the nervous systems of Muslims were resistant to syphilis. He edited, with **Henry Reboul**, the report on the "Assistance of Lunatics in the Colonies" for the 1912 Tunis Congress, with **Antoine Porot** working as general secretary of the Congress.

Richardot, Armand: French doctor; worked as an intern at the Civil Hospital of Mustapha in Algiers. Medical dissertation on "Medical Practices of Native Algerians" at the University of Toulouse in 1896.

Rolland, J. L.: French psychiatrist and psychoanalyst, who lived in Morocco from 1953 to 1967. Built a psychiatric service in Salé. In 1955 he became Chief Physician of the Neuropsychiatric Hospital of Berrechid after **R. P. Poitrot**. In 1955 he wrote, together with Poitrot and Poitrot's predecessor **C. A. Pierson**, an article on "Psychiatric Assistance in Morocco".

Sauzay, Paul: Born in Algiers; French psychiatrist. Psychiatric dissertation on the "Assistance of Psychopaths (Alienated or Non-Alienated) in Algeria" at the University of Algiers in 1925; student of **Antoine Porot**. In his dissertation, he described the inadequacy of colonial mental patients being shipped to France.

Sérieux, Paul: 1864–1947; French psychiatrist. Psychiatric dissertation on "Anomalies of the Sexual Instinct" at the University of Paris in 1888. Worked as an intern at the asylums of the Department of the Seine; Chief Physician of the Saint-Anne Asylum in Paris. He was, together with **Solomon Lwoff**, Chief Physician of the asylums of the department of the Seine. Both were sent on a "mission" to Morocco by the Ministry of the Interior and the Ministry of Public Education in 1910. They then published a series of articles on their experiences: for example on "Lunatics in

---

17 Information was taken from the obituary for Maurice Porot's father, Antoine Porot, written by Michaux. Michaux, Professeur Antoine Porot (1876–1965), 71 f.

18 Discussion du rapport d'assistance psychiatrique, 183 f.

Morocco. Moristans and Prisons" in 1911 and a "Note on the Organisation of the Assistance of Lunatics in Morocco" in 1913. In 1922, Sérieux was commissioned by the Tunisian government to build an asylum in Tunis, which opened in 1931/1932 as the Manouba Psychiatric Hospital.

Sicard, Georges: Born in Tizi-Ouzou, Algeria; French psychiatrist. Psychiatric dissertation on the "Frequency of Nervous Disorders among Native Algerian Muslims" at the University of Lyon in 1907; student of Paul Moreau de Tours (**Jacques-Joseph Moreau de Tours**' son). Worked as an intern in the hospitals of Algiers.

Si Hassen, Abdennour: Algerian psychiatrist; worked at Blida Psychiatric Hospital. Wrote an article with **François-Georges Marill** on "Progressive General Paralysis in Native Muslims of North Africa" in 1951.

Soumeire, Henri: French psychiatrist; worked as an extern at the hospitals of Marseille. Medical dissertation on "Murder among the Indigenous Mad in Algeria" at the University of Marseille in 1932. Plagiarised in his dissertation large parts from **Henri Bouquet**'s 1909 dissertation.[19]

Susini, Paul: French doctor; worked in the hospitals in Paris; studied at the Institute of Colonial Medicine in Paris. Medical dissertation on "Syphilis in the Natives of Algeria" at the University of Paris in 1920, under the supervision of **Édouard Jeanselme**.

Susini, Robert: Born in Algiers; French psychiatrist; worked as an intern in the hospitals of Algiers. Medical dissertation on the "Clinical Aspects of Hysteria in the North African Native (in the Military Milieu)" at the University of Algiers in 1947; student of **G.-A. Manceaux**. He wrote a number of articles in collaboration with other members of the *École d'Alger*: in 1947, for example, he wrote an article on "Hysteria in the Native Algerian" together with G.-A. Manceaux and **Charles Bardenat**, and one in 1959 on "Nuptial Psychoses in Algerian Muslims" together with Jean Sutter, **Yves Pélicier** and **Gérard Pascalis**.

Sutter, Jean: 1911–1998; born in Algiers; French psychiatrist. Psychiatric dissertation on "Mental Epilepsy in the North African Native" at the University of Algiers in 1937; student of **Antoine Porot**. Worked at the Civil Hospital of Mustapha; Chief Physician of one of the four divisions of Blida Psychiatric Hospital, together with **Charles Bardenat, Maurice Porot** and **Jean Olry**. Fought in World War II and was wounded. In 1959, he succeeded **G.-A. Manceaux** as Professor of Clinical Neurology and Psychiatry at the University of Algiers, where he stayed until the independence of Algeria in 1962. After moving to France, he was Professor of Clinical Psychiatry at the University of Marseille from 1964 to 1980. He wrote widely on topics relevant to the ideology of the *École d'Alger*: His most important contribution to this school was his 1939 article on the "'Primitivism' of North African Natives", written in collaboration with Antoine Porot. In 1959, the year he became professor in Algiers, he published two papers: one with Maurice Porot and **Yves Pélicier** on "Algerian Aspects of Mental Pathology" and one with **Robert Susini**, Yves Pélicier and **Gérard Pascalis** on "Nuptial Psychoses in Algerian Muslims", which still advocated the theories of the *École d'Alger*. He was also fascinated by new treatments, collaborating, for

---

19   Compare for example: Bouquet, Aliénés en Tunisie, 22 f.; Soumeire, Meurtre, 18.

example, on the article "Reflexions on 3,000 Electroshocks Performed in the Psychiatric Services of Algeria", published in 1942.[20]

Taïeb, Suzanne Rachel: 1907–?; born in Tunisia to a Jewish family; French psychiatrist. Psychiatric dissertation on "Ideas Influencing the Mental Pathology of the Native North African" at the University of Algiers in 1939; student of **Antoine Porot**. Worked as an intern at Blida Psychiatric Hospital between 1936 and 1939; spoke fluent Arabic. She emigrated to France after World War II, where she worked as a general practitioner. She and **Michèle Chappert** were the only female clinical psychiatrists who could be found working in colonial North Africa during the research for this book.[21]

Thierry, H.: French doctor in Morocco; medical dissertation on the "Medical Practices and Superstitions of the Moroccans and the Influence of French Medicine in Morocco" at the University of Paris in 1917.

Thierry, Michel-Jacques: 1924–?; born in Casablanca; French doctor. Student at the School of Health of the Navy and of the Colonial Troops. Medical dissertation on the "French Medical Oeuvre in Morocco" at the University of Bordeaux in 1953.

Trenga, Victor: Born in Algeria, third generation; French psychiatrist. Psychiatric dissertation on "Psychoses in the Jews of Algeria" at the University of Lyon in 1902. Wrote a book entitled "The Arab-Berber Soul. A Sociological Study on the Muslim North African Society" in 1913.

Vadon, Raoul: French psychiatrist; psychiatric dissertation on the "Medical Assistance of Psychopaths in Tunisia" at the University of Marseille in 1935. Worked as an intern at the hospitals of Clermont-Ferrand; diploma of Colonial Hygiene and Medicine.

Variot, Gaston: 1855–1930; French doctor and professor, focusing on childcare. He was one of the founders of the *puériculture* movement in France. In 1881, he visited the newly founded Sadiki General Hospital in Tunis and published a report in the *Revue Scientifique de la France et de l'Étranger* entitled "A Visit to the Arab Hospital in Tunis".

Villot, Charles: Worked for the French administration and military intelligence (the so-called "*bureaux arabes*") in Algeria and wrote a book on "Mores, Customs and Institutions of the Natives in Algeria" in 1875.

Voisin, Auguste-Félix: 1823–1898; French psychiatrist; student of **Louis Jean François Delasiauve** and **Jacques-Joseph Moreau de Tours**. Succeeded his grandfather, the prominent French psychiatrist Félix-Auguste Voisin, to the post of director of Bicêtre in 1865. Two years later he became director of the Salpêtrière.[22] He visited the lunatic ward of the Civil Hospital of Mustapha in Algiers and presented an account of his experiences at the *Medico-Psychological Society* in 1873,[23] which led to an official commission being sent to Algeria, consisting of the three inspectors

---

20   Details have been taken from the obituary for Jean Sutter, written by Jean-Claude Scotto: Scotto, Hommage au professeur Jean Sutter.

21   On Suzanne Taïeb, see also: Faranda, La signora di Blida.

22   Morel, Dictionnaire, 244.

23   Lunier, Aliénés en Algérie, 335.

general, **Augustin Constans**, **Lunier Ludger** and **Dumesnil**. In 1896 he travelled to Tunisia for the 24th session of the *French Association for the Advancement of Sciences* in Tunis and published an account of his journey ("Souvenirs of a Visit to Tunisia") in the *Annales Médico-Psychologiques* that same year. The conference involved an organised visit to the Sadiki General Hospital in Tunis; Voisin greatly regretted the conditions he found there.

Warnock, John: British psychiatrist in Egypt from 1895 to 1923; reformed the psychiatric system in Egypt in his capacity as Director of the Lunacy Division, Egyptian Ministry of the Interior, and as Director of the ʿAbbāsiyya Hospital for the Insane in Cairo. In addition to yearly reports on the situation in Egypt, he published an article on "Insanity from Hasheesh" in the *Journal of Mental Science* in 1903 and his memoires "Twenty-Eight Years' Lunacy Experience in Egypt (1895–1923)" in 1924.

Wolters, L.: French doctor; worked as an extern at the Civil Hospital of Mustapha in Algiers and as an intern in the Hospital of Constantine. Medical dissertation on the "Role of the Teacher in Kabylia. From the Standpoint of Colonial Medicine" at the University of Toulouse in 1902.

Woytt-Gisclard, Alix: French jurist; legal dissertation on the "Assistance of Muslim Natives in Morocco" at the University of Paris in 1936, in which the question of the treatment of the insane in pre-colonial Morocco was pursued.

Appendix B:
Representation of Colonial Statistics

Fig. 1: Colonial Patients in French Asylums, 1874–1909

The y-axis shows the patient numbers, while the x-axis shows the years.
Information taken from: 1874–1903 – Reboul/Régis, Assistance, 50; 1909 – Livet,
Aliénés algériens, 34.

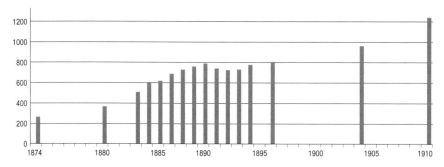

Fig. 2: Demographic Development in Algeria, 1856–1954

The y-axis shows the general population in Algeria, while the x-axis shows the years.
Information taken from: Maison, Population de l'Algérie, 1080 ff.

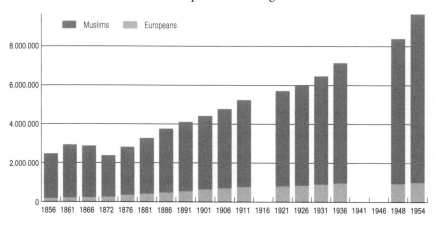

Fig. 3: Patients admitted into the Manouba Psychiatric Hospital, 1931–1971, and into Blida Psychiatric Hospital, 1948–1968

The y-axis shows the patient numbers, while the x-axis shows the years.
Information taken from: Ammar, Hôpital, 663; Hôpital psychiatrique de Blida, 824.

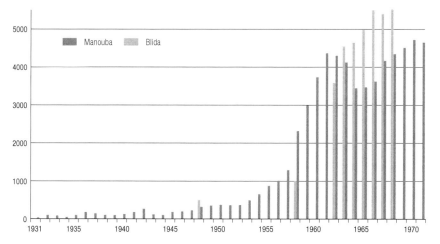

Fig. 4: Distribution of Europeans, Muslims and Jews in French Colonial Asylums and Psychiatric Institutions

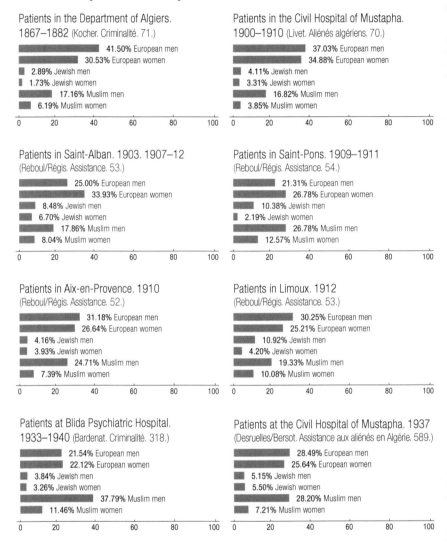

Patients in the Department of Algiers.
1867–1882 (Kocher. Criminalité. 71.)

41.50% European men
30.53% European women
2.89% Jewish men
1.73% Jewish women
17.16% Muslim men
6.19% Muslim women

0   20   40   60   80   100

Patients in the Civil Hospital of Mustapha.
1900–1910 (Livet. Aliénés algériens. 70.)

37.03% European men
34.88% European women
4.11% Jewish men
3.31% Jewish women
16.82% Muslim men
3.85% Muslim women

0   20   40   60   80   100

Patients in Saint-Alban. 1903. 1907–12
(Reboul/Régis. Assistance. 53.)

25.00% European men
33.93% European women
8.48% Jewish men
6.70% Jewish women
17.86% Muslim men
8.04% Muslim women

0   20   40   60   80   100

Patients in Saint-Pons. 1909–1911
(Reboul/Régis. Assistance. 54.)

21.31% European men
26.78% European women
10.38% Jewish men
2.19% Jewish women
26.78% Muslim men
12.57% Muslim women

0   20   40   60   80   100

Patients in Aix-en-Provence. 1910
(Reboul/Régis. Assistance. 52.)

31.18% European men
26.64% European women
4.16% Jewish men
3.93% Jewish women
24.71% Muslim men
7.39% Muslim women

0   20   40   60   80   100

Patients in Limoux. 1912
(Reboul/Régis. Assistance. 53.)

30.25% European men
25.21% European women
10.92% Jewish men
4.20% Jewish women
19.33% Muslim men
10.08% Muslim women

0   20   40   60   80   100

Patients at Blida Psychiatric Hospital.
1933–1940 (Bardenat. Criminalité. 318.)

21.54% European men
22.12% European women
3.84% Jewish men
3.26% Jewish women
37.79% Muslim men
11.46% Muslim women

0   20   40   60   80   100

Patients at the Civil Hospital of Mustapha. 1937
(Desruelles/Bersot. Assistance aux aliénés en Algérie. 589.)

28.49% European men
25.64% European women
5.15% Jewish men
5.50% Jewish women
28.20% Muslim men
7.21% Muslim women

0   20   40   60   80   100

Fig. 5: Ratio of European Women to European Men in French Colonial Asylums and Psychiatric Institutions

Department of Algiers.
1867–1882
(Kocher. Criminalité. 70.)

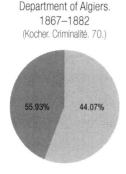

55.93%   44.07%

Civil Hospital of Mustapha.
Algiers. 1898–1909
(Bouquet. Aliénés en Tunisie. 34.)

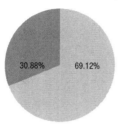

30.88%   69.12%

Civil Hospital of Mustapha.
Algiers. 1900–1910
(Livet. Aliénés algériens. 70.)

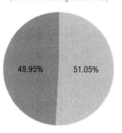

48.95%   51.05%

Asylum of Saint-Alban. 1903.
1907–1912
(Reboul/Régis. Assistance. 53.)

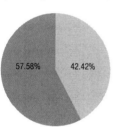

57.58%   42.42%

Asylum of Aix-en-Provence.
1910
(Reboul/Régis. Assistance. 52.)

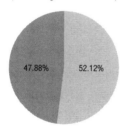

47.88%   52.12%

Asylum of Saint-Pons.
1909–1911
(Reboul/Régis. Assistance. 54.)

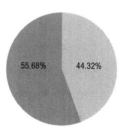

55.68%   44.32%

Asylum of Limoux.
1912
(Reboul/Régis. Assistance. 53.)

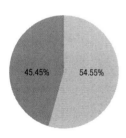

45.45%   54.55%

Blida Psychiatric Hospital.
1933–1940
(Bardenat. Criminalité. 318.)

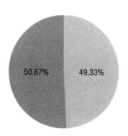

50.67%   49.33%

Civil Hospital of Mustapha.
Algiers. 1937
(Desruelles/Bersot. Assistance aux aliénés en Algérie. 589.)

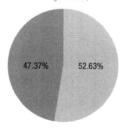

47.37%   52.63%

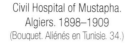

European women

European men

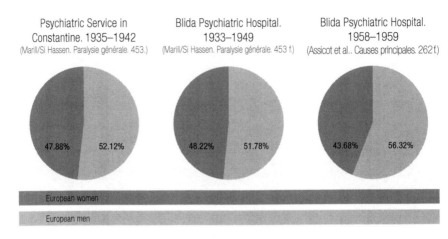

Psychiatric Service in
Constantine. 1935–1942
(Marill/Si Hassen. Paralysie générale. 453.)

Blida Psychiatric Hospital.
1933–1949
(Marill/Si Hassen. Paralysie générale. 453 f.)

Blida Psychiatric Hospital.
1958–1959
(Assicot et al.. Causes principales. 262 f.)

47.88% 52.12%   48.22% 51.78%   43.68% 56.32%

European women

European men

Fig. 6: Ratio of Muslim Women to Muslim Men in French Colonial Asylums and Psychiatric Institutions

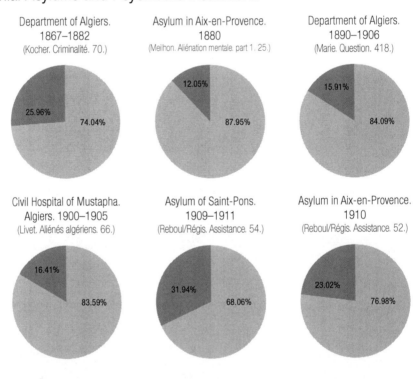

Department of Algiers.
1867–1882
(Kocher. Criminalité. 70.)

Asylum in Aix-en-Provence.
1880
(Meilhon. Aliénation mentale. part 1. 25.)

Department of Algiers.
1890–1906
(Marie. Question. 418.)

25.96% 74.04%   12.05% 87.95%   15.91% 84.09%

Civil Hospital of Mustapha.
Algiers. 1900–1905
(Livet. Aliénés algériens. 66.)

Asylum of Saint-Pons.
1909–1911
(Reboul/Régis. Assistance. 54.)

Asylum in Aix-en-Provence.
1910
(Reboul/Régis. Assistance. 52.)

16.41% 83.59%   31.94% 68.06%   23.02% 76.98%

European women

European men

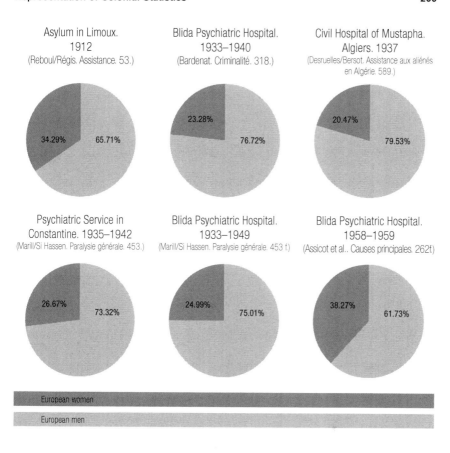

Fig. 7: Ratio of Muslim Women to Muslim Men in the Published Case Studies

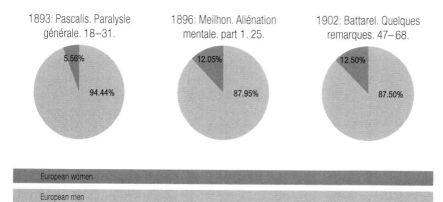

1907: Gervais.
Contribution. 36.

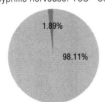

1907: Sicard. Étude.
17–47.

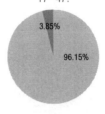

1926: Arrii. Impulsivité
criminelle. 84–7.

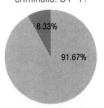

1926: Goëau-Brissonnière.
Syphilis nerveuse. 103–60.

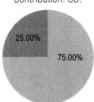

1927: Benkhelil. Contribution.
67–90.

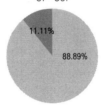

1932: Porot/Arrii. Impulsivité
criminelle. 591–609.

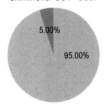

1932: Soumeire. Meurtre.
43–75.

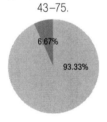

1937: Sutter. Épilepsie mentale.
128–213.

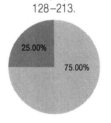

1939: Taïeb. Idées d'influence.
85–146.

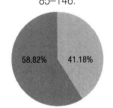

1940: Olry. Paralysie générale.
39–61.

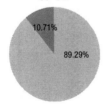

1961: Assicot et al., Causes
principales. 266–84

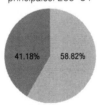

European women

European men

Fig. 8: Distribution of Diseases

Fig. 8a: Department of Algiers, between 1867 and 1882

Information taken from: Kocher, Criminalité, 70.

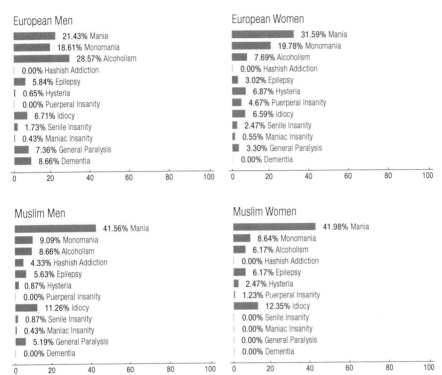

European Men

- 21.43% Mania
- 18.61% Monomania
- 28.57% Alcoholism
- 0.00% Hashish Addiction
- 5.84% Epilepsy
- 0.65% Hysteria
- 0.00% Puerperal Insanity
- 6.71% Idiocy
- 1.73% Senile Insanity
- 0.43% Maniac Insanity
- 7.36% General Paralysis
- 8.66% Dementia

0   20   40   60   80   100

European Women

- 31.59% Mania
- 19.78% Monomania
- 7.69% Alcoholism
- 0.00% Hashish Addiction
- 3.02% Epilepsy
- 6.87% Hysteria
- 4.67% Puerperal Insanity
- 6.59% Idiocy
- 2.47% Senile Insanity
- 0.55% Maniac Insanity
- 3.30% General Paralysis
- 0.00% Dementia

0   20   40   60   80   100

Muslim Men

- 41.56% Mania
- 9.09% Monomania
- 8.66% Alcoholism
- 4.33% Hashish Addiction
- 5.63% Epilepsy
- 0.87% Hysteria
- 0.00% Puerperal Insanity
- 11.26% Idiocy
- 0.87% Senile Insanity
- 0.43% Maniac Insanity
- 5.19% General Paralysis
- 0.00% Dementia

0   20   40   60   80   100

Muslim Women

- 41.98% Mania
- 8.64% Monomania
- 6.17% Alcoholism
- 0.00% Hashish Addiction
- 6.17% Epilepsy
- 2.47% Hysteria
- 1.23% Puerperal Insanity
- 12.35% Idiocy
- 0.00% Senile Insanity
- 0.00% Maniac Insanity
- 0.00% General Paralysis
- 0.00% Dementia

0   20   40   60   80   100

Fig. 8b: Asylum in Aix-en-Provence, 1880

Information taken from: Meilhon, Aliénation mentale, part 2, 191.

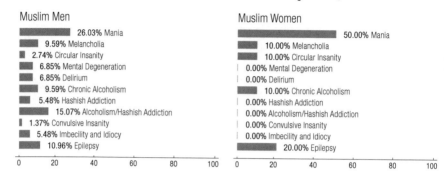

Fig. 8c: Civil Hospital of Mustapha, between 1900 and 1910

Information taken from: Livet, Aliénés algériens, 70; Reboul/Régis, Assistance, 51.

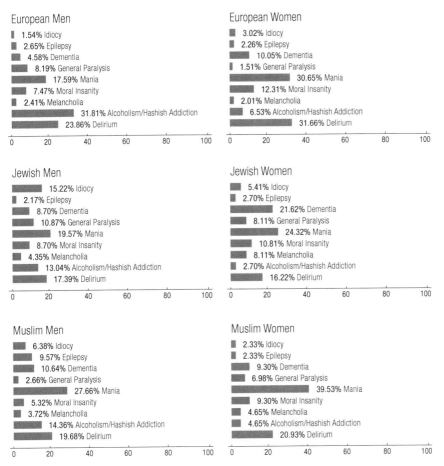

European Men
- 1.54% Idiocy
- 2.65% Epilepsy
- 4.58% Dementia
- 8.19% General Paralysis
- 17.59% Mania
- 7.47% Moral Insanity
- 2.41% Melancholia
- 31.81% Alcoholism/Hashish Addiction
- 23.86% Delirium

European Women
- 3.02% Idiocy
- 2.26% Epilepsy
- 10.05% Dementia
- 1.51% General Paralysis
- 30.65% Mania
- 12.31% Moral Insanity
- 2.01% Melancholia
- 6.53% Alcoholism/Hashish Addiction
- 31.66% Delirium

Jewish Men
- 15.22% Idiocy
- 2.17% Epilepsy
- 8.70% Dementia
- 10.87% General Paralysis
- 19.57% Mania
- 8.70% Moral Insanity
- 4.35% Melancholia
- 13.04% Alcoholism/Hashish Addiction
- 17.39% Delirium

Jewish Women
- 5.41% Idiocy
- 2.70% Epilepsy
- 21.62% Dementia
- 8.11% General Paralysis
- 24.32% Mania
- 10.81% Moral Insanity
- 8.11% Melancholia
- 2.70% Alcoholism/Hashish Addiction
- 16.22% Delirium

Muslim Men
- 6.38% Idiocy
- 9.57% Epilepsy
- 10.64% Dementia
- 2.66% General Paralysis
- 27.66% Mania
- 5.32% Moral Insanity
- 3.72% Melancholia
- 14.36% Alcoholism/Hashish Addiction
- 19.68% Delirium

Muslim Women
- 2.33% Idiocy
- 2.33% Epilepsy
- 9.30% Dementia
- 6.98% General Paralysis
- 39.53% Mania
- 9.30% Moral Insanity
- 4.65% Melancholia
- 4.65% Alcoholism/Hashish Addiction
- 20.93% Delirium

Fig. 8d: Asylum of Saint-Alban, 1903, 1907–1912

Information taken from: Reboul/Régis, Assistance, 53.

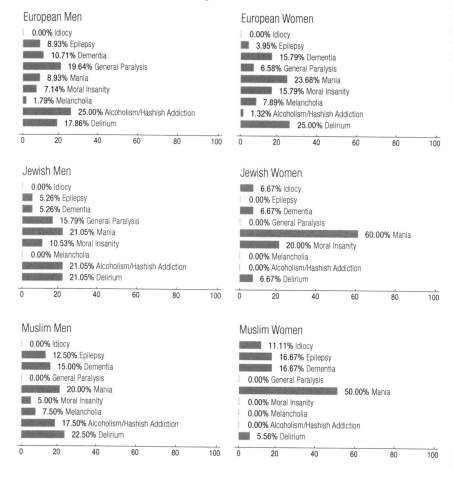

Fig. 8e: Asylum of Saint-Pons, 1909–1911

Information taken from: Reboul/Régis, Assistance, 54.

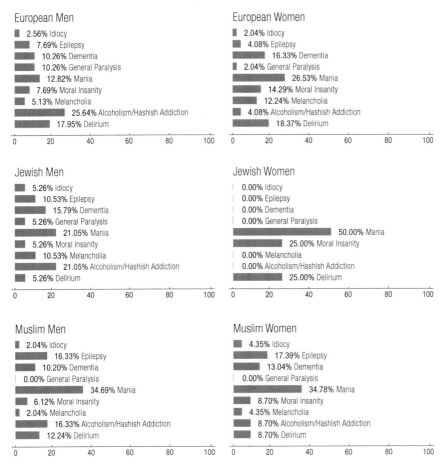

European Men
- 2.56% Idiocy
- 7.69% Epilepsy
- 10.26% Dementia
- 10.26% General Paralysis
- 12.82% Mania
- 7.69% Moral Insanity
- 5.13% Melancholia
- 25.64% Alcoholism/Hashish Addiction
- 17.95% Delirium

European Women
- 2.04% Idiocy
- 4.08% Epilepsy
- 16.33% Dementia
- 2.04% General Paralysis
- 26.53% Mania
- 14.29% Moral Insanity
- 12.24% Melancholia
- 4.08% Alcoholism/Hashish Addiction
- 18.37% Delirium

Jewish Men
- 5.26% Idiocy
- 10.53% Epilepsy
- 15.79% Dementia
- 5.26% General Paralysis
- 21.05% Mania
- 5.26% Moral Insanity
- 10.53% Melancholia
- 21.05% Alcoholism/Hashish Addiction
- 5.26% Delirium

Jewish Women
- 0.00% Idiocy
- 0.00% Epilepsy
- 0.00% Dementia
- 0.00% General Paralysis
- 50.00% Mania
- 25.00% Moral Insanity
- 0.00% Melancholia
- 0.00% Alcoholism/Hashish Addiction
- 25.00% Delirium

Muslim Men
- 2.04% Idiocy
- 16.33% Epilepsy
- 10.20% Dementia
- 0.00% General Paralysis
- 34.69% Mania
- 6.12% Moral Insanity
- 2.04% Melancholia
- 16.33% Alcoholism/Hashish Addiction
- 12.24% Delirium

Muslim Women
- 4.35% Idiocy
- 17.39% Epilepsy
- 13.04% Dementia
- 0.00% General Paralysis
- 34.78% Mania
- 8.70% Moral Insanity
- 4.35% Melancholia
- 8.70% Alcoholism/Hashish Addiction
- 8.70% Delirium

Fig. 8f: Asylum of Aix-en-Provence, 1910

Information taken from: Reboul/Régis, Assistance, 52.

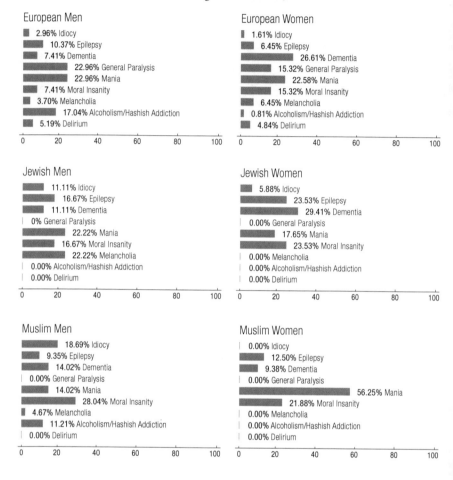

Fig. 8g: Asylum of Limoux, 1912

Information taken from: Reboul/Régis, Assistance, 53.

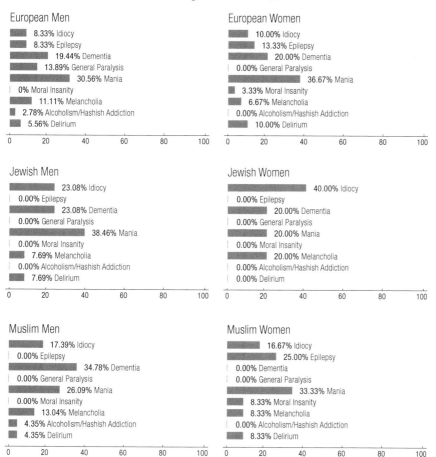

European Men

- 8.33% Idiocy
- 8.33% Epilepsy
- 19.44% Dementia
- 13.89% General Paralysis
- 30.56% Mania
- 0% Moral Insanity
- 11.11% Melancholia
- 2.78% Alcoholism/Hashish Addiction
- 5.56% Delirium

European Women

- 10.00% Idiocy
- 13.33% Epilepsy
- 20.00% Dementia
- 0.00% General Paralysis
- 36.67% Mania
- 3.33% Moral Insanity
- 6.67% Melancholia
- 0.00% Alcoholism/Hashish Addiction
- 10.00% Delirium

Jewish Men

- 23.08% Idiocy
- 0.00% Epilepsy
- 23.08% Dementia
- 0.00% General Paralysis
- 38.46% Mania
- 0.00% Moral Insanity
- 7.69% Melancholia
- 0.00% Alcoholism/Hashish Addiction
- 7.69% Delirium

Jewish Women

- 40.00% Idiocy
- 0.00% Epilepsy
- 20.00% Dementia
- 0.00% General Paralysis
- 20.00% Mania
- 0.00% Moral Insanity
- 20.00% Melancholia
- 0.00% Alcoholism/Hashish Addiction
- 0.00% Delirium

Muslim Men

- 17.39% Idiocy
- 0.00% Epilepsy
- 34.78% Dementia
- 0.00% General Paralysis
- 26.09% Mania
- 0.00% Moral Insanity
- 13.04% Melancholia
- 4.35% Alcoholism/Hashish Addiction
- 4.35% Delirium

Muslim Women

- 16.67% Idiocy
- 25.00% Epilepsy
- 0.00% Dementia
- 0.00% General Paralysis
- 33.33% Mania
- 8.33% Moral Insanity
- 8.33% Melancholia
- 0.00% Alcoholism/Hashish Addiction
- 8.33% Delirium

Fig. 9: Distribution of Races and Genders among the Different Diagnoses, Tunis Congress 1912

Compiled information on the patients in the Civil Hospital of Mustapha, 1900–1910 (Livet, Aliénés algériens, 70; Reboul/Régis, Assistance, 51); on the patients in the Saint-Alban asylum, 1903, 1907–1912 (Reboul/Régis, Assistance, 53); on the patients in the Saint-Pons asylum, 1909–1911 (Reboul/Régis, Assistance, 54); on the patients in Aix-en-Provence, 1910 (Reboul/Régis, Assistance, 52); and the patients in Limoux, 1912 (Reboul/Régis, Assistance, 53).

Fig. 9a: General Population

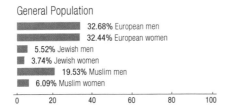

General Population

- 32.68% European men
- 32.44% European women
- 5.52% Jewish men
- 3.74% Jewish women
- 19.53% Muslim men
- 6.09% Muslim women

0   20   40   60   80   100

Fig. 9b: Different Diseases

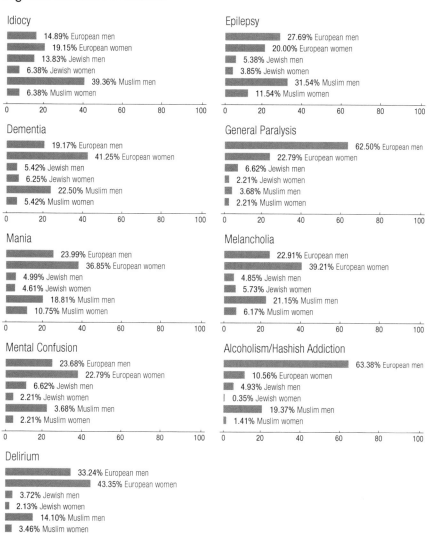

Idiocy

- 14.89% European men
- 19.15% European women
- 13.83% Jewish men
- 6.38% Jewish women
- 39.36% Muslim men
- 6.38% Muslim women

0 20 40 60 80 100

Epilepsy

- 27.69% European men
- 20.00% European women
- 5.38% Jewish men
- 3.85% Jewish women
- 31.54% Muslim men
- 11.54% Muslim women

0 20 40 60 80 100

Dementia

- 19.17% European men
- 41.25% European women
- 5.42% Jewish men
- 6.25% Jewish women
- 22.50% Muslim men
- 5.42% Muslim women

0 20 40 60 80 100

General Paralysis

- 62.50% European men
- 22.79% European women
- 6.62% Jewish men
- 2.21% Jewish women
- 3.68% Muslim men
- 2.21% Muslim women

0 20 40 60 80 100

Mania

- 23.99% European men
- 36.85% European women
- 4.99% Jewish men
- 4.61% Jewish women
- 18.81% Muslim men
- 10.75% Muslim women

0 20 40 60 80 100

Melancholia

- 22.91% European men
- 39.21% European women
- 4.85% Jewish men
- 5.73% Jewish women
- 21.15% Muslim men
- 6.17% Muslim women

0 20 40 60 80 100

Mental Confusion

- 23.68% European men
- 22.79% European women
- 6.62% Jewish men
- 2.21% Jewish women
- 3.68% Muslim men
- 2.21% Muslim women

0 20 40 60 80 100

Alcoholism/Hashish Addiction

- 63.38% European men
- 10.56% European women
- 4.93% Jewish men
- 0.35% Jewish women
- 19.37% Muslim men
- 1.41% Muslim women

0 20 40 60 80 100

Delirium

- 33.24% European men
- 43.35% European women
- 3.72% Jewish men
- 2.13% Jewish women
- 14.10% Muslim men
- 3.46% Muslim women

0 20 40 60 80 100

Bibliography

Sources

Articles, Reports and Monographies

Abadie, Jean. Report on the XXII Congrès des Médecins Aliénistes et Neurologistes de France des Pays de Langue Française. Tunis, 01.–07.04.1912. In: Presse Médicale. 20th Year, No 29 (10.04.1912). 293 ff. And: 20th Year, No 35 (30.04.1912). 378–83.

Abbasîya and Khanka. In: Journal of Mental Science. Vol. 71 (Oct. 1925). 794 f.

Abbatucci, S. Assistance et hygiène mentales aux colonies. In: Presse Médicale. 34th Year, No 41 (22.05.1926). 652 f.

Alliez, Joseph/Decombes, Henri. Réflexions sur le comportement psycho-pathologique d'une série de nord-africains musulmans immigrés. In: Annales Médico-Psychologiques. 110th Year, Vol. 2 (June–Dec. 1952). 150–6.

Amat, Charles. Le M'zab et les M'zabites. Paris 1888.

Ammar, Sleïm. L'assistance aux aliénés en Tunisie (quelques étapes). In: L'Information Psychiatrique. 31st Year, 4th Series, No 1 (Jan. 1955). 24–7.

Armand, Adolphe. L'Algérie médicale. Topographie, climatologie, pathogénie, pathologie, prophylaxie, hygiène, acclimatement et colonisation. Paris 1854.

Assicot, Michel/Dequeker, J./Faure/Lemaire/Lotiron/Maudoux, S./Soubrier/Maudoux, M./Vasan. Causes principales de morbidité psychiatrique chez les musulmans algériens. In: L'Hygiène Mentale. 50th Year, No 3 (1961). 261–86.

Aubin, Henri. Brèves réflexions sur l'assistance psychiatrique dans nos territoires d'outre-mer. In: L'Information Psychiatrique. 31st Year, 4th Series, No 1 (Jan. 1955). 8 ff.

Aubin, Henri/Gachkel/Zangerlin/Gallo. Les troubles mentaux dans la fièvre récurrente. In: Algérie Médicale. 50th Year, No 5 (May 1947). 408–16.

Aubin, Henri. Indigènes Nord-Africains (Psychopathologie des). In: Porot, Antoine (ed.). Manuel alphabétique de psychiatrie clinique et thérapeutique. Paris 1954. 292.

Aubin, Henri. Introduction à l'étude de la psychiatrie chez les noirs. In: Annales Médico-Psychologiques. 15th Series, 97th Year, Vol. 1 (Jan. 1939). 1–29. And: 15th Series, 97th Year, Vol. 1 (Feb. 1939). 181–213.

Aubin, Henri. L'assistance psychiatrique indigène aux colonies. Congrès des Médecins Aliénistes et Neurologistes de France et des Pays de Langue Française. 42nd Session, Algiers (06.–11.04.). Paris 1938. 147–76.

Auclert, Hubertine. Les femmes arabes en Algérie. Paris 1900.

Barbier. Les fous et le mal de mer. In: Journal de Médecine et de Pharmacie de l'Algérie. Vol. 9 (Oct. 1884). 227 ff.

Bardenat, Charles. Criminalité et délinquance dans l'aliénation mentale chez les indigènes algériens. In: Annales Médico-Psychologiques. 106th Year, Vol. 2 (June 1948). 317–33; 468–80.

Battarel, E. Les aliénés à l'hôpital civil de Mustapha. In: Bulletin Médical de l'Algérie. 2th Series, No 7 (July 1902). 244 f.

Benabud, Ahmed. Aspects psychopathologiques du cannabisme au Maroc: données statistiques pour l'année 1956. In: Bulletin des Stupéfiants. Vol. 9, No 4 (Oct.–Dec. 1957). 1–27.

Bertherand, Alphonse. Mémoire de médecine et chirurgie médicale. Paris 1842.

Bertherand, Émile-Louis. Le suicide chez les musulmans de l'Algérie. In: Annales Médico-Psychologiques. 5th Series, 33rd Year, Vol. 14 (1875). 153–5.

Bertherand, Émile-Louis. Médecine et hygiène des arabes. Études sur l'exercice de la médecine et de la chirurgie chez les musulmans de l'Algérie, leurs connaissances en anatomie, histoire naturelle, pharmacie, médecine légale, etc., leurs conditions climatériques générales, leurs pratiques hygiéniques publiques et privées, leurs maladies, leurs traitements les plus usités. Paris 1855.

Bertholon, Lucien. Esquisse de l'anthropologie criminelle des Tunisiens musulmans. In: Archives d'Anthropologie Criminelle et des Sciences Pénales. Vol. 4, No 22 (1889). 389–439.

Blancardi, C./Ferrand, G./Moulinie, P. Sur la syphilis nerveuse du Marocain musulman. Deux observations de Tabès. In: Maroc Médical. 28th Year, No 287 (April 1949). 226 f.

Bloch, Iwan. Das erste Auftreten der Syphilis (Lustseuche) in der europäischen Kulturwelt. Gewürdigt in seiner weltgeschichtlichen Bedeutung, dargestellt nach Anfang, Verlauf und voraussichtlichem Ende. Jena 1904.

Boigey, Maurice. Le mariage dans les tribus musulmanes de l'Afrique. In: Presse Médicale. 19th Year, Annexe, No 102 (23.12.1911). 1185–8.

Boigey, Maurice. Comment accouchent les Sahariennes. In: Presse Médicale. 15th Year, Annexe, No 47 (12.06.1907). 377 ff.

Boigey, Maurice. Étude psychologique sur l'Islam. In: Annales Médico-Psychologiques. 9th Series, 66th Year, Vol. 8 (1908). 5–14.

Boigey, Maurice. L'assistance hospitalière en pays musulman. In: Presse Médicale. 15th Year, Annexe, No 76 (21.09.1907). 609 ff.

Bouquet, Henri. Médecine et colonisation. In: El Medico Colonial. Feuilleton du Temps. 23.07.1931. No page numbers.

Bousquet, Georges-Henri. La morale de l'Islam et son éthique sexuelle. Paris 1953.

B., R. La médecine au Maroc. In: Presse Médicale. 19th Year, Annexe, No 33 (26.04.1911). 381 ff.

Brault, Jules François Marie Joseph. Pathologie et hygiène des indigènes musulmans d'Algérie. Algiers 1905.

Brierre de Boismont, Alexandre. Rapport sur la candidature de M. le docteur Mongeri, médecin en chef de l'asile de Suléimanié à Constantinople, au titre de membre associé étranger de la Société médico-psychologique. In: Annales Médico-Psychologiques. 4th Series, 24th Year, Vol. 7 (1866). 69–80.

Brierre de Boismont, Alexandre. Review of d'Escayrac de Lauture. De la Turquie et des États musulmans en général. Paris 1858. In: Annales Médico-Psychologiques. 3rd Series, Vol. 5 (1859). 147–54.

Brissot, F. Propos sur la mentalité des musulmans nord-africains. In: Annales Médico-Psychologiques. 117th Year, Vol. 1 (1959). 495–504.

Brunswic-Le Bihan. Hôpital Sadiki. L'assistance médicale des indigènes de Tunisie et les auxiliaires médicaux. Communication faite au Congrès de Géographie. Tunis 1904.

Brunswic-Le Bihan. L'hôpital Sadiki et l'assistance médicale indigène en Tunisie. In: Presse Médicale. 13th Year (17.06.1905). 377 ff.

Bugéja, Marie. Nos sœurs musulmanes. Algiers 1931.

Burdett, Henry C. Hospitals and Asylums of the World: Their Origin, History, Construction, Administration, Management and Legislation; with Plans of the Chief Medical Institutions accurately drawn to a Uniform Scale, in Addition to those of all the Hospitals of London in the Jubilee Year of Queen Victoria's Reign. London 1891.

Campbell Clark, Archibald. Aetiology, Pathology and Treatment of Puerperal Insanity. In: Journal of Mental Science. Vol. 33, No 142 (July 1887). 169–89. Vol. 33, No 143 (Oct. 1887). 372–9. Vol. 33, No 144 (Jan. 1888). 487–96.

Camuset, L. Review of Kocher, A. De la criminalité chez les Arabes au point de vue de la pratique médico-judiciaire en Algérie. Paris 1884. In: Annales Médico-Psychologiques. 7th Series, 43rd Year, Vol. 1 (1885). 345 ff.

Carothers, John Colin. A Study of Mental Derangements in Africans, and an Attempt to Explain its Peculiarities, more Especially in Relation to the African Attitude to Life. In: Journal of Mental Science. Vol. 93 (1947). 548–97.

Carothers, John Colin. Frontal Lobe Function and the African. In: Journal of Mental Science. Vol. 97 (Jan. 1951). 12–48.

Ceillier, André. Report on the Meeting of the Société de Psychiatrie. 20.10.1927. Paralysie générale chez un Arabe. In: Presse Médicale. 35th Year, No 89 (05.11.1927). 1353.

Celarié, Henriette. Un mois au Maroc. Paris 1923.

Charbonneau, Pierre. L'assistance et la prévoyance sociale au Maroc. In: Maroc Médical. Part 1: 33rd Year, No 350 (July 1954). 731–52. Part 2: 33rd Year, No 351 (Aug. 1954). 790–800. Part 3: 33rd Year, No 352 (Sept. 1954). 881–92. Part 4: 33rd Year, No 355 (Dec. 1954). 1134–61. Part 5: 34th Year, No 356 (Jan. 1955). 75–96. Part 6: 34th Year, No 358 (March 1955). 288–318.

Charbonneau, Pierre. Le climat pathologique de l'enfance marocaine. In: Maroc Médical. 32nd Year, No 338 (July 1953). 655–72.

Charcot, Jean-Martin. Leçon d'ouverture. In: Progrès Médical. 06.05.1882. 336.

Charcot, Jean-Martin. Leçons sur les maladies du système nerveux faites à la Salpêtrière. 1872/1873.

Charles, Raymond. L'âme musulmane. Casablanca 2007 (first published 1958).

Charpentier, René. Comptes Rendus. Congrès des Médecins Aliénistes et Neurologistes de France des Pays de Langue Française. 37th Session. Rabat (07.–13.04.). Paris 1933.

Chellier, Dorothée. Voyage dans l'Aurès. Notes d'un médecin envoyé en mission chez les femmes arabes. Tizi-Ouzou 1895.

Chérif, Ahmad. Étude psychologique sur l'Islam. In: Annales Médico-Psychologiques. 9th Series, 67th Year, Vol. 9 (1909). 353–63.

Clinique de M. Chomel. Hystérie compliquée d'accidents épileptiformes. Réflexions sur l'influence des rapports sexuels sur l'hystérie. (23.02.1843). In: Annales Médico-Psychologiques. Vol. 2 (1843). 105–9.

Collomb, Henri/Robert, P. Le thème d'homosexualité chez le nord-africain musulman. In: Annales Médico-Psychologiques. 116th Year, Vol. 1 (1958). 531–5.

Comby, Jules. La médecine française en Tunisie. In: Presse Médicale. 30th Year, Annexe, No 47 (24.06.1922). 977–92.

Comby, Jules. Un voyage médical au Maroc. In: Presse Médicale. 31st Year, Annexe, No 55 (11.07.1923). 1145–53. 31st Year, Annexe, No 57 (18.07.1923). 1188–1205. 31st Year, Annexe, No 59 (25.07.1923). 1229–38.

Constans, Augustin/Lunier, Ludger/Dumesnil. Rapport sommaire sur le service des aliénés en 1877. In: Annales Médico-Psychologiques. 6th Series, 38th Year, Vol. 1 (1879). 82–95.

Couderc, L. Conséquences des conditions actuelles d'assistance psychiatrique en Algérie. In: L'Hygiène Mentale. 50th Year, No 3 (1961). 250–60.

Couderc, L. L'assistance psychiatrique dans le département d'Oran (Algérie). In: L'Information Psychiatrique. 31st Year, 4th Series No 1 (Jan. 1955). 19–23.

Courbon, Paul. Review of Porot, Antoine/Sutter, Jean. Le primitivisme des indigènes nord-africains. In: Sud Médical et Chirurgical. 15.04.1939. In: Annales Médico-Psychologiques. 15th Series, 97th Year, Vol. 2 (1939). 440.

D'Arlach, H. Le Maroc en 1856. Paris 1856.

Delasiauve, Louis Jean François. Review of Collardot. De l'opportunité de créer un établissement spéciale d'aliénés en Algérie. In: Journal de Médecine Mentale. Vol. 5 (1865). 115–9.

Dequeker, J./Fanon, Frantz/Lacaton, R./Micucci, M./Ramée, F. Aspects actuels de l'assistance mentale en Algérie. In: L'Information Psychiatrique. Vol. 31, No 4 (Jan. 1955). 11–8. Also in: L'Information Psychiatrique. Vol. 51, No 10 (Dec. 1975). 1107–13.

Desruelles, Maurice/Bersot, Henri. L'assistance aux aliénés chez les Arabes du VIIIe au XIIe siècle: Contribution à l'histoire de l'assistance aux aliénés. In: Annales Médico-Psychologiques. 15th Series, 96th Year, Vol. 2 (1938). 689–709.

Desruelles, Maurice/Bersot, Henri. L'assistance aux aliénés en Algérie depuis le XIXe siècle. In: Annales Médico-Psychologiques. 15th Series, 97th Year, Vol. 2 (1939). 578–96. Also in: History of Psychiatry. Vol. 7 (1996). 549–61.

Desruelles, Maurice/Bersot, Henri. Note sur les origines arabes de l'assistance aux aliénés. In: Congrès des Médecins Aliénistes et Neurologistes de France et des Pays de Langue Française. 42nd Session, Algiers (06.–11.04.). Paris 1938. 304–9.

Desruelles, Maurice/Bersot, Henri. Note sur l'histoire de l'assistance aux aliénés en Algérie depuis la conquête. In: Congrès des Médecins Aliénistes et Neurologistes de France et des Pays de Langue Française. 42nd Session, Algiers (06.–11.04.). Paris 1938. 310–4.

Dilhan, Aug(uste?). Ethnographie de la Tunisie. In: Mémoires de la Société d'Ethnographie. Vol. 12 (1873). 167–212.

Discussion du rapport d'assistance psychiatrique. In: Congrès des Médecins Aliénistes et Neurologistes de France et des Pays de Langue Française. 42nd Session, Algiers (06.–11.04.). Paris 1938. 177–97.

Donnadieu, André. L'alcoolisme mental dans la population indigène du Maroc. In: Maroc Médical. 20th Year, Vol. 214 (Nov.–Dec. 1940). 163–5.

Donnadieu, André. Situation actuelle de la syphilis nerveuse indigène à forme mentale. In: Maroc Médical. 19th Year, No 207 (Sept. 1939). 315–9.

Duclaux, H. Report on the Meeting of the Société de Médecine de Paris. 25.11.1922. Paralysie générale des Arabes. In: Presse Médicale. 30th Year, No 97 (06.12.1922). 1056.

Dumesnil/Pons. A. R. Urquhart and William Samuel Tuke. Deux visites à l'asile du Caire, 1877 and 1878. In: Annales Médico-Psychologiques. 6th Series, 40th Year, Vol. 7 (1882). 154 f.

Dumolard, L. Au sujet de l'assistance psychiatrique en Algérie: La situation véritable. Mise au point. In: L'Hygiène Mentale. 21st Year, No 1 (Jan. 1926). 16 ff.

Dumolard, L. Au sujet de l'assistance psychiatrique en Algérie. In: L'Hygiène Mentale. 21st Year, No 6 (June 1926). 144 f.

Dupouy, Roger. Chronique. Le XXIIe Congrès des Médecins Aliénistes et Neurologistes de France des Pays de Langue Française – Tunis, avril 1912. In: Annales Médico-Psychologiques. 10th Series, 70th Year, Vol. 1 (1912). 513–47.

Fabre, Paul. De l'hystérie chez l'homme. In: Annales Médico-Psychologiques. 5th Series, 33rd Year, Vol. 13 (1875). 354–73.

Fanon, Frantz/Azoulay, Jacques. La socialthérapie dans un service d'hommes musulmans. Difficultés méthodologiques. In: L'Information Psychiatrique. Vol. 30, No 9 (1954). 349–61. Also in: L'Information Psychiatrique. Vol. 51, No 10 (1975). 1095–1106.

Fanon, Frantz/Géronimi, Charles. Le T. A. T. chez les femmes musulmanes. Sociologie de la perception et de l'imagination. In: Congrès des Médecins Aliénistes et Neurologistes de France et des Pays de Langue Française. 54th Session, Bordeaux (30.08.–04.09.). Paris 1956. 364–8.

Fanon, Frantz. Les damnés de la terre. Paris 2002 (first published in 1961).

Fanon, Frantz. Le 'syndrome nord africain'. In: Esprit. Vol. 20, No 2 (Feb. 1952). 237–51. Also in: Ibid. Pour la révolution africaine. Écrits politiques. Paris 1964. 13–25.

Fanon, Frantz. L'hospitalisation de jour en psychiatrie. Valeur et limites. In: Tunisie Médicale. 37th Year, No 10 (1959). 689–732. Also in: L'Information Psychiatrique. Vol. 51, No 10 (Dec. 1975). 1117–30.

Fanon, Frantz. Racisme et culture. In: Présence Africaine. June–Nov. 1956. Also in: Ibid. Pour la révolution africaine. Écrits politiques. Paris 1964. 39–51.

Fanon, Frantz/Sanchez, François. Attitude du musulman maghrébin devant la folie. In: Revue Pratique de Psychologie de la Vie Sociale et d'Hygiène Mentale. Vol. 1 (1956). 24–7.

Fréquence des maladies nerveuses chez les Arabes. In: Archives de Neurologie. 2nd Series, Vol. 22 (1906). 49.

Freud, Sigmund. Allgemeines über den hysterischen Anfall (1909 [1908]). In: Ibid. Hysterie und Angst. Studienausgabe. Frankfurt am Main 1970. 197–203.

Freud, Sigmund/Breuer, Joseph. Studien über Hysterie. Frankfurt am Main 1970, unabridged version (first published in 1895).

Freud, Sigmund. Bruchstück einer Hysterieanalyse (1905 [1901]). In: Ibid. Hysterie und Angst. Studienausgabe. Frankfurt am Main 1970. 83–186.

Freud, Sigmund. Hysterische Phantasien und ihre Beziehung zur Bisexualität (1908). In: Ibid. Hysterie und Angst. Studienausgabe. Frankfurt am Main 1970. 187–95.

Freud, Sigmund. Über den psychischen Mechanismus hysterischer Phänomene (1893). In: Ibid. Hysterie und Angst. Studienausgabe. Frankfurt am Main 1970. 9–24.

Freud, Sigmund. Zur Ätiologie der Hysterie (1896). In: Ibid. Hysterie und Angst. Studienausgabe. Frankfurt am Main 1970. 51–81.

Frey, F. Évolution, après le retour en Algérie, des maladies mentales contractées en métropole par les travailleurs musulmans. In: L'Hygiène Mentale. 50th Year, No 3 (1961). 244–9.

Fribourg-Blanc, A. L'état mental des indigènes de l'Afrique du Nord et leurs réactions psychopathiques. In: L'Hygiène Mentale. 22nd Year, No 9 (Nov. 1927). 135–44.

Gillot, Victor. Quelques considérations sur la pathologie des Arabes en Algérie. In: Lyon Médical. No 44 (1902). 864 ff.

Green, E. M. Psychoses among Negroes – a Comparative Study. In: Journal of Nervous and Mental Disorder. Vol. 41, No 11 (Nov. 1914). 697–708.

Hadida, Elie/Marill, François-Georges/Porot, Maurice. Sur l'augmentation apparente de la fréquence de la neuro-syphilis parenchymateuse chez l'indigène nord-africain. In: Congrès des Médecins Aliénistes et Neurologistes de France et des Pays de Langue Française. 53rd Session, Nice (05.–11.09.). Paris 1955. 466–71.

Henry, J./Assicot, Michel. Le 7044 RP dans des psychoses chroniques et en particulier dans la schizophrénie. In: Algérie Médicale. 63rd Year, No 7 (July 1959). 691–5.

Humann. Troubles mentaux des indigènes du Sahara algérien. In: Presse Médicale. 42nd Year, No 53 (04.07.1934). 1084 ff.

Ibsen, Henrik. Peer Gynt. Translated by Hermann Stock. Stuttgart 1953.

Idanof, D. Contribution à l'étiologie de la folie puerpérale. In: Annales Médico-Psychologiques. 7th Series, 51st Year, Vol. 17 (1893). 161–91.

Igert, Maurice. Introduction à la psychopathologie marocaine. In: Maroc Médical. 34th Year, No 365 (Oct. 1955). 1309–32.

Igert, Maurice. Milieu culturel marocain et névroses. In: Maroc Médical. 34th Year, No 360 (May 1955). 648–55.

Igert, Maurice/Viaud, L. Bilan d'une année d'électrochocs. In: Maroc Médical. 28th Year, No 287 (April 1949). 217 ff.

Issa Bey, Ahmed. Histoire des bimaristans (hôpitaux) à l'époque islamique. In: Congrès International de Médecine Tropicale et d'Hygiène. Dec. 1928, Cairo. Vol. 2 (1929). 81–209.

Jayle, F. La faculté de médecine et l'hôpital de Mustapha. In: Presse Médicale. 42nd Year, No 5 (17.01.1934). 97–101.

Jeanselme, Édouard. La condition des aliénés dans les colonies françaises, anglaises et néerlandaises d'Extrême-Orient. In: Presse Médicale. 13th Year (09.08.1905). 497 f.

Jobert, A. Du projet de créer un établissement spécial d'aliénés en Algérie. In: Gazette Médicale de l'Algérie. 1868. 13–16; 61 ff.

Jude/Assad Hakkim. Les troubles mentaux les plus généralement observés à Damas. In: L'Hygiène Mentale. 22nd Year, No 9 (Nov. 1927). 125–35.

Lacapère, Georges. Vue d'ensemble de la syphilis tertiaire chez les indigènes du Maroc. In: Presse Médicale. 26th Year, No 16 (18.03.1918). 146 ff.

La civilisation est-elle cause des maladies nerveuses? In: Annales Médico-Psychologiques. 7th Series, 51st Year, Vol. 17 (1893). 505.

Laforgue, René. De l'aspect psychosomatique des névroses. In: Maroc Médical. 32nd Year, No 336 (May 1953). 473–6.

Laignel-Lavastine. Review of Sicard, Georges. Étude sur la fréquence des maladies nerveuses chez les indigènes musulmans d'Algérie. In: Presse Médicale. 15th Year, No 78 (28.09.1907). 624.

Lambo, Thomas Adeoye. The Role of Cultural Factors in Paranoid Psychoses Among the Yoruba Tribe of Nigeria. In: Journal of Mental Science. Vol. 101, No 423 (April 1955). 239–66.

Lasnet, Alexandre/Porot, Antoine. L'organisation de l'assistance psychiatrique en Algérie. In: Congrès des Médecins Aliénistes et Neurologistes de France et des Pays de Langue Française. 36th Session, Limoges, 25.–30.07.). Paris 1932. 385–90.

Legey, Françoise. Essai de folklore marocain. Paris 1926.

Lemanski, Witold. Hygiène du colon, ou vade-mecum de l'européen aux colonies. Paris 1902.

Lemanski, Witold. Mœurs arabes. Scènes vécues. Paris 1913.

Lemanski, Witold. Psychologie de la femme arabe. In: Revue Tunisienne. 7th Year, No 25 (Jan. 1900). 87–94.

Le quartier réservé de Casablanca. In: Presse Médicale. 34th Year, No 79 (02.10.1926). 1245.

Les aliénés dans les hôpitaux de Constantinople. In: Annales Médico-Psychologiques. 7th Series, 44th Year, Vol. 3 (1886). 499–502.

Les aliénés en liberté. Tentatives d'homicide. In: Annales Médico-Psychologiques. 9th Series, 67th Year, Vol. 9 (1909). 173 f.

Levet. L'assistance des aliénés algériens dans un asile métropolitaine. In: Annales Médico-Psychologiques. 9th Series, 67th Year, Vol. 9 (1909). 45–67; 239–49.

Lévy-Bruhl, Lucien. La mentalité primitive. Paris 1922.

L'hôpital arabe de Tunis. In: Annales Médico-Psychologiques. 6th Series, 40th Year, Vol. 7 (1882). 174 ff.

Linas, A. Les aliénés en Algérie. In: Annales Médico-Psychologiques. 5th Series, 31st Year, Vol. 9 (1873). 491 f.

Luccioni, Joseph. Les maristanes du Maroc. Le nouveau maristane de Sidi-Fredj à Fès. In: Bulletin Economique et Social du Maroc. Vol. 16, No 58 (1953). 461–70.

Lunier, Ludger. De l'augmentation progressive du chiffre des aliénés et ses causes. In: Annales Médico-Psychologiques. 5th Series, 27th Year, Vol. 3 (1870). 20–33.

Lunier, Ludger. Des aliénés en Algérie. In: Annales Médico-Psychologiques. 5th Series, 40th Year, Vol. 11 (1874). 335.

Lunier, Ludger. Review of Les aliénés en Algérie. From: Gazette Hebdomadaire. 05.11.1875. In: Annales Médico-Psychologiques. 5th Series, 34th Year, Vol. 15 (1876). 160.

Lwoff, Solomon/Sérieux, Paul. Les aliénés au Maroc. In: Annales Médico-Psychologiques. 9th Series, 69th Year, Vol. 13 (1911). 470–9.

Lwoff, Solomon/Sérieux, Paul. Note sur l'organisation de l'assistance des aliénés au Maroc. In: Annales Médico-Psychologiques. 10th Series, 71st Year, Vol. 3 (1913). 694–700.

Manceaux, G.-A./Bardenat, Charles/Susini, Robert. L'hystérie chez l'indigène algérien. Quelques aspects de ses manifestations en milieu militaire. In: Annales Médico-Psychologiques. 105th Year, Vol. 2 (1947). 1–34.

Manceaux, G.-A./Bardenat, Charles/Sutter, Jean-M./Escoutte, R. Intérêt diagnostique et pronostique du choc à la méthédrine. In: Congrès des Médecins Aliénistes et Neurologistes de France et des Pays de Langue Française. 53rd Session, Nice (05.–11.09.). Paris 1955. 301–9.

Manceaux, G.-A./Sutter, Jean-M./Bardenat, Charles/Pélicier, Yves/Counillon, G. L'héroïnomanie dans la région algéroise. In: Congrès des Médecins Aliénistes et Neurologistes de France et des Pays de Langue Française. 53rd Session, Nice (05.–11.09.). Paris 1955. 294–300.

Manceaux, G.-A./Sutter, Jean-M./Pélicier, Yves. Les états mélancoliques chez l'indigène nord-africain. A propos de cent nouvelles observations. In: Congrès des Médecins Aliénistes et Neurologistes de France et des Pays de Langue Française. 52nd Session, Liège (19.–26.07.). Paris 1954. 270–3.

Marcel, Ch. De la fréquence comparée dans nos colonies et en France de maladies non spéciales aux pays chauds. In: Presse Médicale. 14th Year, Annexe (02.05.1906). 278.

Marcé, Louis-Victor. Études sur les causes de la folie puerpérale. In: Annales Médico-Psychologiques. 3rd Year, Vol. 3 (1857). 562–84.

Maréschal, Pierre/Ben Soltane, Tahar/Corcos, Victor. Résultats du traitement par l'électro-choc appliqué à 340 malades à l'Hôpital Psychiatrique de La Manouba (Tunisie). In: Congrès des Médecins Aliénistes et Neurologistes de France et des Pays de Langue Française. 43rd Session, Montpellier (28.–30.10.) Paris 1942. 341–6.

Maréschal, Pierre/Chaurand. La paralysie générale en Tunisie. In: Congrès des Médecins Aliénistes et Neurologistes de France et des Pays de Langue Française. 41st Session, Nancy (30.06.–03.07.). Paris 1937. 247–54.

Maréschal, Pierre/Lamarche. L'assistance médicale aux aliénés en Tunisie. In: Congrès des Médecins Aliénistes et Neurologistes de France et des Pays de Langue Française. 41st Session, Nancy (30.06.–03.07.). Paris 1937. 393–401.

Maréschal, Pierre. L'héroïnomanie en Tunisie. In: Congrès des Médecins Aliénistes et Neurologistes de France et des Pays de Langue Française. 41st Session, Nancy (30.06.–03.07.). Paris 1937. 255–9.

Maréschal, Pierre. Réflexions sur vingt ans de psychiatrie en Tunisie. In: La Raison. Vol. 15 (1956). 69–79.

Mares, J./Barre, R. Quelques aspects des accidents psychiatriques de la puerpéralité en milieu musulman algérien. In: Annales Médico-Psychologiques. 120th Year, Vol. 1 (Jan. 1962). 31–49.

Margain, Louis. De l'aliénation mentale aux colonies et pays de protectorat. In: Revue Indigène. Vol. 23 (1908). 87–97.

Marie, Auguste. Immigration et hygiène mentale. Remarques à propos de l'article du docteur Martial. In: L'Hygiène Mentale. 29th Year, No 2 (Feb. 1934). 25–32.

Marie, Auguste/Godin, Pierre. Les malades musulmans à Paris. A propos de l'assistance aux psychopathes étrangers. Le problème des malades musulmans à Paris. In: L'Hygiène Mentale. 29th Year, No 2 (Feb. 1934). 33–44.

Marie, Auguste. La question de l'asile colonial. À propos des asiles indigènes égyptiens. In: Presse Médicale. 15th Year, Annexe, No 52 (29.06.1907). 417 f.

Marie, Auguste. Sur quelques aspects de la question des aliénés coloniaux. In: Bulletin de la Société de Médecine Mentale de Belgique. Dec. 1905. 754–77.

Marie, Auguste (ed.). Traité international de psychologie pathologique. 3 Volumes. Paris 1910/1911/1912.

Marill, François-Georges/Si Hassen, Abdennour. La paralysie générale progressive chez l'indigène musulman de l'Afrique du Nord. In: Annales Médico-Psychologiques. 109th Year, Vol. 1 (Jan.–May 1951). 435–64.

Maupassant, Guy de. La vie errante. Paris 1900.

Maurin, Amédée. La saison d'hiver en Algérie. Paris 1873.

Mazel, Jean de Labretoigne du. Visite au maristan de Sidi Fredj à Fez. Marseille 1922. No page numbers.

Meilhon, Abel-Joseph. Contribution à l'étude de la paralysie générale considérée chez les Arabes. In: Annales Médico-Psychologiques. 7th Series, 49th Year, Vol. 13 (1891). 384–97.

Meilhon, Abel-Joseph. L'aliénation mentale chez les Arabes: Études de nosologie comparée. In: Annales Médico-Psychologiques. 8th Series, 54th Year, Vol. 3 (1896). Part 1: 17–32. Part 2: 177–207. Part 3: 364–77. 8th Series, 54th Year, Vol. 4 (1896). Part 4: 27–40. Part 5: 204–20. Part 6: 344–63.

Menouillard, H. Mœurs indigènes: mejnoun (les possédés). In: Revue Tunisienne. 12th Year, No 54 (Nov. 1905). 477 ff.

Mignot, Roger. Les journées médicales tunisiennes et l'assistance des aliénés en Tunisie. In: L'Hygiène Mentale. 21st Year, No 6 (June 1926). 159–64.

Montpellier, J. Le problème de l'orientation de la syphilis chez les Nord-Africains. In: Presse Médicale. 34th Year, No 29 (10.04.1926). 451 f.

Moreau de Tours, Jacques-Joseph. Du hachisch et de l'aliénation mentale: Études psychologiques. Paris 1845.

Moreau de Tours, Jacques-Joseph. La psychologie morbide. Paris 1859.

Moreau de Tours, Jacques-Joseph. Recherches sur les aliénés, en Orient. In: Annales Médico-Psychologiques. Vol. 1 (1843). 103–32.

Moreau de Tours, Paul. Notes sur les asiles d'aliénés en Orient. In: Annales Médico-Psychologiques. 7th Series, 45th Year, Vol. 5 (1887). 307–12.

Morel, Bénédict-Augustin. Traité des dégénérescences physiques, intellectuelles, et morales de l'espèce humaine. Paris 1857.

Nicole, M. G. La prostitution en Egypte. In: Annales d'Hygiène Publique et de Médecine Légale. 2nd Series, Vol. 50 (July 1878). 206–15.

P(orot?), A(ntoine?). Review of Aubin, Henri. L'homme et la Magie. In: Algérie Médicale. 57th
    Year, No 1 (Jan. 1953). 93 f.

Parant, Victor. La folie puerpérale. Sa nature et ses origines d'après de récents travaux. In: Annales
    Médico-Psychologiques. 7th Series, 46th Year, Vol. 8 (1888). 62–82.

Parant, Victor. Review of Warnock, John. La folie par le hachich. From: Journal of Mental Science.
    Jan. 1903. In: Annales Médico-Psychologiques. 9th Series, 63rd Year, Vol. 2 (1905). 454 f.

Payn. Les pénitenciers indigènes et la rareté du suicide en Algérie. In: Annales Médico-Psychologiques.
    5th Series, 35th Year, Vol. 17 (1877). 300 ff.

Périale, Marise. Le maristane de Sidi Benachir appelé communément 'l'asile des fous'. In: Bulletin
    de l'Enseignement Public au Maroc. No 135, 21st Year (Nov. 1934). 383–91.

Peyre, E.-L. Les maladies mentales aux colonies. In: L'Hygiène Mentale. 29th Year, No 8 (Sept.-
    Oct. 1934). 185–212.

Pierron. Précis de jurisprudence musulmane, rite malékite. Translation of Khalil Ibn Ishaq. 6 Vol-
    umes. Paris 1852.

Pierson, C. A. Editorial. L'assistance psychiatrique au Maroc. In: Maroc Médical. 28th Year, No 287
    (April 1949). i–iv.

Pierson, C. A. Paléophrénie réactionnelle: Psycho-pathologie de l'impulsion morbide en milieu
    Nord-Africain. In: Maroc Médical. 34th Year, No 360 (May 1955). 642–7.

Pierson, C. A./Poitrot, R. P./Rolland, J. L. L'assistance psychiatrique au Maroc. In: L'Information
    Psychiatrique. 31st Year, 4th Series, No 1 (Jan. 1955). 30–7.

Piessac, Jean de. Le devoir social. L'œuvre du médecin colonial. 01. 10. 1931. No page numbers.

Poitrot, R. P. Influences climatiques à l'hôpital neuro-psychiatrique de Berrechid. In: Maroc Médi-
    cal. 32nd Year, No 342 (Nov. 1953). 1254.

Poitrot, R. P. Statistiques et remarques concernant la syphilis nerveuse au Maroc. In: Maroc Médi-
    cal. 29th Year, No 306 (Nov. 1950). 1069 f.

Porot, Antoine. Allocution de M. le Professeur Porot. In: Congrès des Médecins Aliénistes et
    Neurologistes de France et des Pays de Langue Française. 36th Session, Limoges (25.–30.07.).
    Paris 1932. 28 ff.

Porot, Antoine/Arrii, Don Côme. L'impulsivité criminelle chez l'indigène algérien. Ses facteurs. In:
    Annales Médico-Psychologiques. 14th Series, 90th Year, Vol. 2 (1932). 588–611.

Porot, Antoine. Au sujet de l'assistance psychiatrique et de l'enseignement en Algérie. In: L'Hygiène
    Mentale. 21st Year, No 3 (March 1926). 67 ff.

Porot, Antoine/Bardenat, Charles. Anormaux et malades mentaux devant la justice pénale. Paris 1960.

Porot, Antoine/Bardenat, Charles. Psychiatrie médico-légale. Paris 1959.

Porot, Antoine/Bardenat, Charles/Sutter, Jean/Porot, Maurice/Léonardon, Pierre/Kammerer,
    Th. Réflexions sur 3 000 électro-chocs pratiqués dans les services psychiatriques de l'Algérie. In:
    Congrès des Médecins Aliénistes et Neurologistes de France et des Pays de Langue Française.
    43rd Session, Montpellier (28.–30.10.) Paris 1942. 329–36.

Porot, Antoine/Bardenat, Charles/Sutter, Jean. Un cas d'échokinésie chez un indigène. In: Congrès des Médecins Aliénistes et Neurologistes de France et des Pays de Langue Française. 42nd Session, Algiers (06.–11.04.). Paris 1938. 205–10.

Porot, Antoine. Chronique algérienne. In: L'Hygiène Mentale. 20th Year, No 9 (Nov. 1925). 269–79.

Porot, Antoine. Dernier mot – en réponse à M. Dumolard – sur l'assistance psychiatrique en Algérie. In: L'Hygiène Mentale. 21st Year, No 6 (June 1926). 145.

Porot, Antoine. L'assistance psychiatrique en Algérie et le futur hôpital psychiatrique de Blida. In: Algérie Médicale. No 65 (May 1933). 86–92.

Porot, Antoine. Les services hospitaliers de psychiatrie dans l'Afrique du Nord (Algérie et Tunisie). In: Annales Médico-Psychologiques. 15th Series, 94th Year, Vol. 1 (1936). 793–803.

Porot, Antoine. L'œuvre psychiatrique de la France aux colonies depuis un siècle. In: Annales Médico-Psychologiques. 101st Year, Vol. 1 (1943). 356–78.

Porot, Antoine (ed.). Manuel alphabétique de psychiatrie clinique, thérapeutique, et médico-légale. Paris 1952.

Porot, Antoine. Notes de psychiatrie musulmane. In: Annales Médico-Psychologiques. 10th Series, 74th Year, Vol. 9 (1918). 377–84.

Porot, Antoine/Sutter, Jean. Le 'primitivisme' des indigènes Nord-Africains. Ses incidences en pathologie mentale. In: Sud Médical et Chirurgical. (15.04.1939). 226–41.

Porot, Antoine. Tunisie. In: Congrès des Médecins Aliénistes et Neurologistes de France et des Pays de Langue Française. 22nd Session, Tunis (01.–07.04.). Paris 1912. 55–75.

Porot, Maurice/Bisquerra, Émile. Note préliminaire sur l'utilisation de l'iodure de succinyl-choline dans la curarisation des malades soumis aux électrochocs. In: Congrès des Médecins Aliénistes et Neurologistes de France et des Pays de Langue Française. 52nd Session, Liège (19.–26.07.). Paris 1954. 890–5.

Porot, Maurice/Cohen-Tenoudji, A. Tuberculose et traitements psychiatriques de choc. In: Annales Médico-Psychologiques. 113th Year, Vol. 1 (Jan.–May 1955). 376–408.

Porot, Maurice/Descuns, Pierre. État actuel de la psycho-chirurgie. In: Afrique Française Chirurgicale. Vol. 13, No 6 (1955). 525–37.

Porot, Maurice/Destaing, Fernand. Streptomycine et troubles mentaux. In: Algérie Médicale. 54th Year, No 10 (Dec. 1950). 515–26.

Porot, Maurice/Duboucher, G. La guérison des alcooliques par l'antabus. Algérie Médicale. 56th Year, No 1 (Jan. 1952). 1–21.

Porot, Maurice/Duboucher, G. Quatre ans après, ou les résultats éloignés du traitement des alcooliques par le Disulfiram (Antabus). In: Algérie Médicale. 58th Year, No 8 (Aug. 1954). 641–4.

Porot, Maurice/Gentile, J. Alcoolisme et troubles mentaux chez l'indigène musulman algérien. In: Bulletin Sanitaire de l'Algérie. 36th Year, No 522 (May 1941). 125–30.

Porot, Maurice/Jouanneau, H. Traitement par la chlorpromazine seule d'un syndrome mélancolique chez une femme enceinte. In: Algérie Médicale. 60th Year, No 5 (May 1956). 395 ff.

Porot, Maurice. La leucotomie préfrontale en psychiatrie. In: Annales Médico-Psychologiques. 105th Year, Vol. 2 (1947). 121–42.

Porot, Maurice. Les retentissements psychopathologiques des évènements d'Algérie. In: Annales Médico-Psychologiques. 114th Year, Vol. 2 (1956). 622–36.

Porot, Maurice/Sutter, Jean/Bardenat, Charles. La tuberculose des aliénés. Organisation du dépistage et des soins antituberculeux dans un hôpital psychiatrique. In: Annales Médico-Psychologiques. 102nd Year, Vol. 2 (June–Dec. 1944). 398–415.

Porot, Maurice. Traitements psychiatriques de choc et grossesse. In: Presse Médicale. 57th Year, No 76 (03.12.1949). 1118 ff.

Potet, H. Au sujet de l'hygiène mentale au Maroc. In: Congrès des Médecins Aliénistes et Neurologistes de France et des Pays de Langue Française. 37th Session, Rabat (07.–13.04.). Paris 1933. 449 ff.

Prix de la société de médecine de Bordeaux pour 1846. In: Annales Médico-Psychologiques. Vol. 9 (1847). 315 f.

Ramée, F./Lacaton, R./Sanchez, François/Boulanger, M. Effets favorables du Largactil dans la pratique psychiatrique algérienne. In: Encéphale. Vol. 45, No 4 (1956). 821–7.

Reboul, Henry/Régis, Emmanuel. L'assistance des aliénés aux colonies. In: Congrès des Médecins Aliénistes et Neurologistes de France et des Pays de Langue Française. 22nd Session, Tunis (01.–07.04.). Paris 1912.

Réceptions et excursions. In: Congrès des Médecins Aliénistes et Neurologistes de France et des Pays de Langue Française. 42nd Session, Algiers (06.–11.04.). Paris 1938. 381–7.

Régis, Emmanuel. Manuel pratique de médecine mentale. Paris 1885.

Report for the Year 1917 from the Lunacy Division, Egypt, being the Twenty-Third Annual Report on the Government Asylum at Abbasiya, and the Sixth Annual Report on the Asylum at Khanka. In: Journal of Mental Science. Vol. 65 (April 1919). 131–5.

Review of Furnari. Voyage médical dans l'Afrique septentrionale. Paris 1845. In: Annales Médico-Psychologiques. Vol. 8 (1846). 148–50.

Rocher, H. L. Maurice Boigey (1877–1952). In: Presse Médicale. 61st Year, No 26 (15.04.1953). 558.

Rouquès, Lucien. Report on the Meeting of the Académie de Médecine. 07.02.1933. Note sur l'hystérie dans le Proche-Orient. In: Presse Médicale. 41st Year, No 15 (22.02.1933). 305.

Sandwith, Fleming Mant. The Cairo Lunatic Asylum, 1888. In: Journal of Mental Science. Vol. 34, No 148 (Jan. 1889). 473–90.

Savage, George H. Lunacy in Egypt, 1918. In: Journal of Mental Science. Vol. 66 (April 1920). 173 ff.

Savage, George H. Report of the Government Asylums for the Insane in Egypt for 1914. In: Journal of Mental Science. Vol. 61 (July 1915). 469 f.

Scherb, G. De la rareté des accidents nerveux chez les indigènes musulmans algériens. In: Comptes Rendus au Congrès Français de Médecine. Vol. 2 (1905).

Seignette, N. Code musulman, rite malékite, statut réel. Translation of Khalil Ibn Ishaq. Paris 1878.

Semalaigne, René. Anatomie pathologique et étiologie de la paralysie générale. In: Annales Médico-Psychologiques. 8th Series, 56th Year, Vol. 7 (1898). 464–84.

Statistique de Bicêtre et de la Salpêtrière. In: Annales Médico-Psychologiques. 3rd Series, Vol. 1 (1855). 178.

Sutter, Jean. Leçon inaugurale. Chaire de clinique neurologique et psychiatrique. In: Algérie Médicale. 63rd Year, No 5 (May 1959). 431–43.

Sutter, Jean. Les nouvelles médications anti-dépressives. In: Algérie Médicale. 66th Year, No 4 (April 1962). 391–8.

Sutter, Jean/Pascalis, Gérard. Effets psychologiques de la chlorpromazine. In: Encéphale. Vol. 45, No 4 (1956). 979–86.

Sutter, Jean/Pélicier, Yves. La crise pubertaire chez le musulman algérien. In: Congrès des Médecins Aliénistes et Neurologistes de France et des Pays de Langue Française. 57th Session, Tours (08.–13.06.). Paris 1959. 514–20.

Sutter, Jean/Porot, Maurice/Pélicier, Yves. Aspects algériens de la pathologie mentale. In: Algérie Médicale. 63rd Year, No 9 (Sept. 1959). 891–6.

Sutter, Jean. Quelques aspects de la psychogenèse en milieu indigène nord-africain. In: Maroc Médical. 28th Year, No 287 (April 1949). 215 f.

Sutter, Jean. Review of Taïeb, Suzanne. Les idées d'influences dans la pathologie mentale de l'indigène nord-africain. Le rôle des superstitions. In: Annales Médico-Psychologiques. 15th Series, 99th Year, Vol. 1 (1941). 55 f.

Sutter, Jean/Susini, Robert/Pélicier, Yves/Pascalis, Gérard. Quelques observations de psychoses nuptiales chez des musulmans d'Algérie. In: Annales Médico-Psychologiques. 117th Year, Vol. 1 (1959). 907–13.

Tablettes. In: Gazette Médicale de l'Algérie. 18th Year (1873). 35; 95.

Teissier, J.-P. Report on the Meeting of the Société de neurologie, 05.07.1906. Fréquence des maladies nerveuses chez les Arabes. In: Presse Médicale. 14th Year (18.07.1906). 459.

The Egyptian Government Hospital for the Insane. In: Journal of Mental Science. Vol. 55 (Jan. 1909). 166–70.

Trenga, Victor. L'âme arabo-berbère. Étude sociologique sur la société musulmane nord-africaine. Algiers 1913.

Tuke, William Samuel. Two Visits to the Cairo Asylum, 1877 and 1878. In: Journal of Mental Science. Vol. 25 (April 1879). 48–53.

Urquhart, A. R. Two Visits to the Cairo Asylum, 1877 and 1878. In: Journal of Mental Science. Vol. 25 (April 1879). 43–8.

Variot, Gaston. Une visite à l'hôpital arabe de Tunis. In: La Revue Scientifique de la France et de l'Étranger. 3rd Series, Vol. 1 (Jan.–July 1881). 537 f.

Vernet, Georges. Chronique. In: Annales Médico-Psychologiques. 9th Series, 63rd Year, Vol. 2 (1905). 5–21.

Villot, Charles. Mœurs, coutumes et institutions des indigènes de l'Algérie. Algiers/Paris 1875.

Vitoux, Georges. Report on the 5th Congrès de Gynécologie, d'Obstétrique et de Pédiatrie. Algiers, 01.04.–16.04.1907. Le service de gynécologie indigène à l'hôpital Zadiki, à Tunis. In: Presse Médicale. 15th Year, No 34 (27.04.1907). 268.

Voisin, Auguste. Souvenirs d'un voyage en Tunisie (1896). In: Annales Médico-Psychologiques. 8th Series, 54th Year, Vol. 4 (1896). 89 f.

Walter, Richard D. What became of the Degenerate? A Brief History of a Concept. In: Journal of the History of Medicine and Allied Sciences. Vol. 11, No 4 (Oct. 1956). 422–9.

Warnock, John. Insanity from Hasheesh. In: Journal of Mental Science. Vol. 49 (Jan. 1903). 96–100.

Warnock, John. The Twenty-First Annual Report on the Government Hospital for the Insane at Abassia, Cairo, and the Fourth Annual Report on the Asylum at Khanka. In: Journal of Mental Science. Vol. 62 (April 1916). 441–5.

Warnock, John. Twenty-Eight Years' Lunacy Experience in Egypt (1895–1923). In: Journal of Mental Science. Vol. 70 (1924). 233–61, 380–410, 579–612.

Westermarck, Edward. Ritual and Belief in Morocco. 2 Volumes. London 1926.

Dissertations

Abadie-Feyguine, Hélène. De l'assistance médicale des femmes indigènes en Algérie. Med. thesis, University of Montpellier 1905.

Aboab, Joseph. Contribution à l'étude de la neurosyphilis des indigènes musulmans de l'Afrique du Nord, basée sur la recherche méthodique du signe d'Argyll-Robertson. Med. thesis, University of Algiers 1921.

Arène, Sextius. De la criminalité des Arabes au point de vue de la pratique médico-judiciaire en Tunisie. Med. thesis, University of Lyon. Valence 1913.

Arrii, Don Côme. De l'impulsivité criminelle chez l'indigène algérien. Med. thesis, University of Algiers 1926.

Astruc, E. J. Les pratiques révulsives chez les Musulmans de l'Afrique du Nord. Med. thesis, University of Toulouse 1912.

Battarel, Pierre. Quelques remarques sur la paralysie générale chez les indigènes musulmans algériens. Étude faite à l'Hôpital de Mustapha (Alger). Med. thesis, University of Montpellier 1902.

Benkhelil, Abdesselam. Contribution à l'étude des affections neuro-psychiques et de la neuro-syphilis chez l'indigène musulman algérien. Med. thesis, University of Algiers 1927.

Borreil, Paul. Considérations sur l'internement des aliénés sénégalais en France. Med. thesis, University of Montpellier 1908.

Bouhadjeb, Hussein. Accouchement et avortement en Tunisie. Med. thesis, University of Bordeaux 1901.

Bouquet, Henry. Les aliénés en Tunisie. Med. thesis, University of Lyon 1909.

Bulliod, Jean. Étude sur la prostitution à Alger. Med. thesis, University of Toulouse 1895.

Chappert, Michèle. Contribution à l'étude des psychoses puerpérales. 80 cas de psychoses du post-partum chez les musulmanes algériennes. Med. thesis, University of Paris 1962.

Chérif, Ahmad. Histoire de la médicine arabe en Tunisie. Med. thesis, University of Bordeaux 1908.

Collomb, Jean-Marie. Essai sur l'hygiène et la pathologie de l'Assam et du Tong-Kin. Med. thesis, University of Lyon 1883.

Coudray, Jean. Considérations sur l'hôpital Sadiki et la pathologie chirurgicale indigène en Tunisie. Med. thesis, University of Montpellier. Tunis 1914.

Demassieux, Eliane. Le service social en psychiatrie. Son application à la clinique psychiâtrique de l'Université d'Alger. Med. thesis, University of Algiers 1941.

Duchêne-Marullaz, Henri. L'hygiène des musulmans d'Algérie. Med. thesis, University of Lyon 1905.

Duplenne, Blanche-Fanny-Marguerite. Étude sur la tuberculose chez les indigènes musulmans en Tunisie. Med. thesis, University of Paris 1927.

Faradj Khan, Emir. Hygiène et islamisme. Med. thesis, University of Lyon 1904.

Gervais, Camille-Charles. Contribution à l'étude du régime et du traitement des aliénés indigènes d'Algérie au point de vue médical et administratif. Med. thesis, University of Lyon 1907.

Goëau-Brissonnière, William. La syphilis nerveuse chez l'indigène musulman algérien. Contribution à l'étude de la syphilis exotique. Med. thesis, University of Algiers 1926.

Gomma, François. L'assistance médicale en Tunisie. Essai sur l'histoire de la médicine et de l'hygiène publiques dans la régence. Med. thesis, University of Toulouse. Bordeaux 1904.

Gournay, Lionel de. Les Arabes et la médecine. Med. thesis, University of Montpellier 1909.

Khiat, Simon. Essai sur le statut personnel des Musulmans. Leg. thesis, University of Aix-en-Provence 1924.

Kocher, Adolphe. De la criminalité chez les Arabes au point de vue de la pratique médico-judiciaires en Algérie. Med. thesis, University of Lyon 1883.

Lacascade, Renée. Puériculture et colonisation. Étude sur la puériculture au Maroc. Aperçu du rôle colonisateur que peut jouer la femme médecin dans les pays d'occupation. Med. thesis, University of Paris 1922.

Lacaze, Henri. De la criminalité féminine en France. Étude statistique et médico-légale. Med. thesis, University of Lyon 1910.

Lafitte, Joseph-Marie-Fernand. Contribution à l'étude médicale de la Tunisie. Climatologie, hydrographie, ethnographie, flore, faune, maladies prédominantes. Med. thesis, University of Bordeaux 1892.

Lataillade, Louis. Coutumes et superstitions obstétricales en Afrique du Nord. Med. thesis, University of Algiers 1936.

Laurens, Étienne-Paul. Contribution à l'étude de la syphilis nerveuse chez les indigènes mahométans de l'Algérie. Med. thesis, University of Algiers 1919.

Lauriol, Louis. Quelques remarques sur les maladies mentales aux colonies. Med. thesis, University of Paris 1938.

Lévy-Bram, Abel. L'assistance médicale des indigènes d'Algérie, particulièrement assistance médicale des femmes et des enfants (Essai sur cette assistance pour les femmes et les enfants). Med. thesis, University of Paris 1907.

Livet, Louis. Les aliénés algériens et leur hospitalisation. Med. thesis, University of Algiers 1911.

Luccioni, Joseph. Le habous ou wakf (rites malékite et hanéfite). Leg. thesis, University of Algiers. Casablanca 1942.

Malmassari, Jean. De l'avortement chez la femme indigène musulmane, principalement en Algérie. Med. thesis, University of Algiers 1934.

Mansouri, Abdallah. Contribution des Arabes au progrès des sciences médicales. Med. thesis, University of Lyon 1923.

Matignon, Raymond-Joseph. L'art médical à Tunis. Med. thesis, University of Bordeaux 1901.

Milliot, Louis. Étude sur la condition de la femme musulmane au Maghreb (Maroc, Algérie, Tunisie). Leg. thesis, University of Paris 1910.

Monnery, Maurice. La pratique de l'hygiène sociale et l'action médicale en Tunisie (Essai d'hygiène sociale). Med. thesis, University of Lyon 1924.

Montaldo, Pierre. Mortalité infantile en Algérie. Polymortalité et hérédo-syphilis chez l'enfant indigène algérien. Med. thesis, University of Algiers 1933.

Naudin, Lucien-Joseph-Victor. La psychiatrie coloniale: Essai clinique et médico-légal. Med. thesis, University of Bordeaux 1913.

Olry, Jean. La paralysie générale chez les indigènes musulmans de Tunisie. Travail de l'Hôpital de la Manouba. Med. thesis, University of Marseille 1940.

Pascalis, Élie. De la paralysie générale chez les Arabes. Med. thesis, University of Montpellier 1893.

Pasqualini, Henri. Contribution à l'étude de la médecine traditionnelle au Maroc. Med. thesis, University of Bordeaux. Rabat 1957.

Perrin, Gabriel. Essai sur la médicine des arabes et l'assistance médicale des indigènes de l'Algérie. Med. thesis, University of Toulouse 1895.

Richardot, Armand. Les pratiques médicales des indigènes de l'Algérie. Med. thesis, University of Toulouse 1896.

Sauzay, Paul. L'assistance aux psychopathes (aliénés et non aliénés) en Algérie. Etat actuel de la question. Med. thesis, University of Algiers 1925.

Sérieux, Paul. Recherches cliniques sur les anomalies de l'instinct sexuel. Med. thesis, University of Paris 1888.

Sicard, Georges. Étude sur la fréquence des maladies nerveuses chez les indigènes musulmans d'Algérie. Med. thesis, University of Lyon. Paris 1907.

Soumeire, Henri. Le meurtre chez les aliénés indigènes en Algérie. Med. thesis, University of Marseille 1932.

Susini, Paul. Quelques considérations sur la syphilis des indigènes d'Algérie. Med. thesis, University of Paris 1920.

Susini, Robert. Aspects cliniques de l'hystérie chez l'indigène nord-africain (en milieu militaire). Med. thesis, University of Algiers 1947.

Sutter, Jean. L'épilepsie mentale chez l'indigène nord-africain (étude clinique). Med. thesis, University of Algiers 1937.

Taïeb, Suzanne. Les idées d'influence dans la pathologie mentale de l'indigène nord-africain. Le rôle des superstitions. Med. thesis, University of Algiers 1939.

Thierry, H. Étude sur les pratiques et superstitions médicales des Marocains et sur l'influence de la médecine française au Maroc. Med. thesis, University of Paris 1917.

Thierry, Michel-Jacques. L'œuvre médicale française au Maroc. Med. thesis, University of Bordeaux 1953.

Tremsal, Jean-Joseph-Marie. Un siècle de médecine coloniale française en Algérie (1830–1929). Contribution à l'étude de l'œuvre médicale française en Afrique du Nord. Med. thesis, University of Algiers. Tunis 1928.

Trenga, Victor. Sur les psychoses chez les Juifs d'Algérie. Med. thesis, University of Montpellier. Lyon 1902.

Vadon, Raoul. L'assistance médicale des psychopathes en Tunisie. Med. thesis, University of Marseille 1935.

Wiehn, Gaston-Edouard-Narcisse-Pierre. Le service médical dans le bled et les internes français des hôpitaux de Tunisie. Med. thesis, University of Bordeaux 1904.

Wolters, L. Du rôle de l'instituteur en Kabylie. Au point de vue de la médecine de colonisation. Med. thesis, University of Toulouse 1902.

Woytt-Gisclard, Alix. L'assistance aux indigènes musulmans au Maroc. Leg. thesis, University of Paris 1936.

Secondary Literature

Adamson, Kay. Approaches to the Study of Women in North Africa: As Reflected in Research of Various Scholars. In: Maghreb Review. Vol. 3, No 7/8 (May–Aug. 1978). 22–31.

Ageron, Charles Robert. Histoire de l'Algérie contemporaine (1830–1970). Paris 1964.

Ahmed, Leila. Western Ethnocentrism and Perceptions of the Harem. In: Feminist Studies. Vol. 8, No 3 (Autumn 1982). 521–34.

Akhmisse, Mustapha. Médecine, magie et sorcellerie au Maroc. Casablanca 2005.

Aldrich, Robert. Colonial Man. In: Forth, Christopher E./Taithe, Bertrand (ed.). French Masculinities. History, Culture and Politics. Basingstoke/New York 2007. 123–40.

Al-Issa, Ihsan/Al-Issa, Brigitta. Psychiatric Problems in a Developing Country: Iraq. In: International Journal of Social Psychiatry. Vol. 16, No 1 (Jan. 1970). 15–22.

Al-Issa, Ihsan. Culture and Mental Illness in Algeria. In: International Journal of Social Psychiatry. Vol. 36, No 3 (1990). 230–40. Also in: Ibid. (ed.). Al-Junūn: Mental Illness in the Islamic World. Madison 2000. 101–19.

Al-Issa, Ihsan. Mental Illness in Medieval Society. In: Ibid. (ed.). Al-Junūn: Mental Illness in the Islamic World. Madison 2000. 43–70.

Al-Issa, Ihsan. Psychiatry in Algeria. In: Psychiatric Bulletin. Vol. 13 (1989). 240–5.

Al-Krenawi, Alean. Explanations of Mental Health Symptoms by the Bedouin-Arabs of the Negev. In: International Journal of Social Psychiatry. Vol. 45, No 1 (March 1999). 56–64.

Al-Krenawi, Alean/Graham, John R. Gender and Biomedical/Traditional Mental Health Utilization among the Bedouin-Arabs of the Negev. In: Culture, Medicine and Psychiatry. Vol. 23 (1999). 219–43.

Al-Krenawi, Alean/Graham, John R./Ophir, Menachim/Kandah, Jamil. Ethnic and Gender Differences in Mental Health Utilization: The Case of Muslim Jordanian and Moroccan Jewish

Israeli Out-Patient Psychiatric Patients. In: International Journal of Social Psychiatry. Vol. 47, No 3 (Sept. 2001). 42–54.

Al-Krenawi, Alean. Women from Polygamous and Monogamous Marriages in an Out-Patient Psychiatric Clinic. In: Transcultural Psychiatry. Vol. 38, No 2 (June 2001). 187–99.

Almeida, Zulmiro de. Les perturbations mentales chez les migrants. In: L'Information Psychiatrique. Vol. 51, No 3 (March 1975). 249–81.

Al-Sawaf, Mona/Al-Issa, Ihsan. Sex and Sexual Dysfunction in an Arab-Islamic Society. In: Al-Issa, Ihsan (ed.). Al-Junūn: Mental Illness in the Islamic World. Madison 2000. 295–311.

Ammar, Sleïm. Aperçu épidémiologique des troubles mentaux en Tunisie. Étude clinique, statistique et socio-culturelle centrée sur la dernière décennie. In: L'Information Psychiatrique. Vol. 48, No 7 (Sept. 1972). 677–718.

Ammar, Sleïm. Ethnopsychiatrie et psychiatrie transculturelle. Introduction à une compréhension en profondeur de la psychopathologie tunisienne. In: Tunisie Médicale. 48th Year, No 4 (July–Aug. 1970). 217–23. 48th Year, No 5 (Sept.–Oct. 1970). 295–309.

Ammar, Sleïm. Ethnopsychiatrie et psychiatrie transculturelle: Introduction aux problèmes posés par l'impact de l'acculturation sur la santé mentale au Maghreb. In: Tunisie Médicale. 53rd Year, No 6 (Nov.–Dec. 1975). 315–30.

Ammar, Sleïm. Histoire de la psychiatrie maghrébine. In: Douki, Saïda/Moussaoui, Driss/Kacha, Farid (ed.). Manuel de psychiatrie du praticien maghrébin. Paris 1987. 1–15.

Ammar, Sleïm. L'assistance psychiatrique en Tunisie. Aperçu historique. In: L'Information Psychiatrique. Vol. 48, No 7 (Sept. 1972). 647–57.

Ammar, Sleïm. Les relations de la psychiatrie tunisienne avec la psychiatrie française. In: Annales de Thérapeutique Psychiatrique. Vol. 4. Baruk, Henri (ed.). La psychiatrie française dans ses rapports avec les autres psychiatries. Paris 1969. 185–93.

Ammar, Sleïm. L'hôpital pour les maladies mentales de la Manouba (l'Hôpital Psychiatrique Rhazi actuel). In: L'Information Psychiatrique. Vol. 48, No 7 (Sept. 1972). 659–74.

Ammar, Sleïm/M'Barek, Ezzeddine. L'hystérie chez la jeune fille et la femme tunisienne. Aspects cliniques, etiopathogéniques, épidémiologiques et évolutifs. A propos de 60 cas. In: Tunisie Médicale. 39th Year, No 4 (July–Aug. 1961). 479–94.

Amster, Ellen. 'The Harem Revealed' and the Islamic-French Family. Aline de Lens and a French Woman's Orient in Lyautey's Morocco. In: French Historical Studies. Vol. 32, No 2 (Spring 2009). 279–312.

Aouattah, Ali. Ethnopsychiatrie maghrébine. Représentations et thérapies traditionnelles de la maladie mentale au Maroc. Paris 1993.

Aouattah, Ali. Maladie mentale et thérapie maraboutique au Maroc. Le cas Bouia Omar. In: Psychopathologie Africaine. Vol. 23, No 2 (1990–91). 173–96.

Arabi, Oussama. The Regimentation of the Subject: Madness in Islamic and Modern Arab Civil Laws. In: Dupret, Baudouin (ed.). Standing Trial: Law and the Person in the Modern Middle East. London/New York 2004. 264–93.

Arnold, David. European Orphans and Vagrants in India in the Nineteenth Century. In: Journal of Imperial and Commonwealth History. Vol. 7, No 2 (1979). 104–27.

Arnold, David. White Colonization and Labour in Nineteenth-Century India. In: Journal of Imperial and Commonwealth History. Vol. 11, No 2 (1983). 133–58.

Baruk, Henri. La psychiatrie française de Pinel à nos jours. Paris 1967.

Bay, Ellen. Islamische Krankenhäuser im Mittelalter unter besonderer Berücksichtigung der Psychiatrie. Med. thesis, University of Düsseldorf 1967.

Bazzoui, Widad/Al-Issa, Ihsan. Psychiatry in Iraq. In: British Journal of Psychiatry. Vol. 112 (1966). 827–32.

Bégué, Jean-Michel. French Psychiatry in Algeria (1830–1962): from Colonial to Transcultural. In: History of Psychiatry. Vol. 7 (1996). 533–48.

Belkamel, Bidaouia/Raouyane, Boujemaa. Les bimaristanes au Maroc. In: Moussaoui, Driss/Roux-Dessarps, Michel (ed.). Histoire de la médecine au Maroc et dans les pays arabes et musulmans. Casablanca 1995. 47–50.

Bennani, Jalil. La psychanalyse au pays des saints. Les débuts de la psychiatrie et de la psychanalyse au Maroc. Casablanca 1996.

Bensmail, B. M./Bencharif, A. K./Bentorki, H. Considérations sur l'assistance et la morbidité psychiatriques dans l'est algérien. In: Tunisie Médicale. 53rd Year, No 6 (Nov.–Dec. 1975). 393–406.

Bensmail, B. Généralités sur les névroses. In: Douki, Saïda/Moussaoui, Driss/Kacha, Farid (ed.). Manuel de psychiatrie du praticien maghrébin. Paris 1987. 101–8.

Berthelier, Robert. À la recherche de l'homme musulman. In: Sud/Nord. Vol. 1, No 22 (2007). 127–46.

Berthelier, Robert. Fanon, psychiatre encore et toujours. In: VST – Vie sociale et traitements. No 89 (2006). 76–84.

Berthelier, Robert. Incidence psychopathologique de la transplantation d'une population musulmane. Med. thesis, University of Lyon 1966.

Berthelier, Robert. L'homme maghrébin dans la littérature psychiatrique. Paris 1994.

Betts, Raymond F. Assimilation and Association in French Colonial Theory, 1890–1914. New York/London 1961.

Boucebci, Mahfoud. Aspects actuels de la psychiatrie en Algérie. In: L'Information Psychiatrique. Vol. 66, No 10 (Dec. 1990). 951–62.

Boucebci, Mahfoud. Aspects de la psychiatrie en milieu traditionnel algérien. In: Psychologie Médicale. Vol. 13, No 10 (1981). 1527–34. Also in: Berthelier, Robert. L'homme maghrébin dans la littérature psychiatrique. Paris 1994. 175–96.

Boucebci, Mahfoud. Aspects du développement psychologique de l'enfant au Maghreb. In: Santé Mentale au Québec. Vol. 18, No 1 (1993). 163–78.

Boucebci, Mahfoud. Le psychiatre et ses questions face aux pratiques traditionnelles au Maghreb. In: Annales Médico-Psychologiques. 143rd Year (1985). 519–40.

Boucebci, Mahfoud. Psychopathologie sociale en Algérie. In: Les Temps Modernes. 39th Year, No 432–33 (July–Aug. 1982). 199–217.

Boucebci, Mahfoud/Yaker, Annie. Aspects généraux et tendances évolutives de la psychiatrie en Algérie. In: Tunisie Médicale. 53rd Year, No 6 (Nov.–Dec. 1975). 355–65.

Bouhdiba, Abdelwahab. Criminalité et changements sociaux en Tunisie: Étude sociologique. Tunis 1965.

Bouricha, H. Le service de neuropsychiatrie de Sfax et les problèmes posés par la décentralisation des établissements et institutions psychiatriques. In: L'Information Psychiatrique. Vol. 48, No 7 (Sept. 1972). 739–48.

Bowlan, Jeanne. Civilizing Gender Relations in Algeria: The Paradoxical Case of Marie Bugéja, 1919–39. In: Clancy-Smith, Julia/Gouda, Frances (ed.). Domesticating the Empire: Race, Gender, and Family Life in French and Dutch Colonialism. Charlottesville/London 1998. 175–92.

Brown, Penelope/Macintyre, Marthe/Morpeth, Rose/Prendergast, Shirley. A Daughter: A Thing to be Given Away. In: Women in Society. Interdisciplinary Essays. London 1981. 127–45.

Bullard, Alice. The Critical Impact of Frantz Fanon and Henri Collomb: Race, Gender, and Personality Testing of North and West Africans. In: Journal of the History of the Behavioral Sciences. Vol. 41, No 3 (Summer 2005). 225–48.

Bullard, Alice. The Truth in Madness. In: South Atlantic Review. Vol. 66, No 2 (Spring 2001). 114–32.

Busfield, Joan. Mental Illness as Social Product or Social Construct: A Contradiction in Feminists' Arguments? In: Sociology of Health and Illness. Vol. 10 (1988). 521–42.

Busfield, Joan. The Female Malady? Men, Women and Madness in Nineteenth-Century Britain. In: Sociology. Vol. 28, No 1 (Feb. 1994). 259–77.

Butts, Hugh F. Frantz Fanon's Contribution to Psychiatry: The Psychology of Racism and Colonialism. In: Journal of the National Medical Association. Vol. 71, No 10 (1979). 1015–8.

Bynum, William F. Rationales for Therapy in British Psychiatry: 1785–1835. In: Medical History. Vol. 18 (1974). 317–34.

Bynum, William F. The Nervous Patient in Eighteenth- and Nineteenth-Century Britain: The Psychiatric Origins of British Neurology. In: Bynum, William F./Porter, Roy/Shepherd, Michael (ed.). The Anatomy of Madness. Essays in the History of Psychiatry. Vol. 1. London/New York 1985. 89–102.

Chakib, Abdelfattah/Battas, Omar/Moussaoui, Driss. Le maristane Sidi-Frej à Fès. In: Histoire des Sciences Médicales. Vol. 28, No 2 (1994). 171–5. Also in: Moussaoui, Driss/Roux-Dessarps, Michel (ed.). Histoire de la médecine au Maroc et dans les pays arabes et musulmans. Casablanca 1995. 59–62.

Chaleby, Kutaiba S. Forensic Psychiatry in Islamic Jurisprudence. Herndon 2001.

Chaleby, Kutaiba S. Psychosocial Stresses and Psychiatric Disorders in an Outpatient Population in Saudis. In: Acta Psychiatrica Scandinavica. Vol. 73, No 2 (Feb. 1986). 147–51.

Chaleby, Kutaiba S. Traditional Arabian Marriages and Mental Health in a Group of Outpatient Saudis. In: Acta Psychiatrica Scandinavica. Vol. 77, No 2 (Feb. 1988). 139–42.

Chaleby, Kutaiba S. Women of Polygamous Marriages in an Inpatient Psychiatric Service in Kuwait. In: Journal of Nervous and Mental Disease. Vol. 173, No 1 (Jan. 1985). 56 ff.

Cherki, Alice. Frantz Fanon, portrait. Paris 2000.

Chinchilla Sánchez, Kattya María. La religión y la salud mental, desde la perspectiva musulmana. In: ILU, Revista de Ciencias de las Religiones. No 9 (2004). 37–68.

Chkili, Taïeb/El Khamlichi, A. Les psychoses puerpérales en milieu marocain (à propos de cent observations). In: Tunisie Médicale. 53rd Year, No 6 (Nov.–Dec. 1975). 375–91.

Clancy-Smith, Julia. Islam, Gender, and Identities in the Making of Colonial Algeria, 1830–1962. In: Clancy-Smith, Julia/Gouda, Frances (ed.). Domesticating the Empire: Race, Gender, and Family Life in French and Dutch Colonialism. Charlottesville/London 1998. 154–74.

Clancy-Smith, Julia. La Femme Arabe. Women and Sexuality in France's North African Empire. In: El Azhary Sonbol, Amira (ed.). Women, the Family, and Divorce Laws in Islamic History. New York 1996. 52–63.

Cloarec, Françoise. Bîmâristâns, lieux de folies et de sagesse: La folie et ses traitements dans les hôpitaux médiévaux au Moyen-Orient. Paris 1998.

Collignon, René. La construction du sujet colonial: le cas particulier des malades mentaux: Difficultés d'une psychiatrie en terre africaine. In: Kail, Michel/Vermès, Geneviève (ed.). La psychologie des peuples et ses dérives. Paris 1999. 165–81.

Collignon, René. La psychiatrie coloniale française en Algérie et au Sénégal. In: Revue Tiers Monde. Vol. 47, No 187 (2006). 527–46.

Collot, Claude. Les institutions de l'Algérie durant la période coloniale (1830–1962). Paris 1987.

Conklin, Alice. A Mission to Civilize: The Republican Idea of Empire in France and West Africa, 1895–1930. Stanford 1997.

Constantinides, Pamela. Women Heal Women: Spirit Possession and Sexual Segregation in a Muslim Society. In: Social Science and Medicine. Vol. 21, No 6 (1985). 685–92.

Crapanzano, Vincent. The Ḥamadsha: A Study in Moroccan Ethnopsychiatry. Berkeley 1973.

Dols, Michael Walters. Historical Perspective: Insanity in Islamic Law. In: Journal of Muslim Mental Health. Vol. 2, No 1 (2007). 81–99.

Dols, Michael Walters. Majnūn: the Madman in Medieval Islamic Society. Oxford 1992.

Dols, Michael Walters. The Origins of the Islamic Hospital: Myth and Reality. In: Bulletin of the History of Medicine. Vol. 61 (1987). 367–90.

Dorph, Kenneth Jan. Islamic Law in Contemporary North Africa: A Study of the Laws of Divorce in the Maghreb. In: Women's Studies International Forum. Vol. 5, No 2 (1982). 169–82.

Douki, Saïda/Ben Zineb, S./Nacef, F./Halbreich, U. Women's Mental Health in the Muslim World: Cultural, Religious, and Social Issues. In: Journal of Affective Disorders. Vol. 102 (2007). 177–189.

Douki, Saïda. Hystérie. In: Douki, Saïda/Moussaoui, Driss/Kacha, Farid (ed.). Manuel de psychiatrie du praticien maghrébin. Paris 1987. 109–19.

Douki, Saïda/Kacha, Farid/Moussaoui, Driss. Introduction. In: Douki, Saïda/Moussaoui, Driss/Kacha, Farid (ed.). Manuel de psychiatrie du praticien maghrébin. Paris 1987. xi f.

Douki, Saïda/Nacef, Fathy/Ben Zineb, Sara. La psychiatrie en Tunisie: une discipline en devenir. In: L'Information Psychiatrique. Vol. 81, No 1 (Jan. 2005). 49–59.

Dowbiggin, Ian. Back to the Future: Valentin Magnan, French Psychiatry, and the Classification of Mental Diseases, 1885–1925. In: Social History of Medicine. Vol. 9, No 3 (Dec. 1996). 383–408.

Dowbiggin, Ian. Degeneration and Hereditarianism in French Mental Medicine 1840–90: Psychiatric Theory as Ideological Adaption. In: Bynum, William F./Porter, Roy/Shepherd, Michael (ed.). The Anatomy of Madness. Essays in the History of Psychiatry. Vol. 1. London/New York 1985. 188–232.

Dowbiggin, Ian. Inheriting Madness: Professionalization and Psychiatric Knowledge in Nineteenth-Century France. Berkeley/Los Angeles/Oxford 1991.

Edgerton, Robert B. Traditional Treatment for Mental Illness in Africa: A Review. In: Culture, Medicine and Psychiatry. Vol. 4, No 2 (1980). 167–89.

El Ayadi, Mohammed. Les maristanes dans le monde arabo-musulman. In: Moussaoui, Driss/Roux-Dessarps, Michel (ed.). Histoire de la médecine au Maroc et dans les pays arabes et musulmans. Casablanca 1995. 19–26.

El-Islam, M. Fakhr. Mental Illness in Kuwait and Qatar. In: Al-Issa, Ihsan (ed.). Al-Junūn: Mental Illness in the Islamic World. Madison 2000. 121–37.

El-Khayat, Ghita. Tradition et modernité dans la psychiatrie marocaine. In: Ethnopsychiatrica. Vol. 1, No 1 (1978). 61–78.

El-Khayat, Ghita. Une psychiatrie moderne pour le Maghreb. Paris 1994.

El-Khayat, Rita. Observations, la pratique. In: El-Khayat, Rita/Goussot, Alain (ed.). Psychiatrie, culture et politique. Casablanca 2005. 13–72.

El Saadawi, Nawal. Women and Islam. In: Women's Studies International Forum. Vol. 5, No 2 (1982). 193–206.

El-Saadi, Hoda. Changing Attitudes towards Women's Madness in Nineteenth-Century Egypt. In: Hawwa. Vol. 3, No 3 (2005). 293–308.

Elsarrag, M. E. Psychiatry in the Northern Sudan: A Study in Comparative Psychiatry. In: British Journal of Psychiatry. Vol. 114 (1968). 945–8.

Ernst, Waltraud. European Madness and Gender in Nineteenth-Century British India. In: Social History of Medicine. Vol. 9. No 3 (Dec. 1996). 357–82.

Ernst, Waltraud. Idioms of Madness and Colonial Boundaries: The Case of the European and 'Native' Mentally Ill in Early Nineteenth-Century British India. In: Comparative Studies in Society and History. Vol. 39, No 1 (Jan. 1997). 153–81.

Everitt, B. S. Statistics in Psychiatry. In: Statistical Science. Vol. 2, No 2 (May 1987). 107–16.

Faranda, Laura. La signora di Blida. Suzanne Taïeb et il presagio dell'etnopsichiatria. Rome 2012.

Fau-Vincenti, Véronique. Vers les UMD, questionnements, tâtonnements et mise en œuvre: Gaillon (1876) et Villejuif (1910). In: Guignard, Laurence/Guillemain, Hervé/Tison, Stéphane (ed.). Expériences de la folie. Criminels, soldats, patients en psychiatrie (XIXᵉ–XXᵉ siècles). Rennes 2013. 69–79.

Fernando, Suman. Mental Health, Race and Culture. New York 1991.

Foucault, Michel. Histoire de la folie à l'âge classique. Paris 1972.

Foucault, Michel. Maladie mentale et psychologie. Paris 2008.

Gallagher, Nancy Elizabeth. Medicine and Power in Tunisia, 1780–1900. New York 1983.

Gates, Henry Louis Jr. Critical Fanonism. In: Critical Inquiry. Vol. 17, No 3 (Spring 1991). 457–70.

Gelfand, Toby. Charcot in Morocco. Introduction, Notes and Translation. Ottawa 2012.

George, Rosemary Marangoly. Homes in the Empire, Empires in the Home. In: Cultural Critique. Vol. 26 (Winter 1993–1994). 95–127.

German, G. Allen. Mental Health in Africa I: The Extent of Mental Health Problems in Africa Today. In: British Journal of Psychiatry. Vol. 151 (Oct. 1987). 435–9. Mental Health in Africa II: The Nature of Mental Disorder in Africa Today. Some Clinical Observations. In: British Journal of Psychiatry. Vol. 151, No 4 (1987). 440–6.

Goldstein, Jan. Console and Classify: The French Psychiatric Profession in the Nineteenth Century. Chicago/London 2001.

Goldstein, Jan. The Hysteria Diagnosis and the Politics of Anticlericalism in Late Nineteenth-Century France. In: Journal of Modern History. Vol. 54, No 2 (June 1982). 209–39.

Gordon, David C. Women of Algeria. An Essay of Change. Cambridge MA 1968.

Gouriou, Fabien. Psychopathologie et migration. Repérage historique et épistémologique dans le contexte français. Psych. thesis, University of Rennes 2008.

Guignard, Laurence. Prémices de la dangerosité. Les 'hommes dangereux' aux Assises avant la Défense social (1860–1880). In: Guignard, Laurence/Guillemain, Hervé/Tison, Stéphane (ed.). Expériences de la folie. Criminels, soldats, patients en psychiatrie (XIXᵉ–XXᵉ siècles). Rennes 2013. 35–45.

Guillemain, Hervé. Le malheur est-il le crime? Aperçus sur les conceptions de la 'fureur' dans l'institution asilaire (1800–1920). In: Guignard, Laurence/Guillemain, Hervé/Tison, Stéphane (ed.). Expériences de la folie. Criminels, soldats, patients en psychiatrie (XIXᵉ–XXᵉ siècles). Rennes 2013. 25–33.

Hakkou, F. Traitements psychopharmacologiques. In: Douki, Saïda/Moussaoui, Driss/Kacha, Farid (ed.). Manuel de psychiatrie du praticien maghrébin. Paris 1987. 243–56.

Hand, D. J. The Role of Statistics in Psychiatry. In: Psychological Medicine. Vol. 15 (1985). 471–6.

Harsin, Jill. Gender, Class, and Madness in Nineteenth-Century France. In: French Historical Studies. Vol. 17, No 4 (Autumn 1992). 1048–70.

Hatem, Mervat. The Politics of Sexuality and Gender in Segregated Patriarchal Systems: The Case of Eighteenth- and Nineteenth-Century Egypt. In: Feminist Studies. Vol. 12, No 2 (Summer 1986). 251–74.

Hughes, Peter. Psychiatry in Sudan: A Personal Experience. In: Psychiatric Bulletin. Vol. 20 (1996). 46 f.

Ifrah, Albert. Le Maghreb déchiré: tradition, folie et migration. Paris 1980.

Jacob, Françoise. La psychiatrie française face au monde colonial au XIXᵉ siècle. In: Découvertes et explorateurs: Actes du Colloque International (Bordeaux, 12.–14. 06. 1992). VIIᵉ Colloque d'Histoire au Présent. Paris 1994. 365–73.

Jordanova, Ludmilla J. Mental Illness, Mental Illness: Changing Norms and Expectations. In: Women in Society. Interdisciplinary Essays. London 1981. 95–114.

Joseph, Suad. Patriarchy and Development in the Arab World. In: Gender and Development. Vol. 4, No 2 (June 1996). 14–9.

Kabbani, Rana. Imperial Fictions. Europe's Myths of Orient. London 2008.

Kamel, Kateb. Population et organisation de l'espace en Algérie. In: L'Espace Géographique. Vol. 32, No 4 (2003). 311–31.

Katchadourian, Herant A. A Survey of Treated Psychiatric Illness in Lebanon. In: British Journal of Psychiatry. Vol. 114 (1968). 21–9.

Keddie, Nikki. Problems in the Study of Middle Eastern Women. In: International Journal of Middle Eastern Studies. Vol. 10, No 2 (May 1979). 225–40.

Keller, Richard Charles. Clinician and Revolutionary: Frantz Fanon, Biography, and the History of Colonial Medicine. In: Bulletin of the History of Medicine. Vol. 81, No 4 (Winter 2007). 823–841.

Keller, Richard Charles. Colonial Madness. Psychiatry in French North Africa. Chicago/London 2007.

Keller, Richard Charles. Madness and Colonization: Psychiatry in the British and French Empires, 1800–1962. In: Journal of Social History. Vol. 35, No 2 (Winter 2001). 295–326.

Keller, Richard Charles. Pinel in the Maghreb: Liberation, Confinement, and Psychiatric Reform in French North Africa. In: Bulletin of the History of Medicine. Vol. 79, No 3 (Autumn 2005). 459–99.

Keller, Richard Charles. Taking Science to the Colonies: Psychiatric Innovation in France and North Africa. In: Mahone, Sloan/Vaughan, Megan (ed.). Psychiatry and Empire. Basingstoke 2007. 17–40.

Kogelmann, Franz. Sidi Fredj: A Case Study of a Religious Endowment in Morocco. Under the French Protectorate. In: Weiss, Holger (ed.). Social Welfare in Muslim Societies in Africa. Stockholm 2002. 66–79.

Labidi, Lilia. Rita El-Khayat on Moroccan Psychiatry and Sexuality. In: Women's History Review. Vol. 15, No 4 (Sept. 2006). 637–49.

L'activité des services de santé mentale dans l'ouest algérien. In: L'Information Psychiatrique. Vol. 45, No 8 (Oct. 1969). 819 ff.

Lazreg, Marnia. Feminism and Difference: The Perils of Writing as a Woman on Women in Algeria. In: Feminist Studies. Vol. 14, No 1 (Spring 1988). 81–107.

Lazreg, Marnia. The Eloquence of Silence: Algerian Women in Question. New York/London 1994.

Leckie, Jacqueline. Unsettled Minds: Gender and Settling Madness in Fiji. In: Mahone, Sloan/Vaughan, Megan (ed.). Psychiatry and Empire. Basingstoke 2007. 99–123.

Léonard, Jacques. Médecine et colonisation en Algérie au XIXᵉ siècle. In: Annales de Bretagne et des Pays de l'Ouest. Vol. 84, No 2 (1977). 481–94.

L'hôpital psychiatrique de Blida de 1961 à 1968. In: L'Information Psychiatrique. Vol. 45, No 8 (Oct. 1969). 823–8.

Limbert, Mandana. Spirit Possession: Arab States. In: Encyclopedia of Women and Islamic Cultures. Vol. 3. Family, Body, Sexuality and Health. Leiden/Boston 2006. 425 f.

Littlewood, Roland/Cross, Sybil. Ethnic Minorities and Psychiatric Services. In: Sociology of Health and Illness. Vol. 2 (02.07.1980). 194–201.

Lorcin, Patricia M. E. Imperial Identities: Stereotyping, Prejudice, and Race in Colonial Algeria. London 1995.

Lorcin, Patricia M. E. Imperialism, Colonial Identity, and Race in Algeria, 1830–1870: The Role of the French Medical Corps. In: Isis. Vol. 90, No 4 (Dec. 1999). 653–79.

Lorcin, Patricia M. E. Rome and France in Africa: Recovering Colonial Algeria's Latin Past. In: French Historical Studies. Vol. 25, No 2 (2002). 295–329.

Louçaief, Moncef. Les manifestations hystériques chez le Tunisien en milieu civil et militaire. A propos de 25 observations. Med. thesis, University of Paris 1965.

Loudon, Irvine. Puerperal Insanity in the 19th Century. In: Journal of the Royal Society of Medicine. Vol. 81 (Feb. 1988). 76–9.

Loukas, M./Shea, M./Shea, C./Lutter-Hoppenheim, M./Zand, P./Tubbs, R. S./Cohen-Gadol, A. A. Jean Baptiste Paulin Trolard (1842–1910): His Life and Contributions to Neuroanatomy. In: Journal of Neurosurgery. Vol. 112, No 6 (June 2010). 1192–6.

Loussaief, Moncef. L'assistance psychiatrique en Tunisie et ses problèmes. In: Tunisie Médicale. 48th Year, No 2 (March–April 1970). 77–85.

Macey, David. The Algerian with the Knife. In: Parallax. Vol. 4, No 2 (1998). 159–67.

Maher, Vanessa. Women and Social Change in Morocco. In: Beck, Lois/Keddie, Nikki (ed.). Women in the Muslim World. Cambridge MA/London 1978. 100–23.

Mahone, Sloan. East African Psychiatry and the Practical Problems of Empire. In: Mahone, Sloan/Vaughan, Megan (ed.). Psychiatry and Empire. Basingstoke 2007. 41–66.

Mahone, Sloan. Psychiatry in the East African Colonies: A Background to Confinement. In: International Review of Psychiatry. Vol. 18, No 4 (Aug. 2006). 327–32.

Mahone, Sloan. The Psychology of Rebellion: Colonial Medical Responses to Dissent in British East Africa. In: Journal of African History. Vol. 47, No 2 (2006). 241–58.

Maison, Dominique. La population de l'Algérie. In: Population. 28th Year, No 6 (1973). 1079–107.

Mallem, Leïla. La folie féminine et ses représentations romanesques dans quelques œuvres algériennes et libanaises. Lit. thesis, University of Paris 1999.

Marland, Hilary. Disappointment and Desolation: Women, Doctors and Interpretations of Puerperal Insanity in the Nineteenth Century. In: History of Psychiatry. Vol. 14, No 3 (2003). 303–20.

Marsot, Afaf Lufti al-Sayyid. The Revolutionary Gentlewomen in Egypt. In: Beck, Lois/Keddie, Nikki (ed.). Women in the Muslim World. Cambridge MA/London 1978. 261–76.

Massad, Joseph A. Desiring Arabs. London 2007.

Maupomé, J.-J. Sur quelques aspects de la psychiatrie marocaine. In: Annales Médico-Psychologiques. 128th Year, Vol. 2 (1970). 33–56.

McClintock, Anne. Imperial Leather: Race, Gender and Sexuality in the Colonial Contest. New York/London 1995.

McCulloch, Jock. Colonial Psychiatry and the African Mind. Cambridge 1995.

McCulloch, Jock. The Empire's New Clothes: Ethnopsychiatry in Colonial Africa. In: History of the Human Sciences. Vol. 6, No 2 (May 1993). 35–52.

Mejda, Cheour/Feten, Ellouze/Anis, Zouari/Afef, Louati/Hedi, Aboub. Histoire de la stigmatisation des malades mentaux en Tunisie. In: L'Information Psychiatrique. Vol. 83, No 8 (Oct. 2007). 689–94.

Mernissi, Fatima. Women, Saints, and Sanctuaries. In: Signs. Vol. 3, No 1 (Autumn 1977). 101–12.

Michaux, Léon. Professeur Antoine Porot (1876–1965). In: Annales Médico-Psychologiques. 123ʳᵈ Year, Vol. 2 (1965). 71 f.

Mills, James H. Re-forming the Indian: Treatment Regimes in the Lunatic Asylums of British India, 1857–1880. In: Indian Economic and Social History Review. Vol. 36, No 4 (Dec. 1999). 407–29.

Mills, James H. The History of Modern Psychiatry in India, 1858–1947. In: History of Psychiatry. Vol. 12 (2001). 431–58.

Mills, James H. The Mad and the Past: Retrospective Diagnosis, Post-Coloniality, Discourse Analysis and the Asylum Archive. In: Journal of Medical Humanities. Vol. 21, No 3 (2000). 141–58.

Möbius, Angela. Zur Entwicklung der Psychiatrie in Tunesien (1956–1997) unter besonderer Berücksichtigung des Lebenswerkes von Sleïm Ammar. Med. thesis, University of Cologne 2001.

Mohsen-Finan, Khadija. La condition des femmes au Maghreb: entre repli et mondialisation. In: Moyen Orient. Vol. 4 (Feb.–March 2010). 81–5.

Morel, Pierre. Dictionnaire biographique de la psychiatrie. Le Plessis-Robinson 1996.

Moussaoui, Driss/El Otmani, Saadeddine. Introduction des hôpitaux dans les pays arabes et musulmans. In: Moussaoui, Driss/Roux-Dessarps, Michel (ed.). Histoire de la médecine au Maroc et dans les pays arabes et musulmans. Casablanca 1995. 13–18.

Okasha, Ahmed. A Cultural Psychiatric Study of El-Zar Cult in U. A. R. In: British Journal of Psychiatry. Vol. 112 (1966). 1217–21.

Okasha, Ahmed. Focus on Psychiatry in Egypt. In: British Journal of Psychiatry. Vol. 185 (Sept. 2004). 266–72.

Okasha, Ahmed/Kamel, M./Hassan, A. H. Preliminary Psychiatric Observations in Egypt. In: British Journal of Psychiatry. Vol. 114 (Aug. 1968). 949–55.

Okasha, Ahmed/Karam, E. Mental Health Services and Research in the Arab World. In: Acta Psychiatrica Scandinavica. Vol. 98, No 5 (1998). 406–13.

Okasha, Ahmed/Lotaif, F. Attempted Suicide: An Egyptian Investigation. In: Acta Psychiatrica Scandinavica. Vol. 60, No 1 (1979). 69–75.

Okasha, Ahmed. Mental Health Services in the Arab World. In: Arab Studies Quarterly. Vol. 25, No 4 (Autumn 2003). 39–52.

Parle, Julie. Witchcraft or Madness? The Amandiki of Zululand, 1894–1914. In: Journal of Southern African Studies. Vol. 29, No 1 (March 2003). 105–32.

Particularités de la pathologie algérienne. In: L'Information Psychiatrique. Vol. 45, No 8 (Oct. 1969). 879–82.

Pedersen, Jean Elisabeth. 'Special Customs': Paternity Suits and Citizenship in France and the Colonies, 1870–1912. In: Clancy-Smith, Julia/Gouda, Frances (ed.). Domesticating the Empire. Race, Gender, and Family Life in French and Dutch Colonialism. Charlottesville/London 1998. 43–64.

Pelis, Kim. Prophet for Profit in French North Africa: Charles Nicolle and the Pasteur Institute of Tunis, 1903–1936. In: Bulletin of the History of Medicine. Vol. 71, No 4 (1997). 583–622.

Pick, Daniel. Faces of Degeneration: A European Disorder, c. 1848–c. 1918. Cambridge 1989.

Pols, Hans. The Development of Psychiatry in Indonesia: From Colonial to Modern Times. In: International Review of Psychiatry. Vol. 18, No 4 (Aug. 2006). 363–70.

Pols, Hans. The Nature of the Native Mind: Contested Views of Dutch Colonial Psychiatrists in the Former Dutch East Indies. In: Mahone, Sloan/Vaughan, Megan (ed.). Psychiatry and Empire. Basingstoke 2007. 153–71. 172–96.

Porter, Roy. Being Mad in Georgian England. In: History Today. Vol. 31, No 12 (Dec. 1981). 42–8.

Porter, Roy. Wahnsinn. Eine kleine Kulturgeschichte. Zürich 2005.

Prestwich, Patricia E. Family Strategies and Medical Power: 'Voluntary' Committal in a Parisian Asylum, 1876–1914. In: Journal of Social History. Vol. 27, No 4 (Summer 1994). 799–818.

Prestwich, Patricia E. Female Alcoholism in Paris, 1870–1920: The Response of Psychiatrists and of Families. In: History of Psychiatry. Vol. 14, No 3 (2003). 321–36.

Pridmore, Saxby/Pasha, Mohamed Iqbal. Psychiatry and Islam. In: Australasian Psychiatry. Vol. 12, No 4 (Dec. 2004). 380–5.

Prochaska, David. Making Algeria French: Colonialism in Bône, 1870–1920. Cambridge/New York 1990.

Pu, Tinnyung/Mohamed, E./Imam, Kareema/El-Roey, Ali M. One hundred Cases of Hysteria in Eastern Libya. A Socio-Demographic Study. In: British Journal of Psychiatry. Vol. 148 (May 1986). 606–9.

Racy, John. Psychiatry in the Arab East. In: Acta Psychiatrica Scandinavica. Vol. 45, Supplement No 211 (Feb. 1970). 11–79.

Rahim, F. M. A./Al-Sabiae, A. Puerperal Psychosis in a Teaching Hospital in Saudi Arabia: Clinical Profile and Cross-Cultural Comparison. In: Acta Psychiatrica Scandinavica. Vol. 84, No 6 (Dec. 1991). 508–11.

Rappel historique de l'assistance psychiatrique en Algérie. In: L'Information Psychiatrique. Vol. 45, No 8 (Oct. 1969). 815 f.

Razanajao, Claudine/Postel, Jacques. La vie et l'œuvre psychiatrique de Frantz Fanon. In: L'Information Psychiatrique. Vol. 51, No 10 (Dec. 1975). 1053–72. Also in: Sud/Nord. Vol. 1, No 22 (2007). 147–74.

Réflexions sur la pathologie mentale féminine en Algérie. In: L'Information Psychiatrique. Vol. 45, No 8 (Oct. 1969). 885 f.

Rogan, Eugene. Madness and Marginality: The Advent of the Psychiatric Asylum in Egypt and Lebanon. In: Rogan, Eugene (ed.). Outside in: On the Margins of the Modern Middle East. London/New York 2002. 104–25.

Sadowsky, Jonathan. Imperial Bedlam. Institutions of Madness in Colonial Southwest Nigeria. Berkeley 1999.

Sadowsky, Jonathan. Psychiatry and Colonial Ideology in Nigeria. In: Bulletin of the History of Medicine. Vol. 71, No 1 (Spring 1997). 94–111.

Said, Edward W. Orientalism. New York 1979.

Salem-Pickartz, Josi Agnes. Mental Health: Arab States. In: Joseph, Suad (ed.). Encyclopedia of Women and Islamic Cultures. Vol. 3. Family, Body, Sexuality and Health. Leiden/Boston 2006. 268–70.

Schwarz, R. Zur Psychiatrie in Algerien. In: Social Psychiatry and Psychiatric Epidemiology. Vol. 11, No 2 (1976). 87–97.

Scotto, Jean-Claude. Hommage au professeur Jean Sutter. In: Confrontations Psychiatriques. Vol. 40 (1999). 235–9.

Scull, Andrew T. Decarceration. Community Treatment of the Deviant: A Radical View. Englewood Cliffs 1977.

Scull, Andrew T. Hysteria: The Biography. Oxford 2009.

Scull, Andrew T. Museum of Madness Revisited. In: Social History of Medicine. Vol. 6, No 1 (April 1993). 3–24.

Showalter, Elaine. The Female Malady. Women, Madness and English Culture, 1830–1980. London 1987.

Sivan, Emanuel. Colonialism and Popular Culture in Algeria. In: Journal of Contemporary History. Vol. 14, No 1 (Jan. 1979). 21–53.

Skultans, Vieda. Introduction. In: Skultans, Vieda (ed.). Madness and Morals: Ideas on Insanity in the Nineteenth Century. London/Boston 1975. 1–28.

Smith-Rosenberg, Carroll. The Hysterical Woman: Sex Roles and Role Conflict in Nineteenth-Century America. In: Social Research. Vol. 39, No 4 (Winter 1972). 652–78.

Sow, Ibrahim. Les structures anthropologiques de la folie en Afrique Noire. Paris 1978.

Stoler, Ann Laura. Carnal Knowledge and Imperial Power: Race and the Intimate in Colonial Rule. Berkeley/Los Angeles/London 2002.

Stoler, Ann Laura. Making Empire Respectable: The Politics of Race and Sexual Morality in 20th-Century Colonial Cultures. In: American Ethnologist. Vol. 16, No 4 (Nov. 1989). 634–60.

Stoler, Ann Laura. Race and the Education of Desire: Foucault's 'History of Sexuality' and the Colonial Order of Things. Durham 1995.

Stoler, Ann Laura. Rethinking Colonial Categories: European Communities and the Boundaries of Rule. In: Comparative Studies in Society and History. Vol. 31, No 1 (Jan. 1989). 134–61.

Studer, Nina S. Die Pathologisierung des Maghrebs: Der Einfluss der französischen Psychiatrie auf koloniale Berichte über schlafende Schwangerschaften. In: Historische Anthropologie. Vol. 21, No 1 (2013). 126–40.

Studer, Nina S. 'Pregnant with Madness': Muslim Women in French Psychiatric Writing about Colonial North Africa. In: The Maghreb Review. Vol. 35, No 4 (2010). 429–52.

Studer, Nina S. The Green Fairy in the Maghreb: Absinthe, Guilt and Cultural Assimilation in French Colonial Medicine. In: The Maghreb Review. To be published in autumn 2015.

Studer, Nina S. ‚Was trinkt der zivilisierte Mensch?' – Teekonsum und morbide Normalität im kolonialen Maghreb. In: Schweizerische Zeitschrift für Geschichte. Vol. 64, No 3 (2014). 406–24.

Summers, Carol. Intimate Colonialism: The Imperial Production of Reproduction in Uganda, 1907–1925. In: Signs. Vol. 16, No 4 (Summer 1991). 787–807.

Sussman, Sarah. Jewish Population of French North Africa. In: Holocaust Encyclopedia. United States Holocaust Memorial Museum. Available at: http://www.ushmm.org/wlc/en/article.php?ModuleId=10007310 [16.04.2012]

Swain, Gladys. Le sujet de la folie: Naissance de la psychiatrie. Toulouse 1977.

Swartz, Sally. Lost Lives: Gender, History and Mental Illness in the Cape, 1891–1910. In: Feminism & Psychology. Vol. 9, No 2 (1999). 152–8.

Swartz, Sally. The Black Insane in the Cape, 1891–1920. In: Journal of Southern African Studies. Vol. 21, No 3 (Sept. 1995). 399–415.

Taithe, Bertrand. Neighborhood Boys and Men: the Changing Spaces of Masculine Identity in France, 1848–71. In: Forth, Christopher E./Taithe, Bertrand (ed.). French Masculinities. History, Culture and Politics. Basingstoke/New York 2007. 67–84.

Tall, Emmanuelle Kadya. L'anthropologue et le psychiatre face aux médecines traditionnelles. Récit d'une expérience. In: Cahiers des Sciences Humaines. Vol. 28, No 1 (1992). 67–81.

Terranti, Idriss. Fanon vu de Blida. In: Sud/Nord. Vol. 1, No 22 (2007). 89–95.

Thompson, Victoria. 'I Went Pale with Pleasure'. The Body, Sexuality, and National Identity among French Travelers to Algiers in the Nineteenth Century. In: Lorcin, Patricia M. E. (ed.). Algeria and France 1800–2000. Identity, Memory, Nostalgia. Syracuse 2006. 18–32.

Tucker, Judith E. Problems in the Historiography of Women in the Middle East: The Case of Nineteenth-Century Egypt. In: International Journal of Middle East Studies. Vol. 15, No 3 (Aug. 1983). 321–36.

Ussher, Jane M. The Madness of Women: Myth and Experience. London/New York 2011.

Vaughan, Megan. Curing their Ills: Colonial Power and African Illness. Cambridge 1991.

Vaughan, Megan. Healing and Curing: Issues in the Social History and Anthropology of Medicine in Africa. In: Social History of Medicine. Vol. 7, No 2 (Aug. 1994). 283–95.

Vaughan, Megan. Idioms of Madness: Zomba Lunatic Asylum, Nyasaland, in the Colonial Period. In: Journal of Southern African Studies. Vol. 9, No 2 (April 1983). 218–38.

Vaughan, Megan. Introduction. In: Mahone, Sloan/Vaughan, Megan (ed.). Psychiatry and Empire. Basingstoke 2007. 1–16.

Wagner, Ewald. Regeln für die alphabetische Katalogisierung von Druckschriften in den islamischen Sprachen (arabisch, persisch, türkisch): Auf Grund von Beratungen eines Gremiums von Fachbibliothekaren. Wiesbaden 1961.

Arabic Glossary

Balad, pl. buldān: country, here countryside; in the colonial sources transcribed as *bled*, which has become part of the French vocabulary.

Baraka: a form of blessing, often with healing properties.

Dawwār: village; in the colonial sources transcribed as *douar*, which has become part of the French vocabulary.

Faqīh, pl. fuqahā': expert of Islamic law.

Ǧinn, pl. ǧunūn: spirit; jinn.

Māristān/bimāristān: traditional Muslim asylum/hospital for the insane and the desolate.

Murābiṭ, pl. murābiṭūn: saint, often said to have healing properties; in the North African dialects *marabout*, which has become part of the French vocabulary.

Qāḍī, pl. quḍāt: judge.

Sayyid, pl. sāda: lord; in the colonial sources transcribed as *sidi*, which has become part of the French vocabulary.

Ṭālib, pl. ṭullāb/ṭālibūn: student, here sorcerer; in the North African dialects *taleb*.

Ṭabīb, pl. aṭibā': medical doctor; in the colonial sources transcribed as *toubib*, which has become part of the French vocabulary.

List of Images

Title page: Photograph of the male Muslim "Dormitory of the Serious Ward" at the Manouba Psychiatric Hospital shortly after its inauguration in 1932. Taken from: Vadon, Assistance, between pages 42 and 43.

Ill. 1, p. 261: The participating neurologists and psychiatrists of the 1933 Congress in Rabat, photographed at the reception at the Kasbah of the Udayas in Rabat. Taken from: Charpentier, Comptes Rendus, between pages 484 and 485, picture A.

Ill. 2, p. 261: The participating neurologists and psychiatrists of the 1933 Congress in Rabat, photographed after the last session of the conference. Taken from: Charpentier, Comptes Rendus, between pages 484 and 485, picture C.

General Index

People Index

Places Index